DUNCAN DANCER

This is a volume in the Books for Libraries collection

DANCE

See last pages of this volume for a complete list of titles.

DUNCAN DANCER

IRMA DUNCAN

BOOKS FOR LIBRARIES
A Division of Arno Press
New York   1980

Editorial Supervision: Janet Byrne

———

Reprint Edition 1980 by Books for Libraries, A Division of Arno Press Inc.

Copyright © 1965, 1966 by Irma Duncan Rogers

Reprinted by permission of Wesleyan University Press

Reprinted from a copy in the Columbia University Library

DANCE
ISBN for complete set: 0-8369-9275-X
See last pages of this volume for titles.

Manufactured in the United States of America

———

Library of Congress Cataloging in Publication Data

Duncan, Irma.
    Duncan dancer.

    (Dance)
    Reprint of the ed. published by Wesleyan University
Press, Middletown, Conn.
    Includes index.
    1. Duncan, Irma. 2. Dancers—United States—Biog-
raphy. I. Title. II. Series.
[GV1785.D79A3 1980]   793.3'2'0924 [B]   79-7759
ISBN 0-8369-9288-1

DUNCAN DANCER

DUNCAN DANCER

An Autobiography by

IRMA DUNCAN

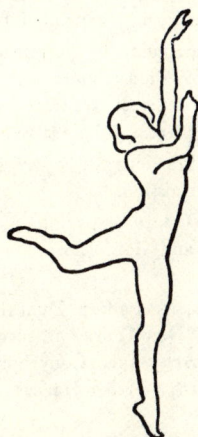

Wesleyan University Press

MIDDLETOWN, CONNECTICUT

This work appeared in condensed form in *Dance Perspectives*, numbers 21 and 22, 1965. The courtesy of the publisher in assigning the copyright is gratefully acknowledged.

Grateful acknowledgment is also made to the proprietors of the rights for their gracious permission to reprint the following materials under their control:

"The Child-Dancers," by Percy MacKaye, copyright © 1914, 1942 Arvia MacKaye Ege and Christy MacKaye Barnes; reprinted by their permission.

"Delight," by John Galsworthy, reprinted by permission of the author, of Charles Scribner's Sons, and of William Heinemann Ltd. United States copyright © 1910 Charles Scribner's Sons, renewal copyright © 1938 Ada Galsworthy; British copyright © 1910 John Galsworthy.

Excerpt from *Isadora*, by Allan Ross Macdougall, copyright © 1960 Thomas Nelson & Sons; reprinted by their permission.

Excerpts from *My Life*, by Isadora Duncan, copyright © 1928, 1955 Liveright Publishing Corporation (Black and Gold Library); reprinted by their permission.

Excerpts from *The Art of the Dance*, by Isadora Duncan, are published by the courtesy of Theatre Arts Books, New York, as successors to the book publishing department of Theatre Arts, Inc. Copyright © 1928 Helen Hackett, Inc.; renewal copyright © 1956 Helen Hackett.

Manufactured in the United States of America
First edition

Contents

vii

PART III. 1921–1933

Illustrations

ix

Foreword

My life with Isadora Duncan dates from 1905, until her untimely end in 1927. This period covers most of my own career as a dancer. During all these vital, creative years of working together, neither of us was able to leave some tangible result of our transient art. This book must therefore remain the sole, abiding record of my work in the world of the dance.

I. D.
Longway, 1966.

NOTE ON SOURCES: Many of the quotations in this book come from papers in the personal collection of Irma Duncan. These materials have been given by Miss Duncan to the Dance Division of the New York Public Library. In some cases, similar statements may be found in published works, but Miss Duncan has used the original sources whenever possible. All translations have been made by the author. References to works frequently cited have been abbreviated: *Life*—Isadora Duncan, *My Life* (New York, 1928); *Art*—Isadora Duncan, *The Art of the Dance* (New York, 1928). Other works cited are acknowledged elsewhere in this volume.

PART I. 1905–1913

Prelude

THE most fateful day of my life, the one destined to make the greatest changes in it, occurred at the end of January, 1905. The sky was dark, for a heavy fog had rolled in from the North Sea during the night, obscuring the streets of Hamburg. I had been born near there in a small town in Schleswig-Holstein, but my mother now lived on the outskirts of this city.

I can see the child I was then, bundled up warm against the damp weather, wearing a velvet bonnet and wool mittens, sitting beside my mother in the electric tramcar that carried me, not only from the quiet suburbs to the busy center of town, but also out of one kind of world into an entirely different one.

As we clanged along the Steindam leading to the more elegant section of Hamburg, I felt a mounting excitement. I was also somewhat frightened at what was about to happen, for I was to audition for a famous dancer to see if I could become a pupil in her school. This had come about because mother had seen an announcement in the newspaper saying that Isadora Duncan, the young American dancer who was then creating a furor in Germany, wanted pupils for her newly founded school in Berlin.

Mother had been dreaming of a stage career for me ever since a neighbor of ours, a music teacher, discovered that I had a good singing voice. This immediately reminded her of Ernestine Schumann-Heink, prima donna of the Hamburg Opera, for mother had come in contact with the glamorous world of the theatre when she acted as governess for the singer's little boy.

The curtain actually rose on my dance career the day before,

3

when mother tried unsuccessfully to enroll me at the Municipal Theatre School. The directress, a dour-looking woman in a tight black dress, poked her head out of the door. When she saw me, she immediately pronounced me too young. "Bring your daughter back when she is twelve years old," she said.

Mother tried hopefully to describe my acting and singing talents, but she cut her short with, "Those are the rules, Madam, goodbye," and shut the door on us.

It was just as well she did, as otherwise I might never have met Isadora Duncan. However, the fates were even then busy weaving the threads that would bring us together.

That same evening mother put me to bed earlier than usual, perhaps to sleep off my supposed disappointment, although the rejection at the Theatre School had actually left no impression on me. She then cleared away the supper dishes from the kitchen table and retired to the front parlour, or *gute Stube,* as they say in Hamburg. She sat down on the mahogany sofa covered with black damask above which hung a picture of my late father with his curly red hair and bristling mustache. On the round mahogany table in front of her, covered with a fringed cloth, she spread the evening newspaper. An old-fashioned oil lamp provided the only illumination. Electricity was a fairly recent convenience that had not as yet penetrated the outskirts of our city to light up the uniformly gloomy row of houses where we lived.

My mother looked old and careworn. Her smooth dark hair was streaked with gray, for she was past fifty. She had worked hard most of her life and didn't really know what leisure meant. My father's death had left us in somewhat straitened circumstances. A Hanoverian by birth, at a time when the elector of that province was also a British royal duke, he owned a small foodstore in Wandsbeck. When mother met him he was a widower with five children, the youngest being a mere infant. Mother took on the job of caring for them all. I was born when my parents were in their late forties. Thus I have no remembrance of mother as a young woman. Of my father I have practically no recollection at all, since I was only four years old when he died. His image is therefore just faintly imprinted in my memory.

Instead of sending her stepchildren to an orphanage as she was advised to do, mother preferred to struggle along as best she could in order to provide a decent home for them, seeing to it that they obtained work when they finished school. By the time I too had reached school age they had all left; only I, mother's one child of her own, remained at home.

Though small of stature and frail in appearance, mother possessed enormous energy and a vast fund of human kindness; always cheerful, she managed to eke out a living.

Perusing the paper now, she came across a startling announcement. It seemed almost miraculous that such a wonderful chance for the advancement of my stage career should present itself so opportunely. The more she read, the more excited she became. A nervous woman and highly emotional, she suddenly jumped up and rushed into the bedroom where I lay fast asleep.

"Irma! Irma dear!" she called. "Wake up, wake up, my child!" I could not immediately figure out what had happened; her voice sounded so urgent. Impatiently she lifted me out of bed. "Come along, I want to read you something wonderful," she said, and carried me into the next room.

Holding me on her lap, mother sat down again. She moved the lamp a little closer, smoothed out the rumpled pages of the newspaper, adjusted the gold-rimmed pince-nez hanging from a black ribbon around her neck, and jerked me into an upright position, all apparently at one and the same time.

"Sit up and listen," she said briskly. Pointing a forefinger at some inky black print, totally indecipherable to me, she began to read aloud.

I sat up and forced myself to listen to the article about a famous "barefoot dancer named Isadora Duncan," of whom I had never heard. It appeared she was then performing with considerable éclat at the Thalia Theatre in Hamburg. She was described as "a slender creature like a Greek goddess come to life."

Pronouncing each word slowly so I could understand, mother read that Isadora Duncan had, only two weeks before, opened a dance school for little girls in Grunewald, near Berlin. And stressing the next words, she said, "Only children aged six to ten are acceptable."

Mother looked at me over her pince-nez. "Did you understand, dear? That means you won't have to wait till you are twelve! Now listen to the description of the school."

The building is a three-story structure with a large basement and top floor. All the rooms are spacious and airy and the many windows allow free access of sunlight and fresh air. On the walls in every room are representations of antique art, and in the dormitories hang Donatello's terra cottas depicting children at play as well as Della Robbia's colorful Madonnas. There are large copies of dancing figures on friezes in the schoolroom, and on a long shelf in the music room is a lovely collection of Tanagra figurines. All these works of art are supposed to give the children a sense and appreciation of beauty, which in turn will influence their dancing, according to Miss Duncan.

The children are boarded and educated free of charge; this includes clothes and other necessities. Besides their dance training personally conducted by Isadora Duncan, the pupils will also receive academic instruction from a competent public school teacher and in addition, in order to stimulate their artistic sensibilities, there will be regular visits to museums with lectures on art. Two governesses are in charge, and the management of the school is in the hands of Miss Isadora's sister, Elizabeth Duncan.

This free, non-profit dance school, founded by Isadora Duncan and entirely supported by her financially, is not a philanthropic institution in the ordinary sense but an enterprise dedicated to the promotion of health and beauty in mankind. Both physically and spiritually the children will here receive an education providing them with the highest intelligence in the healthiest body.

"How wonderful!" mother exclaimed. "Irma, how would you like to be a dancer?"

I did not know what to say. The only dancing I had done was at Hallowe'en. After dark, with the other children in our block, I would skip joyfully along the street with a colored paper lantern on a stick. Holding it high up in the air I would sing a little German rhyme:

> Lanterne! Lanterne!
> Sonne, Mond und Sterne
> Macht aus euer Licht,
> Macht aus euer Licht,
> Aber loescht mir meine Lanterne nicht!

Little did I then realize how extraordinarily symbolic that simple gesture of holding high the torch while dancing would be for me in the future.

When mother asked if I wanted to be a dancer, my answer could not have been too enthusiastic. She tried to arouse my interest by sounding very enthusiastic herself.

"Here, Irma, listen to this! 'In the summertime the pupils will take their lessons out of doors. Clad only in a light, short tunic and with bare feet, they will be taught to move freely in harmony with nature. They will learn to express their own childlike feelings in the dance. . . .'"

"Just think how wonderful that must be!" mother said, thinking no doubt of all the summer days I was forced to spend playing on the dusty street or in our cheerless back yard. "If I send you to that school, who knows . . . perhaps some day . . . you too will be a famous dancer!" She laughed and hugged me tight. "Tell me, darling, would you like to try this school?"

"I don't know," I said hesitatingly, for the thought of leaving home for a distant city frightened me. "Why do I have to decide tonight?" I felt very sleepy. "Can't we wait till tomorrow?"

"No!" Mother explained we had to decide tonight because the dancer was giving only one more tryout early tomorrow morning. After further persuasion I agreed to go. Mother at once carried me back to bed. In the dark bedroom, while tucking me in, she said in a strangely serious voice:

"Just one more thing, darling, before you go to sleep. I must tell you that the pupils are required to remain at the school till they have reached their eighteenth year. That means we shall be separated for a long, long time."

I sat bolt upright and blurted out, "No, I don't want to go!" and straightway felt much relieved. Mother pushed me back onto the pillows. Calmly she reminded me of the wonderful things I would receive at that school—things she could not provide. And she promised to visit me often, which reassured me somewhat. And so, tired of this long discussion in what seemed to me the middle of the night, I once more agreed to attend the tryout.

I had no sooner closed my eyes when I heard mother murmur as if to herself, "What a dreadfully long time to be separated. Oh, how I shall miss you. Darling, will you miss me?"

Alarmed at her emotional outburst, I started to cry. I threw my arms about her and sobbed, "O Mama, I shall miss you too!"

Mother stroked my head. "Go to sleep now, for we shall have to get up very early to be there on time. . . ."

And here we were, on our way to meet the "barefoot dancer," who they said looked like a Greek goddess come to life. The tramcar stopped in front of the Hamburger Hof, our destination. By the big clock over the front desk, mother noticed with a start that we were late for the audition. She asked hastily for Miss Duncan's suite and on being informed clutched my hand, racing me quickly up the carpeted stairs. The sound of music on the third floor led us directly to the right door. Mother knocked repeatedly, but there was no answer. When the music stopped, she knocked again. A maid in black uniform with crisp white cap and apron opened the door. She said curtly, "Sorry, the tryout is over." She was about to close the door again when mother intervened.

"Won't you announce us anyway?" she inquired.

"I have orders not to admit any more applicants," the maid said primly.

"Oh please," mother pleaded, "we have come a long way. Our connections were bad, and my little girl will be so disappointed. Please explain this to Miss Duncan."

The maid looked down at me for a minute. She must have seen a small pale face with two big blue-green eyes staring back at her. Perhaps she was touched by my solemn expression as I clung tightly to mother's hand, for she said in a friendlier tone, "Wait here while I go and inquire."

Mother immediately bent down to straighten my bonnet and retie the satin bow under my chin. With nervous gestures she straightened her own hat and veil, reminding me for the tenth time to be sure to make a nice *knicks* for the lady when we shook hands.

How often since have I recalled that moment! And I always remember with a feeling of profound gratitude that the door did open to me, for through it I passed into a world of wider horizons. But most of all I offer thanks to a kind Providence that made it possible for me to meet the remarkable woman who was to mean so much to me. And I still hear those words that opened the fateful door:

"Enter, please. Madame will receive you!"

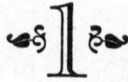

1

Follow Me

Our momentous meeting took place in a room full of people—parents and their children—who had come for the tryout. But because I arrived too late, I received special attention.

On entering the famous dancer's room, I felt a pleasant sensation of warmth and the fragrance of numerous vases and baskets of fresh flowers. The instant she stepped forward to greet me, in bare feet and ankle-length white tunic, looking indeed like a Greek goddess come to life, I had eyes only for her. With childish pleasure I noticed the white ribbon she wore in her light brown hair. I had never seen anyone so lovely and angelic-looking or anyone dressed in that way. Beside mother's long black dress made in the Victorian fashion, Isadora's simple attire gave her the appearance of a creature from another planet. I fell completely under the charm of her sweet smile when she bent down to take my hand while I curtsied.

In a soft voice, speaking in halting German, she told mother that the tryout was over. Mother once again made her excuses, and Isadora must have relented, for she told her to remove my clothes quickly so she could have a look at me. Mother knelt down and promptly started to undress me, right there in front of all those people. It happened so quickly I didn't have time to be scared. In her haste to comply with Isadora's request, mother had difficulty with the many hooks and buttons that encumbered even children's clothing in those days.

After she had removed the black stockings, the high-buttoned shoes, and the last petticoat, I stood exposed in a cotton camisole and a pair of lace-edged underpants, from which dangled long black garters. I felt terribly ashamed when, thus accoutred, I was made to stand alone in the center of the room. But not for long. The lovely vision in the Greek tunic returned and asked my name.

"Come and stand here in front of me, Irma, and do exactly as I do."

The soft strains of Schumann's *Träumerei* came floating to my ears as Isadora Duncan slowly began to raise her bare arms to the music. She watched me closely as I imitated her gesture and then, after a while, she seemed no longer to pay attention to me. A faraway look had come into her eyes as, lost in the music, she raised her beautiful arms and with a swaying motion of her body moved them gently from side to side like the branches of a tree put in motion by the wind. How well I was going to know that expression! She once said, "Like, swelling sails in the wind, the movements of my dance carry me onward and upward and I feel the presence of a mighty power within me."

And how much would I learn to feel that power growing steadily in all the years we worked together. This is how we first came in contact with each other—the great teacher and her small pupil—standing face to face, oblivious of the other people present, moving in unison to the music in our first dance together. With what poignancy I would recall this scene toward the end.

A nod to the musician at the upright piano, and the tempo changed to a lighter rhythm, an allegretto. She swiftly changed the mood and darted away, skipping gracefully around the room. All eyes, I was fascinated watching her circle about me like a bird. She reminded me of the sea gulls I had often observed skimming across the big lake directly in front of the hotel. Uncertain what to do next, I remained where I was. Still dancing, she beckoned to me and called out gaily, "Follow me! Follow me!"

Her radiant personality was contagious. I lost my self-consciousness and bravely skipped after her, trying my best to do exactly as she did. I undulated my little arms in emulation of her for all I was worth. But, in that absurd déshabille with the long black garters flapping against my legs at every step, I must have looked comical. I heard her laugh when she stopped abruptly and said, "That is enough, my dear. Go and put on your things."

While mother dressed me, I kept looking back over my shoulder at the lovely vision in white who had cast such a spell over me. She slowly went from one child to another of the many assembled there and deliberately made her choice as if picking flowers. "I shall take you and you," I heard her chant, "and you and you. . . ."

I glanced with envy at the girls she had chosen. Would she want me too? I wondered, secretly yearning to go with her wherever she went, for this was something I now wanted to do more than anything else. However, she passed me by. She turned instead with sudden animation and interest toward a young man, sketchbook and pencil in hand, who had been quietly sitting in the background observing. He whispered a few words, which caused Isadora to turn around and look at me. She came over to where I stood beside mother, anxiously waiting for her to notice me. She smiled, took my hand in hers and, leading me to the group of girls she had selected, gently said, "And Irma, I will take you, too."

I had no idea then of the role the young artist had played for me. When years later I once asked Isadora what exactly had prompted her to choose me for her pupil, she appeared surprised at my question.

"Why, don't you know? It was Gordon Craig. He said to me, 'Take her, she has the eyes!'"

"Of course I said that about you to Isadora," Gordon Craig told me recently when I inquired. In answer to my letter, he wrote from Vence in the south of France where he now resides:

Dear Irma:

So once again I find you, don't doubt if I remember you. But to get your letter is perhaps the best thing which has happened to me for many years—and no 'perhaps' at all. . . . I look on you as you were, small and holding up your hands as in the picture and your blessed heart is just the same as it was when a child, I feel this.

The Hamburger Hof, do I remember that! Yes, and it was a foggy week—dark by day. I drew a poor sketch of the side of the hotel from my window and some lights. . . . The date I was in Hamburg with her was January 24th to 31st, 1905.

And that is how I became Isadora Duncan's pupil. The chances of our ever meeting had been very slim. Was it hazard or destiny—who can tell?

"Follow me, follow me!" she had said when first we met. And follow her I did, from then on to the end.

There were five of us when we children gathered the next morning at her hotel to be attired in our new school uniform consisting of tunic and sandals and a little hooded woolen cape. Dressed alike, we looked like sisters. I distinctly recall the sense of freedom I experienced in those light and simple clothes, which were the distinctive Duncan uniform and which would henceforth set us apart from other people. Goodbye petticoats and cumbersome dresses with bothersome hooks and high-buttoned shoes. We children, strangers only a moment ago, now timidly smiled at each other in a new-found comradeship.

We were soon on our way to the station. I had never traveled in a train before. In all the excitement I completely lost track of mother. Accompanied by Isadora's maid, we settled ourselves in a second-class compartment in the train for Berlin when, amidst all the confusion, I heard someone tap on the window. It was mother. She tried bravely to smile, but her eyes were red from weeping. I did not immediately understand why she should be crying, since I was on my way to that marvelous school she had told me about, where I would soon be happily playing and dancing with my schoolmates. Why wasn't she happy too? Poor mother! She still had her stepchildren, but I was the only child of her own. Did she have a premonition? Though I would see her again, the bond would never be the same. How could she possibly imagine that her daughter was leaving her, not for a few years as she believed, but that an inscrutable destiny was taking her away practically forever. I leaned out the open window and kissed mother goodbye. She clung to my hand. A sudden shrill blast of the train whistle and we slowly moved out of the station. Mother kept pace with the moving train to the end of the platform. My last glimpse of her showed a weeping black-robed figure with a small bundle, my discarded clothes, pressed tightly to her breast.

A few hours later we arrived in Berlin. A pale winter sun brightened the city. The maid shepherded her small flock to the exit where our new guardian awaited us. She sat in a closed carriage, looking very beautiful. To my childish imagination she represented the legendary Fairy Queen in her coach, carrying me and my companions off to her enchanted castle in the forest.

"Come and sit here beside me," she said sweetly as I climbed in. I was thrilled!

The horses rapidly traversed the long chaussée leading to the Grunewald. Filled with expectation, we all sat quiet as mice. When the carriage at last stopped in front of a yellow stucco villa with a tall picket fence, she said, "Here is the school!"

We all got out. Wide-eyed with curiosity about what awaited us within, I climbed the many stairs to the entrance. Never was I so surprised as when the door opened and there right in front of me stood the seminude statue of a Greek Amazon on a pedestal, her head nearly touching the ceiling! We all gaped with astonishment. When I recovered from my initial shock, I turned to look for an explanation from the beautiful lady who had brought us here. But the Fairy Queen had vanished—coach and all.

Left alone in these strange surroundings and frightened, we children instinctively drew closer together. A curious odor of bay leaves pervaded the hall, emanating from the dried laurel wreaths that decorated the walls. I had the sensation of having entered a chapel. We remained there waiting for what seemed an unconscionable time.

Then something happened. Over to one side some sliding doors opened a crack, and out peered a small monkeylike face, brown and wrinkled. This face stared at us for a minute; then the doors opened wider, and a small woman stepped out. Outlandishly attired in a long red Chinese coat embroidered all over with flowers and parrots, this strange apparition mysteriously approached, limping slightly. She slowly circled around the little group, huddled close together for protection. She kept her hands hidden Chinese-fashion in her voluminous sleeves.

We did not know what to make of it. Who was this?

Without a kind word of greeting to the pathetic little group in her house, this odd creature poked her funny face into each one of our faces for a silent scrutiny and then disappeared as mysteriously as she had come, closing the sliding doors behind her.

I suddenly longed for the comforting arms of my mother. The others must have had similar reactions, for Erica—the youngest, a mere tyke of four—suddenly burst into loud, heartrending wails. We all were about to join her when, luckily, two nursemaids appeared.

"Ah! here they are, our little Hamburgers!" they exclaimed. With pleasant grins lighting up their young faces, they said, "Welcome to the Duncan School!" and in a cheerful, lively manner hustled us off.

Chatting all the way downstairs, they hurried us to the large, airy basement, where they helped us remove our newly acquired white woolen coats with pink-lined hoods and our winter overshoes. "What you children need is some nice hot tea and bread and butter," one of them said. "That will cheer you up."

"And then you are going to meet all your new playmates," the other one grinned and jerked her thumb in the direction of the nearby dining hall. "Listen to them! They have just come back from their daily outing."

The loud hubbub of children's voices resounded in the basement. It stopped suddenly, the moment we newcomers entered the room.

"Meet our little Hamburgers!" one of the nurses called out. "You all have time to get acquainted before tea."

Being an only child and having played mostly solitary games at home, I always felt shy when confronted with a mass on-slaught of other children. But this group looked like a cheerful, friendly lot, with their cheeks red from the wintry air and out-of-doors activities, and their eyes shining. They pushed forward for a closer view of us. A pretty, dark-haired girl with round rosy cheeks and small chocolate-brown eyes, older and taller than myself, made her way through the crowd and grasped my hand. "My name is Anna," she said sweetly. "What is yours?"

I introduced myself and she immediately made me feel at home by saying, "I want you to meet my friend Theresa," and she put her arm around the waist of a girl who was her opposite in coloring, with blue eyes, blonde hair, and a lot of freckles on her tiny nose. They made a charming pair. Anna, who apparently loved to get things organized, then drew out a darling little girl nearer my own age and size. She had a dainty heart-shaped face with hazel eyes and dark lashes. I especially admired her dark, naturally wavy hair. Anna introduced us, stating importantly, "This is Temple. She is Miss Isadora's niece!" (the daughter of her brother Augustin, as I later learned).

Temple said, "Hello!" and stared at me with lips half-open in an expectant sort of way, which I soon found out was a little habit she had. I didn't say anything but thought, What luck! to be the niece of a Fairy Queen! I could not get further acquainted with her, for Anna, who had taken me in tow, had more girls to introduce, mainly the younger ones. There was

Lisel with the pretty golden curls and the large brown eyes of a startled deer. And beside her, little Gretel with violet eyes, ash-blonde hair, and the delicate look of a Dresden china doll. There were many more—Isabelle, Gerda, Marta, Stephanie— too many names to remember all at once. When we sat at the long refectory table, I counted twenty girls. I discovered later they came from every part of Germany, some from Belgium, Holland, Switzerland, and Poland; Temple was the only American.

"I do not know exactly how we chose those children," Isadora once said. "I was so anxious to fill the Grunewald and the forty little beds, that I took the children without discrimination, or merely on account of a sweet smile or pretty eyes; and I did not ask myself whether or not they were capable of becoming future dancers." *

I asked Anna, who took her seat beside me at tea, how she liked it here. She didn't answer directly but inquired, "Have you met Tante Miss?"

"Tante who?" I was puzzled. "Who is that?"

"Didn't you see her upstairs?"

"Oh, you mean the one in the funny red coat with the parrots on it?"

Anna nodded eagerly, a mischievous twinkle in her eyes. "What do you think of her?"

"I was so scared."

Anna whispered, "We are all a bit frightened of her. She is Miss Duncan, Miss Isadora's older sister. We call her Tante Miss." And with the superior air of one who had been enrolled at the school for the space of a whole week before I arrived, she added, "But everybody else is very nice here, you'll see!"

"Attention everyone!" One of the nursemaids at the end of the table clapped her hands for silence. "I am going to take the new ones upstairs to bed. The rest of you stay down here and don't make too much noise. Is that understood?"

* *Life*, p. 177.

A shout by many throats in the affirmative answered her. "Well then, come with me, all you little Hamburgers. You must be tired from the trip and the excitement. Early to bed and early to rise for you five, and tomorrow you'll be fresh and rested and can have a good time with the other children."

With these words she marched us upstairs to the dormitory, where five white beds, with blue satin coverlets and muslin canopies tied with blue ribbon at the top, awaited us. The winter's pale setting sun cast a pink glow over the pretty white and blue room. It struck me as peculiar having to go to bed in daylight, but I didn't mind in the least as soon as I saw the canopied bed that was to be mine. In Germany we call this a *Himmelbett*, or "heavenbed," associated always with children of the rich. The average child merely dreamed of such a heavenly bed, curtained in flowing white muslin and covered in satin, fit for a princess. I could hardly wait, after I had folded my Duncan uniform on the white chair at the foot and placed my sandals neatly underneath, as I had been shown, to climb into my *Himmelbett* and pull the silk coverlet up to my chin, finding that my dream had come true.

While some of the other children dawdled and little Erica, the baby of the school, had to be undressed and put to bed by "Fräulein" (as we were told to call her), I glanced about the room. On the wall directly opposite hung the most appealing picture: a large Madonna and Child in ceramic on an azure background, framed in a garland of fruit and flowers in glazed colors, so natural they looked real. At home in our dark, damp bedroom I had only a dull framed proverb. Here, in the Duncan School, everything was different!

But the picture that pleased me most was the small reproduction of an angel playing the viol that was attached to the bedstead above my head. The other beds had similar Renaissance pictures, each one representing an angel playing a different instrument. But I liked mine the best; the face of my guardian angel, framed in dark curls and inclined over the instrument,

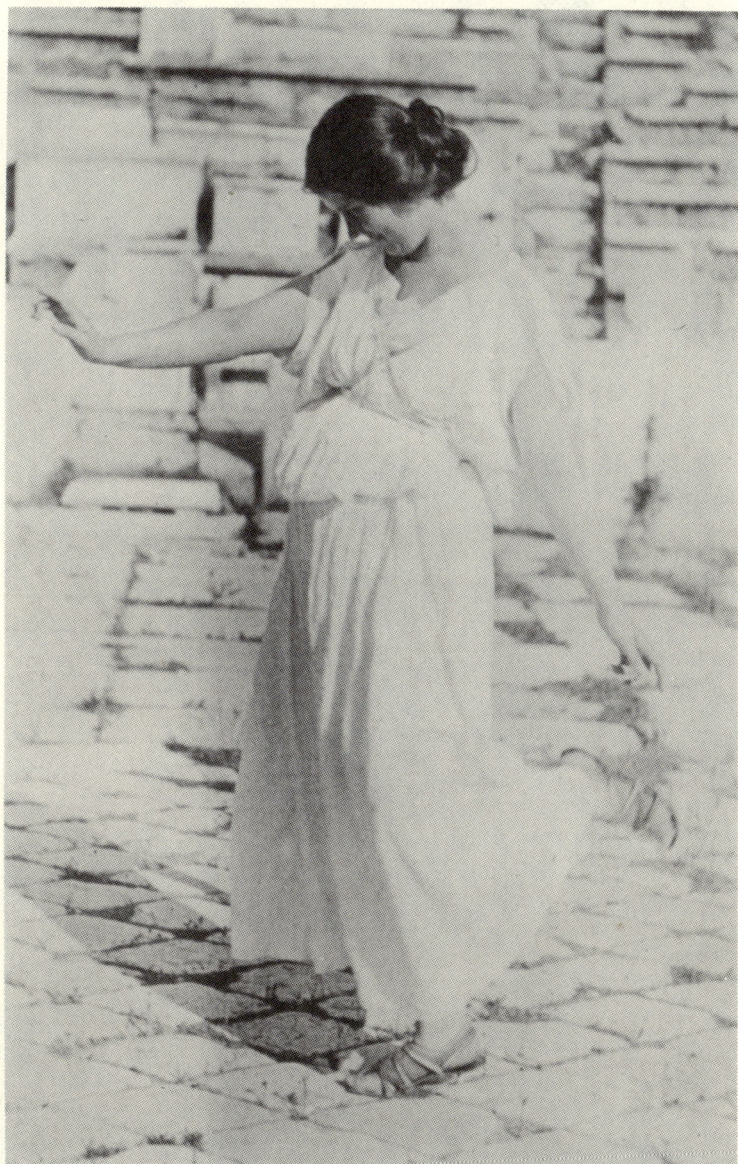

Isadora Duncan at the Theatre of Dionysus, Athens, 1904.

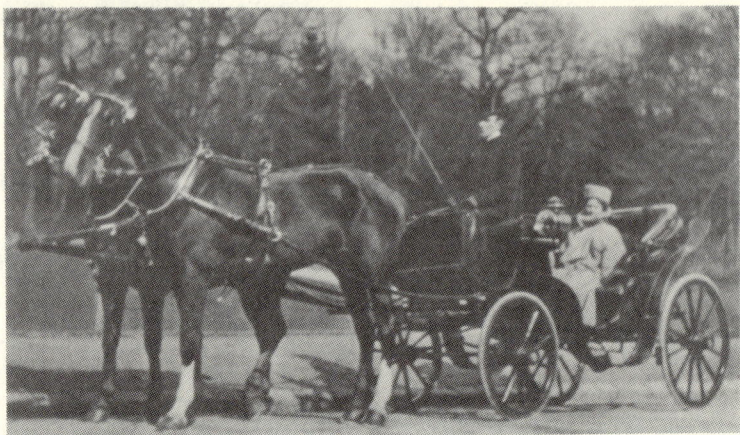

Isadora in her own equipage, Berlin, 1905.

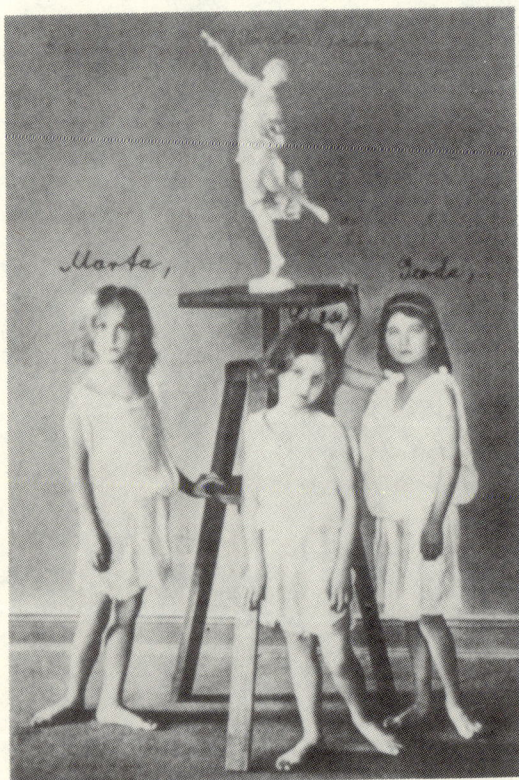

Marta, Lisa, and Gerda before a statuette of
Isadora, Grunewald, 1905.

had so divine an expression that one could almost hear the melody. When Fräulein closed the Venetian blinds, curtailing my observation, I stretched out with contentment and tried to go to sleep.

It was not easy. All the fresh impressions and strange sights that had crowded these last three days tumbled through my mind. The pine-scented air of the nearby forest filled the room with fragrance. Through the open window I could hear the distant rumble of the *Rundbahn* passing by. The melancholy hoot of the locomotive, a sound forever afterward evoking memories of my childhood, made me feel drowsy. Still I could not relax into sleep. Something was missing. What I longed for was not the comforting arms of my own mother giving me a goodnight kiss. It was just one more sight, before I dozed off, of the beautiful Fairy Queen, who had brought us here to her enchanted castle in the woods. She and her coach seemed to have disappeared completely.

I began to fear I would never see her again when I noticed a shadowy vision tiptoeing silently from bed to bed, bending over each child. At last she reached me. It was the Fairy Queen! She placed a cookie between my lips and kissed me. "Good night, darling, sleep well," she murmured, and was gone. I sighed happily and fell into a peaceful slumber on the threshold of a bright new world.

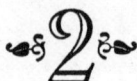

Dancer of the Future

THE year she established her first school, Isadora was basking in new-found fame and popularity. It was Germany's privilege in the opening years of the twentieth century to offer the comparatively unknown American dancer both serious recognition and lucrative success. She chose Germany, she once remarked, "as the centre of philosophy and culture which I then believed it to be, for the founding of my school." *

Germany, at that period still an empire, had for the last three decades enjoyed a state of uninterrupted peace. The liberal arts and sciences flourished. It was no wonder, then, that when Isadora arrived with her dances inspired by Hellenic ideals, the artists and intelligentsia of Germany saw in her some divine manifestation. She in turn—her imagination kindled by the great masters of German music—started a bold new venture in dance history when she created her own choreography to Beethoven's Seventh Symphony, the one that Wagner had labeled "the Apotheosis of Dance." It was animated by her desire to weld the two sister arts, music and dance, closer together. Such a venture created a sensation among music lovers, who tangled in hot debates as to whether or not the music of Beethoven needed this visualization. But she had no choice, for only in great music did she find the source of inspiration that harmonized with her lofty ideals.

To fully comprehend and appreciate her epoch-making contribution to the history of the dance, it is imperative to recall the primitive, stagnant state in which that art was then floundering.

* *Life,* p. 177.

The so-called "classical" ballet was an uninspiring and uninteresting acrobatic exercise which, as one contemporary critic observed, "had no validity other than a mere diversion. No one who considered himself an intellectual gave the dance as it was then serious consideration." Not until Isadora Duncan arrived on the scene and gave the dance new form and life did she, according to the same source, "help us to realize that the dance can be an art."

Another spectator, who described her as being "tall, graceful and slender with a small oval face, good features and a mass of dark hair; who is beautiful on the stage and has particularly graceful arms and hands," saw in the California girl "a dancer of remarkable skill, whose art . . . has a wonderful eloquence of its own. It is as far from the acrobatics of the opera dancer as from the conventional tricks by which the pantomimists are wont to express the more elementary human emotions." To the above quoted reviews of a German and an English writer should be added the impression of a contemporary French journalist, who describes a rehearsal he once attended in a theatre in France. On a bare stage a troupe of girls in pink tights, tutus and ballet slippers, with woolen shawls across their shoulders to keep them warm on that drafty stage, evolve slowly under the direction of a ballet master.

> The ballet master, bustling about, made the troupe repeat the same movement a dozen times. But it never seemed quite right. He got very angry and stormed at them. The stick with which he beat time, tapping it against the floor, frequently struck the legs in pink tights. This whole set-up had something infinitely sinister about it, something very sad. All this inanimate gymnastic had only a very faint resemblance to what one imagines the dance to be. The dance must after all express something. It is not enough to execute movements with the legs alone, the whole body must participiate. The entire being must express some feeling. Our ballerinas are for the most part marvelously articulated dolls whose grace we can admire but whose pointes and jetés

battues cannot be considered anything more than choreographical exercises. It will be the glory of Isadora Duncan, that wanting to renew the art of the dance, she drew her inspiration from ancient Greece and revived for us again that epoch of beauty.

Isadora's appearance on the stage in a simple chiton "à la greque" and sans pink tights (a shocking sight to the prudish element in society) led people to believe that she wanted to revive the Greek dance. Yet she herself categorically stated, "My dance is not Greek. I am not a Greek. I am American." She felt her dance had sprung from the roots of life as her Irish pioneer ancestors lived it in a covered wagon traversing the wide spaces of the West on their way to California in '49. "All this my grandmother danced in the Irish jig," she told her pupils, "and I learned it from her and put into it my own aspiration of young America." *

With the same enterprising spirit that had animated her pioneer ancestors, she undertook the formidable task of establishing her long-dreamed-of school. I know of no other precedent in modern times where a young artist, at the start of a promising career, is moved to invest hard-won earnings in a philanthropical enterprise simply to gratify some lofty ideal. But Isadora Duncan did just that. Rather than invest her money in diamonds and costly furs and expensive mansions and other luxuries so many women crave, she spent every penny she earned on the upkeep of her school. "I had no wish for the triumphal world tours" (which her manager urged on her), Isadora, the idealist, explained. "I wanted to study, continue my researches, create a dance and movements which then did not exist, and the dream of my school which had haunted all my childhood, became stronger and stronger." †

Months before she founded her school late in December 1904, Isadora was walking with a friend when they happened

* Cf. *Life,* p. 340.
† *Life,* p. 141.

upon a group of girls doing calisthenics with dumbbells in an open courtyard. The girls, dressed in black woolen bloomers, long-sleeved middy blouses, black stockings and shoes, went through their exercises in a lifeless manner. Isadora, bent on reform, not only in the art of dance but also in dress, said to her companion, "Consider these poor girls trying to exercise with all those horrible clothes on! One of these days I am going to change all that."

"How are you going to bring that about?" Her friend reminded her of the age they lived in and the ingrained prudishness of centuries. "It would be a miracle." Isadora answered with conviction,

"I am determined to found a school, where children will walk barefoot in sandals the same as I do and wear short, sleeveless tunics so they can move in utter freedom and be a fine example to all the other children in the world. They shall learn not to be ashamed to expose their limbs to the rays of the health giving sun. And I shall teach them to dance; not in the stilted, outworn tradition of either a fairy, a nymph, or a coquette, as I found when I was a child and took dancing lessons, but in harmony with everything that is beautiful in nature."

Ardently wishing to share her revelation of truth and beauty with others, she spared no time or expense. Engaged in this laudable endeavor for the benefit of children in general and the good of her future little charges in particular, she had to overcome much antagonistic opposition from all those who live like ants in an anthill, greeting every advanced idea with ridicule. Many critics were then barking at her heels, trying to disparage her efforts and ridicule her art. One deluded member of that confraternity went so far as to question whether she could dance at all! Comparing her technique unfavorably with that of the contemporary ballet, he declared her lacking in both the correct physical requirements for a dancer and the required technique to establish a new art form. He proposed that the question of her qualifications be placed before the ballet masters of the world. "Let them be the judge!" he sneered, little realizing that he hurled this jeer at the woman destined to raise the dance to a level equal with all the other arts.

Isadora, who had concentrated on proving the obsolescence of the ballet, declaring that "the principles of the ballet school are in direct opposition to what I am aiming at," did not let the insult go unchallenged. In January or February 1903, she sent a typical reply to the offending newspaper, the *Morgen Post:*

I was very much embarrassed on reading your esteemed paper to find that you had asked of so many admirable masters of the dance to expend such deep thought and consideration on so insignificant a subject as my humble self. I feel that much literature was somewhat wasted on so unworthy a subject. And I suggest that instead of asking them "Can Miss Duncan Dance?" you should have called their attention to a far more celebrated dancer —one who has been dancing in Berlin for some years before Miss Duncan appeared. A natural dancer who also in her style (which Miss Duncan tries to follow) is in direct opposition to the school of the ballet of today.

The dancer I allude to is the statue of the dancing Maenad in the Berlin Museum. Now will you kindly write again to the admirable masters and mistresses of the ballet and ask them— "Can the dancing Maenad dance?"

For the dancer of whom I speak has never tried to walk on the end of her toes. Neither has she spent time in the practice of leaping in the air in order to find out how many times she could clap her heels together before she came down again. She wears neither corset or tights and her bare feet rest freely in her sandals.

I believe a prize has been offered for the sculptor who could replace the broken arms in their original position. I suggest it might be even more useful for art of today to offer a prize for whoever could reproduce in life the heavenly pose of her body and the secret beauty of her movement. I suggest that your excellent paper might offer such a prize, and the excellent masters and mistresses of the ballet compete for it.

Perhaps after a trial of some years they will have learned something about human anatomy, something about the beauty, the purity, the intelligence of the movements of the human body. Breathlessly awaiting their learned reply, I remain, sincerely yours,

Isadora Duncan

In her concentrated studies of the origin of movement (which the ballet claims starts at the hips) the truth was inevitably revealed to her. When she declared, "Every movement starts from within, from here," placing both hands on her chest to illustrate to her pupils, she had the centrality of the solor plexus in mind. From there the nerve signals of the brain generate the impetus that must precede every movement. She soon discovered that there exists a Science of Movement—something that no one had discovered before. When medical scientists of today tell us that there is a right and a wrong to every movement we make, it is a fact that Isadora discovered over a half-century ago. And she proceeded to teach and demonstrate this truth through her dancing. Her entire technique was based on this idea. Endowed with nature's rarest gift—genius—she possessed a strong, prophetic vision of her own important mission in life. In a lecture delivered before the Press Association in Berlin at the outset of her career she stated it eloquently:

The dancer of the future will be one whose body and soul have grown so harmoniously together that the natural language of that soul will have become the movement of the body. The dancer will not belong to a nation but to all humanity.

Oh, what a field is here awaiting her! Do you not feel that she is near, that she is coming, this dancer of the future? She will help womankind to a new knowledge of the possible strength and beauty of their bodies, and the relation of their bodies to the earth nature and to the children of the future. She will dance, the body emerging again from centuries of civilized forgetfulness, emerging not in the nudity of primitive man, but in a new nakedness, no longer at war with spirituality and intelligence, but joining with them in a glorious harmony.

This is the mission of the dancer of the future. . . . Let us prepare the place for her. I would build for her a temple to await her. Perhaps she is yet unborn, perhaps she is now a little child. Perhaps, oh blissful! it may be my holy mission to guide her first steps, to watch the progress of her movements day by day until, far outgrowing my poor teaching, her movements will become godlike, mirroring in themselves the waves, the winds, the movements of growing things, the flight of birds, the passing of clouds, and finally the thought of man in relation to the universe.

Oh, she is coming, the dancer of the future! The free spirit who will yet inhabit the body of new woman; more glorious than any woman that has yet been; more beautiful than the Egyptian, than the Greek, the early Italian, than all women of past centuries—the highest intelligence in the freest body! *

Inscrutable fate propelled me, wrapped in childish insouciance, to become the unwitting pawn for an idealistic experiment. I was chosen to play my part in two pioneering projects that resulted in considerable benefit to mankind.

First: I was to be initiated into a completely novel mode of dance expression, based on an entirely novel technique; the foundation of a newly created dance form composed of movements and gestures never employed before by any dancer, anywhere, that did not come to life until my great teacher, Isadora Duncan, invented them.

Second: my schoolmates and I would henceforth be compelled, *nolens volens*, to take an active part in the promotion of the dress reform that was innovated and designed by Isadora. By dint of our courageous example, a general adoption (with minor modifications) of this sane, simple, and beautiful fashion came about.

It was an ambitious program and one we undertook wholeheartedly in the first instance, but with certain reservations and many misgivings in the second. I can still see the shocked ex-

* Reconstructed from notes in 1903 copybook.

pressions among the local population, especially women, when we Duncan pupils first appeared in broad daylight with the coming of spring, appareled in tunics and with our bare feet in sandals, on the open streets of Berlin. Pitying exclamations like, "Oh, you poor, poor, little children! Why, you must be freezing to death with so little on!" engulfed us. Approaching our innocent governess with threatening gestures and looks, they shouted after her, "It's cruelty, that's what it is! We ought to get the police after you. Cruel! Cruel! Cruel!"

Unfortunately, that wasn't by any means the end of it. No one had reckoned with the other children of the neighborhood, mostly boys, who subjected us poor victims to what amounted to a minor persecution. Like the Christian martyrs of old, we were actually stoned. Frequently (and this was most humiliating) the children pelted us—in this era of horse-drawn carriages—with something else entirely! In this way we were continually forced to dodge either stones that hurt or filth that besmirched. We often panicked, despite heroic efforts on the part of our chaperone to fend off these wild hordes of insult-screaming juveniles.

How I dreaded those daily outings! They made me feel ashamed to be exposing my bare limbs in public, and they instilled in me an unreasonable complex, which I later had great difficulty in overcoming, about not dressing like other human beings. New ideas always frighten people. But it hardly seems credible that, in the first decade of this atomic century, the pupils of Isadora Duncan should have been stoned because of their unconventional dress. But a novel idea was on the march and nothing could stop its progress.

My education as a dancer of the future was purposely delayed until I had mastered the minutiae of daily school routine. My first lesson, for instance, had nothing to do with dancing. For identification's sake, we had each been provided with a number. Mine was 16. The day after my arrival I was handed a length of white tape with red numbers, which I was taught to sew neatly into every piece of clothing. There happened to be something symbolic about mine. The street number of the Duncan School was also 16. In my childish fashion I took great pride in that fact, together with a sort of proprietary interest.

It was not easy to adjust to a school discipline that demanded lining up in pairs every time we walked up and down the stairs to go from one classroom to another and even on our daily promenade. There were long periods every day when we were not allowed to speak, and infraction of that strict rule meant punishment. Then I was forced to eat food I didn't like. But hardest of all was getting up at 6:30 every morning to go through an hour's exercise *before* breakfast. Clad only in blue one-piece bathing suits (years before Annette Kellerman made her sensational appearance in one!), we held onto rails along the wall and went through a series of limbering-up exercises we children used to call *Beinschwingen* and *Kniebeugen*. When Isadora said, "Gymnastics must come before dancing," she never meant before breakfast. That was strictly the Spartan idea of Elizabeth Duncan, not the Athenian ideal of her sister.

The rest of the morning was taken up by schoolwork presided over by a regular public school teacher supplied by the German government. Dancing and music or singing lessons occupied the afternoon hours. Fresh in my memory is the unforgettable occasion of my first lesson in our dance room, standing there in bare feet and wearing a short white tunic made of cheesecloth. The room seemed very large to me, although it could not have measured more than twenty-five by eighteen feet. Empty except for a few benches ranged along a wall and a brown felt carpet tacked to the floor, it had many windows and a glass-enclosed porch off to one side, from which a door opened onto a flight of iron stairs leading down into the garden. Sliding doors on the opposite wall connected with the spacious music room, where a grand piano (an Ibach) occupied the semicircular space formed by a large bay window.

Here, as everywhere else in the house, antique bas-reliefs formed the decorative motif. I principally remember the large one of a Nike tying her sandals; she was minus a head but had beautifully flowing draperies. I was fortunate enough nearly two decades later to admire the original in Greece. However much I admired these works of art, none could compare to the small statuette of our own goddess of the dance gracefully poised on a tripod in one corner of the dance room. It inspired and helped me more to understand Isadora's art than all the archaic Greek representations. Whenever the guiding spirit of our school was absent—and that occurred more frequently than we liked—her adoring youthful pupils would gather in front of it and offer a silent prayer, as to a votive statue, wishing for her speedy return. For it was in this room that she initiated us into the fundamental principles of her dance, teaching us to walk in harmony and beauty with arms raised to the light. With the intuition of a true artist, she knew how to impart an understanding of her aims to her young disciples—a feat that her older sister, who took over when Isadora left, was never able to accomplish.

It seems strange that a woman suffering from a defect, which made one leg slightly shorter than the other, should have been put in charge of our basic dance instruction. But such was the case. As we grew up, we learned to accept with equanimity Isadora's unpredictable nature. But for a long time I puzzled, trying to figure out how Isadora expected us to learn to dance from her lame sister, who not once appeared in a dance tunic or demonstrated a movement for the pupils. She always wore the voluminous Chinese coat, which helped to hide her defect and restricted her teaching to simple dance steps. She taught us the waltz, the polka, and the mazurka—all of them popular dances in her youth—for she had conducted social dancing classes in America. She would lift her skirt a few inches and demonstrate the step; that was all. Now and then she would roll up her long, loose-hanging sleeves and illustrate a series of arm movements devoid of any expression or meaning, merely to impart suppleness. Her method of teaching had nothing in common with Isadora's, which relied a great deal on inspirational technique. Thus, under Elizabeth's guidance, we at first learned to dance rather perfunctorily. Somehow, however, we acquired enough basic knowledge and made sufficient progress for Isadora to work with us. One lesson from her made up for all of Tante Miss's routine. According to her own precepts, Isadora taught us simple, rhythmic movements—walking, running, skipping— movements that come naturally to children.

European children have the quaint custom of calling grownups with whom they come in close contact by the courtesy title of Aunt or Uncle. When we called her "Tante Isadora," she acted horrified. She said, "Now that you are my pupils, you may call me Isadora, or darling Isadora, but never, never call me Auntie!" On the contrary, her sister, who was twelve years older than she, did not object to the somewhat incongruous appellation of Tante Miss, which was given her when the German pupils in the beginning thought the prefix "Miss" was her name. Somehow or other, it suited her perfectly. Tante Miss, who lived in the school, we saw every day. Isadora, who had an apartment on the Hardenbergstrasse in Charlottenburg, we saw seldom.

Of the three Americans who instructed us in the arts of dance and music, Professor Passmore, our singing teacher, impressed us most as an American. Mr. Passmore, who looked like a cartoon of Uncle Sam with his beard and side whiskers, had his own method of teaching singing. A cheerful gentleman who liked to laugh a lot, he placed us in a semicircle, with hands resting on top of our heads, and made us vocalize to the words "Santa Barbara a Santa Clara." That this curious, outlandish incantation, repeated at every lesson, held an important message concerning my future could not of course be guessed. Santa Barbara, the first American city whose name I learned to pronounce and sing, would turn out to be the birthplace of the man I was to marry. Dear Professor Passmore—had he only known! "The Jay is a jolly old bird, heigh-ho!"—that was the first song in American he taught us—a composition of his own—and that is how we children regarded him—as a "Jolly Old Bird." After his Wednesday and Friday singing lessons he would drink a cup of tea with Tante Miss in the music room as he conversed animatedly with her and his long black beard had a funny way of moving up and down, much to our amusement. He was, in fact, a skillful vocal instructor, guiding our voices gently into their natural pitch and emphasizing breath control. This was a technique we were grateful for later, when we had to sing and dance at the same time.

Learning something new every day, the time passed swiftly and I had no chance to suffer from those attacks of *Heimweh* that were shortly to reduce the number of pupils in the Grunewald school to fifteen. Mother had decided that I should try out the school thoroughly before making up my mind whether or not to stay. Just before Easter she wrote me to stay on if I wished. I still have the letter I wrote to her in reply. My first letter was dated April 30, 1905. I wrote with the steep, large lettering of an eight-year-old that I was glad she had decided to leave me at school.

To make absolutely sure that I was in good hands, mother had repeatedly tried to get permission to visit me. Her many requests were refused by Elizabeth under the pretext that insufficient time had elapsed for me to become acclimatized. These refusals, made without Isadora's knowledge, angered mother. As soon as Isadora appeared again in Hamburg, mother went to see her. Isadora received her very kindly, immediately assuring her that she could visit me whenever she wanted. Graciously, she invited mother to stay at the school during her visit.

I had no idea mother was coming. One morning, when we

descended to the basement dining hall, lined up in pairs as usual and holding hands, not allowed to speak a single word, I suddenly saw mother. I was even more speechless than before. Dressed in a mauve silk negligée, her hair still in braids and quickly pinned up, she stood beside a narrow iron cot in a corner. The moment she saw me, she held out her arms and came rushing to me for an emotional embrace. As she pressed me to her breast, she called out endearments in her native Schleswig-Holstein dialect. This embarrassed me in front of the others. Most of them had never seen mother, and I wanted terribly for her to make a good impression. She clung so long to me that Fräulein thought discipline was being impaired. She called out, "Now Irma, sit down and eat your breakfast first and visit with your mother afterward."

The other children were already seated, a big steaming bowl of hot porridge in front of each of them. But no one ate. Fascinated, they just stared at my mother. Their eyes filled with longing as they thought of their own mothers, whom they had not seen for months. Mother spoke to them gently, giving each a smile, trying to make their acquaintance. By her mere presence she spread a sort of homey *Gemütlichkeit,* a tenderness only mothers know how to bestow. Hearing her speak in the familiar, clipped North German accent, the girls from Hamburg became so homesick they started to cry. Later, except for little Erica and myself, they all returned home.

I had permission to skip school and spend the entire day with mother. I remember sitting in a coffee shop where she let me stuff myself with pastry and hot chocolate, something I hadn't tasted since I entered the school. While I was eating, she pumped me further about the food I was getting there.

"Tell me frankly," she said, "how you like it."

"Oh, so so. Not the way you cook, Mama."

"What do they give you? Tell me in detail."

"Vegetables," I said, making a wry face.

"What else? That can't be all?"

"Macaroni . . . you know, that sort of stuff."

"No meat?"

"No meat."

Mother looked worried. At home I had eaten meat every day, and sometimes she would give me raw chopped meat with onions on black bread and plenty of salt and pepper, which I actually ate with relish. Naturally, after that kind of fare, our vegetarian diet was unappetizing and tasteless. There was no use complaining; the school physician, Dr. Hoffa, had ordered it. I loathed it with all my heart and stomach, and never had enough to eat. But I did not say this to mother. I did not want to upset her.

"And for dessert—you do get dessert, don't you?" she asked hopefully.

"Yes, prunes."

"Prunes every day?"

"No, sometimes we get sago pudding."

When she learned that we had five meals a day—breakfast, second breakfast, luncheon, tea, and supper—she was satisfied that I wasn't starving. She promised to send me some homemade cake as soon as she got back. She still looked worried. "Are you sure they are treating you all right and that you really like it there?" she wanted to know.

"I like it fine, Mama," I assured her. "The people are very nice . . . some nicer than others."

I thought of Isadora. And suddenly, out of the blue, it struck me how much of a stranger mother had become. In the short span of three months, I had somehow grown away from her, as if I had entered another world. And of course I had. Being educated far in advance of ordinary children, dressing differently from them, we Duncan pupils had indeed been set apart. Like members of a religious community, under the benediction of some holy influence, we became an ever more dedicated group as we were further initiated into the secrets of Isadora's art. This was a world that no outsider could enter, nor could he ever fathom the depths of understanding and spiritual communion that existed amongst us whenever we worked or danced together with Isadora. That was a secret known to ourselves alone.

I had known Isadora so far only as a teacher. That spring for the first time I had the joy of seeing her perform on the stage. Sitting in a box with her other pupils, I watched her give a program called *Dance Idylls* which she originally performed in 1900, at the New Gallery in London under the patronage of H.R.H. the Princess Christian of Schleswig-Holstein. It contained a group of dances set to early Italian music, with costumes and dance motifs copied from Renaissance paintings. In those early days she made use of whatever stage décor was available, such as a sky-blue panorama in the background and tree groupings for the wings on either side. Later she adopted those tall, blue-gray curtains of her own design (though this was disputed by Gordon Craig), which she used henceforth exclusively. Those famous tall curtains subsequently became standard equipment, in one color or another, at every theatre, concert hall, school auditorium, or television set—wherever a neutral background was required.

On that memorable day when we first saw her perform, Isadora's dancing, lively and beautiful with all her youthful charm, was a revelation to her pupils. One particular dance made the most indelible impression on my childish mind. It was called "Angel Playing the Viol," to cello music by Peri. In this dance, in which she did not move her feet at all, I saw before my astonished eyes my guardian angel come to life. It was the one in the picture above my bed. Ever afterward, when I looked at this picture, it was Isadora's face I saw.

Of this performance Karl Federn, the German writer who instructed her in Nietzsche's philosophy, wrote:

> A simple scene . . . a green carpet and a spacious gray-blue backdrop . . . almost childish and laughable seems this stage

décor until she appears, for then the scene changes with each of her dances and becomes real. So powerful is the mood she creates that we can see meadows and the flowers she gathers . . . hear the waves break against the shore and surmise the approach in the distance of a fleet of ancient ships with billowing sails.

Her entrance, her walk, her simple gesture of greeting are movements of beauty. She wears no tights, no frilled ballet skirts, her slender limbs gleam through the veils and her dance is religion. . . . She appears as the Angel with Viol out of the painting by Ambrosio di Predis. A long violet garment worn over grayish veils floats down to her bare feet. In her hair, which hangs loosely to her shoulders, she wears a crown of white and red roses. And the Quattrocento comes alive again before us with all its innocence and deep religious feeling.

Pan and Echo—a short Greek tunic, her hair tied into a knot. We ask ourselves: Can this possibly be the same creature? With wonderful gestures expressive of the antique ideal, she resurrects the nostalgia of Hellas. How many statues have come to life in her! In a heavily draped Greek attire, she mourns to music of Gluck over the death of Eurydice, in rhythmic, measured, ceremonious grief that mounts and mounts until she sinks to the ground in despair. And then she appears again—this time the scene is darker, wrapped in sombre shadows, and her gown is colorless and floating like the shadows, and her movements are rapid and ghostlike: the shadows of the underworld listening to Orpheus. Suddenly the scene is bright again and everything is joy and contentment—Orpheus has found his Eurydice.

She has a dance without music, awesome and very gripping, called "Death and the Maiden" . . . as in Maeterlinck's "Intruse," death announces itself unseen but intensely apprehended. . . . The spectator feels a cold shiver run up and down his spine. Everyone has sensed the awesome presence of the destroyer.*

* From *Nach Fünfundzwansig Jahren*, dated 1928, in Isadora Duncan's *Der Tanz der Zukunft* [*The Dance of the Future*] *Eine Vorlesung* [Jena, 1929] iii–iv.

(Isadora once remarked that she did not call this dance "Death and the Maiden" when she composed it, but that she had some vague idea of it as Maiden and brutal reality, and it was the audience who named it Death. If one recalls her own tragic end, the dance seems almost prophetic.)

The unusual gift of the great artist to make others see the things born of her imagination gave depth and significance to everything Isadora created. She knew how to dance with such commanding authority that those who saw her perform were impressed even when they did not comprehend the meaning of her art. Few dancers possess such insight into music that the dance seems to express exactly what the composer intended. Richard Wagner has said: "The most genuine of all art forms is the dance. Its artistic medium is the living human being, and not merely one part of it but the whole body from the soles of the feet to the top of the head. For anyone completely sensitive to art, music and poetry can only truly become comprehensible through the art of the dance-mime." And with every gesture Isadora Duncan revealed herself as a supreme dance-mime. She was the prototype of her own inspired vision of the Dancer of the Future—whose dance belongs to no one nation but to all of humanity.

3

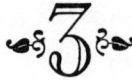

The Greatest Thing in Life

"WE must adopt more children and build an addition to the school!" Isadora exclaimed enthusiastically when she saw the progress we had made during her five months' absence. Returning from one of her protracted tours in the latter part of June that same year, she was filled with plans for the future, not counting the expense. Her sister was more practical. "Where will the money come from? As it is, we are living way beyond our budget."

"I have an idea!" Never at a loss to make life more exciting, Isadora said, "We'll give a benefit performance and show the children off to the public for the first time. That will surely arouse sufficient interest. We will ask everybody we know to subscribe."

"That's an excellent idea," Elizabeth agreed, since she had already enlisted the aid of several Berlin society ladies to act as patronesses of the school. She added, "Princess Henry of Reuss was here a few days ago and saw the pupils dance. She was enchanted."

Princess Henry VII of Reuss, whose principality in Thuringia was a small one, possessed, nevertheless, enormous wealth. A woman close to the Imperial court, she could be useful in getting other influential ladies to join.

"I shall write to her immediately," Isadora said, and she composed the following letter:

Dear Princess:
For the last eight months twenty little girls have been living together in my school in Grunewald creating much joy to them-

37

selves, a delight to all who have seen them, and a radiant hope for the future of the Art of the Dance.

I wish to take twenty-five more next winter. This will necessitate a new building erected on the vacant plot next door. As you know, I have given my entire earnings to the maintenance of the school and am most pleased to do so in the future. But they are not enough for the new ground and erection of the second building to be connected by a passageway with the old one. So I am giving a benefit at Kroll's Opera House on July 20th, as a means of raising money for it.

Of course we do not expect people who are out of town to be present but that they may subscribe and give their tickets to artists, etc. All the artists who have visited the school have been enthusiastic in their praises for the lovely dancing of the little girls and are unanimous in their belief in the value of the school to art and the state.

I myself am delighted with the progress of my pupils and am convinced that almost every child has more or less talent for the dance if directed along natural channels; and that the dancing of these little girls will be a source of much joy to the public in the years to come. For this reason I do not hesitate to ask for help in the advancing of my idea and feel sure my request will meet with your sympathy.

Isadora Duncan

Among the various artists she mentions as visiting the school was an unknown Swiss musician called Jaques-Dalcroze. He witnessed a lesson once, and I recall the occasion vividly because of his infectious enthusiasm and constant interruptions. What fascinated him most were the kinetics involved in what Isadora called the "scale of movements," which started with a slow walk, gradually accelerating into a fast and faster pace till it evolved into a run, and from there by degrees reverted to a slow walk again.

"Ha!" he exclaimed, jumping up from his seat in great agitation; and he inquired of Tante Miss, "May I have your permission to improvise at the piano for a repetition of this exercise?" Permission granted, he proceeded to improvise for us. When he left, he signed the guest book, which was always on top of the piano. A few years later, he founded his whole system of Eurythmics on what he had seen that day at our school.

Such things occurred so frequently with people interested in the new dance form Isadora had invented that it was no wonder she should constantly voice the complaint, "Everybody is running off with my ideas!" Unfortunately, they could not be patented. If they could have been, what royalties she might have collected from her millions of imitators, including the Russian ballet!

It so happened that the well-known German composer Engelbert Humperdinck lived next door to us on Trabenerstrasse. Famous for his universally beloved children's opera *Hänsel and Gretel,* he headed the committee for the support of our school. One afternoon we all went to have tea with him and his family. A man of about fifty, he regaled us by playing music from his opera such as the "Knusper-Waltzer" and the lively, tuneful "Rosenringel" and "Tanzreigen." Appropriately enough for our youthful years, Isadora taught us a dance to the last two compositions. Humperdinck often played his tunes for us to get the right tempo and feeling. He played them with such verve that we children responded with natural spontaneity and put all we had into the charming dance.

The subscription list mounted daily, with Princess Reuss contributing a thousand goldmarks; Princess von Meiningen, a hundred; Frau von Mendelsohn of the banking family, also a thousand; Countess Harrach, a lady-in-waiting to the Kaiserin, five hundred; Siegfried Wagner, son of Richard Wagner of Bayreuth, a thousand; and so forth down the list to Frau Begas, the wife of Reinhold Begas, the famous German sculptor, who created the national monument to Emperor William I as well as many of the principal statues of Berlin. Isadora gave us new silk tunics in pastel shades of blue, pink, and yellow to wear for the occasion, making us discard the cheesecloth ones entirely. Also we had small wreaths of rosebuds for our hair.

Then came the big day. The excitement of that moment can never be repeated. Here I was, after only seven months of apprenticeship, ready to make my stage debut. Such a thrill comes to few children, and when it does they are never afterwards the same. A marvelous ingredient, a wonderful feeling of accomplishment, is then added to the ordinary routine of daily existence. This is something that the average child does not experience.

We were to appear at the very end of Isadora's performance. Quietly, we entered the stage door of the big Opera House late at night. We had slept all afternoon and early evening so as to be fresh and bright. I had an awesome sensation as I mounted the stairs to the dressing rooms while the performance was in progress. The sound of the orchestra playing faintly reached my ears. The curious, indefinable smell of backstage familiar to every performer, mixed with the unseen but nevertheless acutely sensed, electrifying presence of the hushed audience out in front, gave me my first attack of stage fright. The stern voice of Tante Miss saying, "Here, sit down in front of me so I can put your make-up on," brought me out of it.

I did as I was told, holding my hair back so she could smear cold cream over my face. When she finished and had applied the lipstick, she said, "There you are! I made you a nice cupid's bow." She surveyed me critically to judge the effect of her handiwork. "Now don't touch your face," she warned. "Who's next?"

This strange, unfamiliar business of make-up completed, I turned to the mirror. A rouged and powdered face stared back, resembling a painted mask; a face that was and yet was not mine. How familiar this pre-curtain ritual was to become in the course of my long theatrical career!

When the other children had been similarly transformed with the aid of *poudre de riz* and Dorin's rouge, and we stood ready in silk tunics and circlets of rosebuds for a final inspection, we all jumped and looked startled when a shrill bell suddenly rang in our dressing room.

"This is it!" Tante Miss said. "Get ready to go downstairs, and don't forget to put on your slippers and woolen shawls." Then, lined up two by two, we were hustled downstairs. With finger on her lips, Tante Miss signaled us to keep quiet and take our places backstage. Excitement took hold of me again, for I was about to experience something completely unknown, like diving into deep water. The orchestra struck up the by-now-familiar melody and, waiting in the wings poised to take off on cue, I summoned up my courage and dashed out onto the vast, empty stage of the Royal Opera House.

Dancing from the encircling shadows into the glaring light, I instantly forgot my previous nervousness, as I lost myself in the music and the dance. What joy, to dance in natural abandon carried along by the beautiful sounds of a symphony orchestra! This utterly entrancing sensation made all of us dance with such spontaneous enjoyment that we must have projected our own happiness across the footlights, for when we finished the audience responded with deafening applause.

The shock of this unexpected noise descended upon us with the suddenness of a thunderclap. We turned for reassurance toward the wings, where, near the proscenium arch, we had espied the lithe figure of our idol, who had been watching our dancing and for whom alone we had danced. Sensing our childish alarm, she quickly advanced toward us smiling, her light draperies floating behind her. Arms filled with long-stemmed roses, she stopped in our midst and took a bow while the gaze of her little pupils turned toward her as flowers toward the sun.

The audience clamored for encores. When the music began again, Isadora quickly whispered to us to dance toward her, one by one, from the opposite corner of the stage. We did so, and as each child skipped up she handed her a pink rose. With the flowers in our hands, we then circled about her as she posed in the center of the stage, arms outstretched as if to embrace us all in a loving, maternal gesture. Happy, laughing children danced a rondo about her, a real "Rosenringel Reigen," and in that ecstatic group was one who wished this happy dance would never, never stop.

In the audience that night in July 1905 was Gordon Craig. He gave his impression later:

> She called her little pupils to come to her and please the public with their little leapings and runnings! as they did, and with her leading them the whole troupe became irresistibly lovely. I suppose some people even then and there began reasoning about it all, trying to pluck out the heart of the mystery. But I and hundreds of others who saw this first revelation did not stop to reason, for we too had all read what the poets had written of life and love and nature, and we did not reason then; we read, we wept and laughed for joy. And to see her shepherding her little flock, keeping them together and especially looking after one very small one of four years old, was a sight no one there had ever seen before and, I suppose, will never see again.*

Whoever would have believed it possible that our innocent dance debut should bring forth wrath from on high? No one less than the German Kaiserin, Auguste Victoria, a pious woman (who inspired her husband's famous remark about its being woman's duty to occupy herself solely with *Kinder, Kirche, Kueche*), pronounced herself outrageously shocked at children performing in bare limbs. Brought up in the Victorian era, when the sight of a woman's ankle was considered daring, she could not look upon children's bare legs without feeling that it was immoral. If the poor Kaiserin could only see her royal descendants today going bare-legged in the summertime, she surely would realize what enormous progress has been made against prudishness through the good example set by that same group of dancing children she once criticized.

Her official utterance condemning the display of bare limbs occasioned wide publicity. It aroused further controversy and

* In a talk for BBC Radio.

also a livelier interest on the part of influential people in Isadora Duncan's school for the education of children along modern lines. It was then the only one of its kind in the world teaching freedom of motion; a sane, healthy attitude toward the human body; and, to complement these two important objectives, an appropriate dress reform. Nothing comparable had been seen in the Occidental world since the Hellenic and Roman civilizations. It was no wonder that under these circumstances the question of the propriety of exposing limbs to public view should be discussed seriously even by learned professors. How much the question was a topic of the day is evident in an article written in 1906:

IN ISADORA DUNCAN'S HOUSE

Several ladies and gentlemen of society recently gathered together in Grunewald to have Isadora's sister Elizabeth Duncan present to them the pupils of the Duncan School.

The interior of Isadora's home breathes the severe style of classical Greece softened by modern conveniences. Everywhere subdued colors and geometric lines and, in all things, from the reliefs of old Italian masters hanging on the walls, to the colorful flowers decorating the tables, a display of good taste. What the visitor is immediately aware of and what helps to dispel any lingering skepticism and calls forth respect is that here are people who have more than a sure sense of good taste. What impresses him is that there is indeed a great idea behind all this—perhaps a way of life.

As we enter the festive hall we behold, in addition to the ancient Greek spirit, the most refreshing youth. We are confronted with what at first impact confuses and leaves one dumbfounded; namely, a group of seventeen little girls in tunics of transparent silk and with hair unbound and carefully adorned with flowers or a simple diadem!

Seventeen youthful dancers, that is a total of thirty-four little dancing legs, bare as bare can be. And here is something curious! However greatly it may contradict one's conventional customs, the spectator is hardly conscious of this bareness of limbs in these surroundings. He does not perceive it as something odd or even offensive but rather as an aesthetic necessity, and he gains the impression that even the smallest sandal would spoil the quiet flow of lines.

One of the little dancers takes a big ball and bounces it onto the floor. She skips around it playfully and continues to bounce the ball with dancing gestures. Never have I seen anything so graceful! Never beheld so harmoniously rounded a dance image that appeared so entirely natural. . . .

How very difficult to achieve, and how very seldom employed in ordinary life, is the beauty of apparently the simplest of human motions. The Duncan sisters are quite right when they regard the walk, the rhythmic stride, as the basis for all dance art. As the most important of the 95,140 combinations of movements which, according to the opinion of the dance theoretician Emanuel of Paris, are possible for the human body to achieve. Whether the little Duncan girls stride ceremoniously in the manner of antique choruses, whether they hop about cheerfully or mime games, always, their every movement seems born out of the spirit of the music. . . . What enjoyment does the sight of a well-proportioned foot and the play of its muscles afford! This wonderful adjunct to the human body has become estranged to modern man. The compulsion of footwear has so pitiably crippled it that it has become almost a shameful thing. These child-dancers have completely normal feet. And since the whole foot and not the toes alone have been designed by nature to support the body's weight, their art does not deteriorate into the mannered offense which is the alpha and the omega of the old-style ballet and which causes those who practice it so much effort and pain. . . .

Better-cared-for children cannot be imagined, and they are all visibly and most lovingly devoted to the cause. Elizabeth Duncan conducted us into the dormitories: a symphony in white and blue bathed in light and fresh air, in an orderliness and cleanliness that conveys an indescribable comfort. The girls are to remain in this house till they are seventeen, thereafter they are going to appear with Isadora Duncan on the stage. It is reassuring to know that this gay but fundamentally serious art of the dance has, in this conception, a future.

When, after two hours which passed like a dream, I stood once more in the tumult of the streets in the midst of hurrying, perspiring, and laborious people, the skeptic stirred again in me and I asked myself: What is the purpose of all this? What benefit is there in it for us modern-machine people living in this era of shrillest disharmonies, in this piece of ancient Greece transplanted to a northern clime? . . . But then, above conflicting sentiments the thought arose, that even if there seems to be no practical use for it, one must admit it really is very nice when, far removed from the monstrous, dusty highroad trodden by millions, there exist a few gardens here and there secluded and filled with "Wunderblumen."

This was not the first skeptic nor the last to ask himself: Of what practical use is all this? He had part of the answer when he surmised that it was "perhaps a way of life." New ideas are seldom of immediate, general benefit to the contemporary generation. Sufficient time must elapse before the seeds start to germinate and take root. Isadora's credo was: "To dance is to live." She said that what she wanted was a *school of life*, for man's greatest riches were in his soul, in his imagination. She called the dance "not a diversion but a religion"; and she taught that idea to the children in her school. "Life is the root and art is the flower." Again and again she would reiterate that dance was the most natural and most beautiful aid to the development of the growing child in its constant movement, and only that education was right which included the dance.*

It is not surprising that intelligent men were somewhat perplexed when they first came in personal contact with a living demonstration of this credo. Isadora Duncan's idea was still above their heads. Cultured Europeans were suddenly confronted with the unusual phenomenon of seeing an American (and a woman at that) bring culture from the New World to the Old. It had always been the reverse. Her unique dance art represented one of the very few genuine, original art forms the

* Cf. *Art*, pp. 88, 141–142.

United States had produced in its less than two hundred years of existence.

Frequent inquiries as to the exact purpose of her dance school came from every direction. In a notebook of this period, she set forth her views:

If the dance is not to come to life again as an art, then far better that its name should rest in the dust of antiquity. . . . I am deeply interested in the question: Is the dance a sister art or not; and if so, how shall it be brought to life as an art? And I put this question quite apart from myself or my dance, which may be nothing—or something—simply as a question which must be of interest to most people.

My dancing is to me an instinctive thing born with me. . . . You call me a barefoot dancer. To me you might as well say a bare-headed or bare-handed dancer. I took off my clothes to dance because I felt the rhythm and freedom of my body better that way. In all ages when the dance was an art, the feet were left free as well as the rest of the body; also, whenever the dance has had an influence on the other arts—as in the beautiful bas-reliefs of dancing figures of the Greeks. . . .

If you would think of this a bit you would see that the conception of a dancing figure as being in light drapery and without shoes is not mine especially, but simply the ideal dancing figure as thought of by all artists of all times. Then you would cease to use the title "barefoot dancer," which I confess I detest; and you would see that in endeavoring to found a school for the renewing of the dance as an art, it is quite natural that the pupils should follow in their dress the hint given them by the Great Masters in portraying the dancing figures. . . .

I have danced before the public continuously since I was a little girl; in all these years, although certainly there has been much blame and discussion, there has been on the whole a general feeling of joyous acclaim and encouragement . . . that has upborne me on my way, for I felt it was a sort of voice from the people that such a dance was wanted, *needed*. . . .

Now I could not think that I could teach another what had been a gradual evolution of my own being and a work of all

my life. But I felt I must give response to all these questionings.
And so the idea gradually came to me . . . to endeavor to
found a school whose object would be the finding of the true
dancing. Not in any way a copy of my dance, but the study of
the dance as an Art.

And in the 1906 prospectus of the Grunewald school, she
stated its purposes clearly:

> To rediscover the beautiful, rhythmical motions of the human
> body, to call back to life again that ideal movement which should
> be in harmony with the highest physical type, and to awaken once
> more an art which has slept for two thousand years—these are the
> serious aims of the school.

Isadora's initial effort to arouse sufficient interest for the financial support of the Grunewald school had not been very
successful. She found herself forced to rely entirely on her own
resources for the ever increasing upkeep of her establishment.
Thereafter, she was kept constantly on the move despite her
wish not to go on triumphal world tours to earn enough money
to feed many little mouths five times a day. This made her
undertake tours lasting so long that her pupils didn't get even a
glimpse of her for months, sometimes an entire year—much to
the regret of her devoted charges, who missed her inspiring
presence and guidance. Tante Miss, who was now in complete
charge, could never fill that void. Neither physically nor in
character did she in the slightest degree resemble her younger,
more talented sister. Less idealistic and of a more pedantic temperament, she proved in the end to be of an infinitely more
practical mind. The enthusiastic response of the public to our
initial performance suggested to her the idea that the school
might help to support itself.

In order to learn from nature, the great teacher, we were
often taken to the woods in summer to observe the waving of
trees, the flight of birds, or the movements of clouds. Learning

to dance from these, we developed a sensitive understanding of nature. Isadora once remarked on how often, returning from these studies to the dance room, we pupils felt in our bodies an irresistible impulse to dance out one or another movement which we had just observed. And thus in time, she thought, some of us would come to the composition of our own dances; but even when we were dancing together, each one, while forming a part of the whole under group inspiration, would preserve a creative individuality.*

Not being a choreographer herself, Tante Miss now thought of following Isadora's suggestion and encouraged us to compose dances. The charming *Kinderscenen* by Schumann easily inspired ideas for this. She employed the method of letting us all improvise together and then, picking the one who had hit on the best interpretation, singling her out to develop her idea. In this ingenious way we composed a whole group of little poems, danced either singly or in group formation. I contributed several compositions. One of them I danced as a solo called "Poor Orphan Child." My dramatic instinct came to the fore as, with hesitant steps, I went from side to side holding out my hand, palm upturned, in a pitiable gesture of begging for alms. Isadora liked it so much she always made me dance this when visitors came to the school.

Tante Miss made all the costumes herself. She was very adept at it. Here was something she apparently enjoyed doing. I once saw her sitting on the floor contentedly pasting tiny golden paillettes one by one onto white silk angel gowns—the ones we wore for Schubert's "Sarabande."

She dearly loved to give us small objects to hold while we danced, probably because we did not always know what to do with our hands and she didn't either. We had a variety of bells, cymbals, hoops, garlands, scarves and even, for the "Italian Marinari" dance, short lengths of genuine seaman's rope, decorated with the national colors of Italy! Isadora, the purist, who

* Cf. *Art*, p. 82.

preferred the Doric to the Ionic style, did not, of course, entirely approve of this. But we children thought most of these
gadgets were fun, except that I didn't care to dance with small
brass cymbals tied to my hands. Isadora herself had discarded
these adjuncts long ago, and we later learned from her how
expressive and varied the gestures of the hands can be when
executed with the artfulness of a master.

One day, at the end of our rehearsal of the program, Tante
Miss said that she had an important communication to make.
We immediately sat hushed and attentive. "We have," she announced, "the great honor of presenting this first program of
dances from our school for the second time in public at the
composer's anniversary." Very composer-conscious ever since we
had met Humperdinck, we wanted to know whether Robert
Schumann was still alive. Tante Miss shook her head. "No,"
she said, "he died half a century ago, and we have been asked to
help commemorate the fiftieth anniversary of his death. So you
must all dance especially well on that day."

We had given the program initially at a Sunday matinee at
the Theater Des Westens in Berlin three months after our debut
at the Opera House. This, our first independent appearance,
was reviewed in the *National Zeitung* dated October 31, 1905:

> As the curtain rose a sweet little child skipped out onto the stage
> to a melody by Schumann in a delicate chiffon tunic. With bare
> feet she tripped lightly and daintily across the carpet . . . and
> soon there came a second, and then a third elfin figure until the
> stage was filled with about twenty similar shapes. The images
> they evoked were of enchanting gracefulness. They floated across
> and chased each other like irridescent butterflies with multicolored
> wings, bending, swaying, springing, and dancing like spirits from
> Oberon's court. . . . At times they resembled allegorical figures
> representing Autumn and Winter, indicating with characteristic
> but simple gestures the disparate moods of nature.
>
> And again they appeared, this time as angels in long white
> gowns and wreaths of flowers in the hair striding gravely about.

Then followed a very frolicsome dance . . . an animated swarm of colors and small shapes as if a storm wind had tossed the flowers in a meadow together.* And then in the next dance the girls would break up into orderly groups, those in the foreground seeming to paraphrase the melody while the taller girls in the background indicated the accompaniment. . . . Almost everything went along with admirable precision, but every now and then the set figures gave way and the little ones would skip about spontaneously, and this especially was delightful and interesting because it demonstrated conclusively how well they have learned to coordinate their movements.

It is important to remark that every form of affectation was avoided. The whole thing gave the impression of having been worked out with the characteristic naturalness of expression peculiar to children. This appears to me to be of primary importance in their work. The public applauded the youthful artists enthusiastically and with great vigor.

Someone on the commemorative committee must have seen this program and invited us to Zwickau, Schumann's birthplace, for the anniversary performance. For our first voyage away from school we had each been supplied with a small wicker suitcase held together by two leather straps. It contained our dance costumes and accessories, including a pair of slippers and a woolen shawl for backstage. I remember with what pride I carried mine, which had the number 16 painted in black on the outside.

It was the middle of summer, and the village made a picturesque sight nestling in a valley at the foot of the Erzgebirge in Saxony. In the market place of this medieval town stood the house where Schumann was born, and nearby was the Gothic merchant's hall, turned into a theatre, where we would dance to his music. Perhaps his spirit watched over us, for the townspeople took us instantly to their hearts.

All sixteen of us had been billeted in the quaint old house

* "Courante" by Corelli; a "Blind-man's-buff," danced and choreographed by Irma.

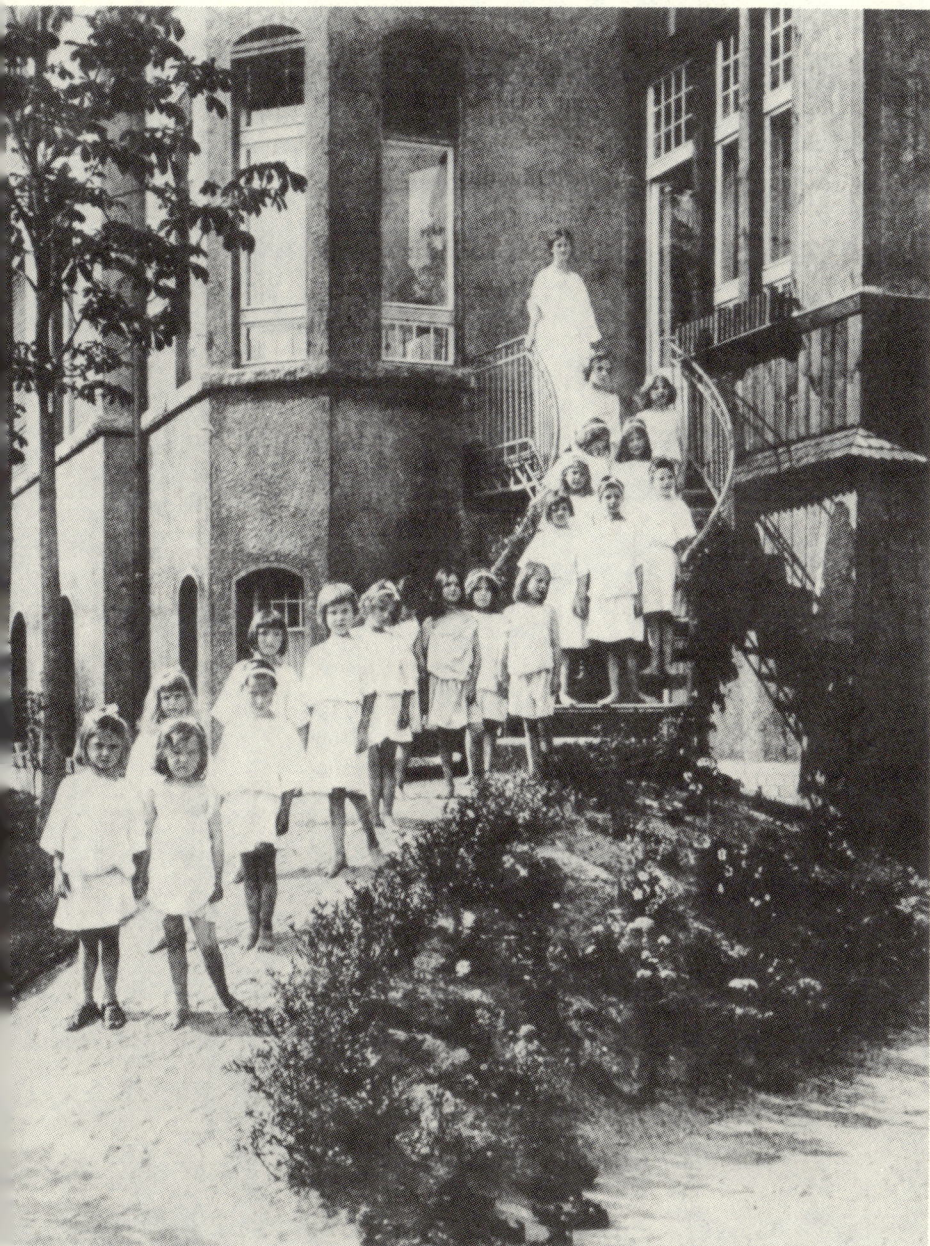

Isadora with Grunewald students, 1905; Irma at right, fifth couple from top.

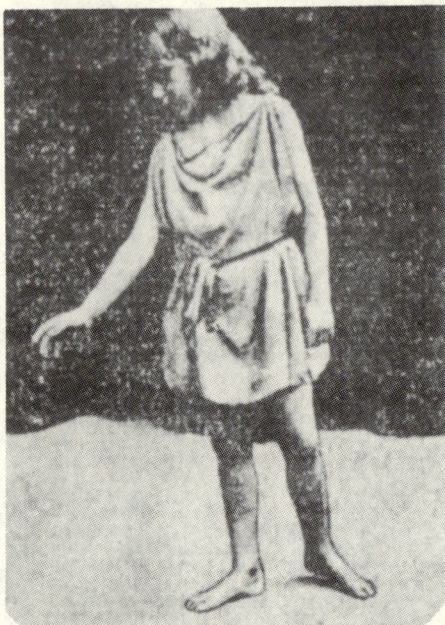
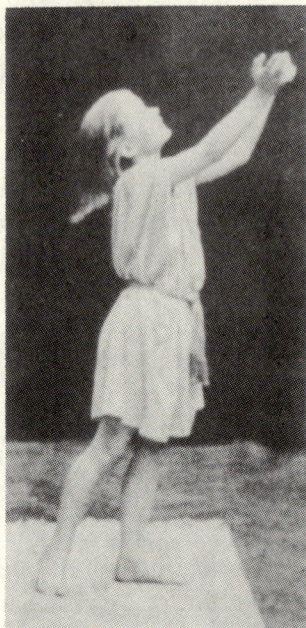

Pupils of the Isadora Duncan School, 1906–1908.
(upper l.) Erica.   (upper r.) Irma.
(lower l.) Theresa.   (lower r.) Anna.

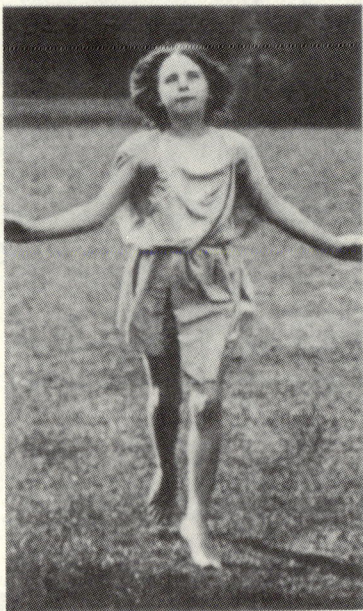
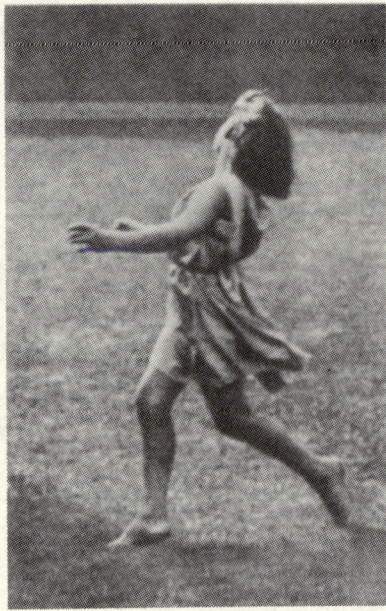

of the local gold-and-silver smith and his friendly young wife. When we left, he presented each child with a small silver chain with a silver pendant. "They were made in my workshop," he said, "and my wife and I would like you to wear them as a memento of Zwickau and Robert Schumann's commemoration festivities." Alas, we wore them only once, for "jewelry" was strictly forbidden. Tante Miss confiscated them and we never saw the little silver chains again.

From Zwickau we proceeded to other cities in Saxony— Dresden, Leipzig, etc.—making a small tour of Germany which lasted till Christmas. Another Christmas away from home. . . . In the library there was a large tree, festooned all over with golden threads and tiny red apples. Small wax candles burned in wire holders that made the golden threads glisten. There was the joy of opening a package from home filled with goodies. Under the tree were paper plates, one for each child, containing gingerbread, assorted nuts, and—in the center—the yearly Christmas symbol, a single orange.

By far the grandest present came from Isadora. Though absent on a tour through Holland and Belgium, she had sent us pretty new dresses and bonnets specially designed by her and made in the Hague. Both the dresses and velvet bonnets were blue and edged with swansdown. Mother had sent me a handsome doll with blond curls and a purple velvet dress. I had loved playing with dolls at home, but now I discovered to my surprise that I had no further interest in them.

To our delight, we received another present from our goldsmith friend—a silver thimble—which we were allowed to keep. For as long as we lived in Germany, each year under the Christmas tree, we found a small silver trinket—a bangle for our hair or a cup—most of which he never knew we were not permitted to keep. Each year we would open his gift eagerly but with sadness, knowing that if only Isadora were present she would never have deprived us of these things.

That winter in Hamburg mother received a letter:

The Isadora Duncan School will appear on Sunday at one o'clock at the Thalia Theater in Hamburg. We have asked the management to place two seats at your disposal. The school will arrive late Saturday night and the directress of the school, Miss Elizabeth Duncan, begs you for the sake of the children's health and peace not, under any circumstances, to visit them either upon arrival or departure. You will have an opportunity to see your little daughter Irma after the performance around three o'clock in the dressing room backstage.

After the performance the children are invited to a tea party given by the local committee for the support of the school. Since the departure is set for six o'clock, it will be impossible for Miss Duncan to permit you to take your little daughter home for the afternoon. The shortness of time and other considerations will make it otherwise difficult for Miss Duncan to keep the necessary control over her charges for whom she is responsible.

As well can be imagined, mother felt like rejecting these demands. The middle-aged spinster who caused them to be written obviously did not understand or sympathize with a mother's feelings. However, not wanting to cause any trouble and familiar with Elizabeth's Spartan tactics, she decided to abide by the rules. Mother came backstage after the matinee, her arms laden with flowers. She handed several small bouquets to her favorites and the biggest one to me. She hugged me and said, "All of you danced so beautifully." Then she kissed me and whispered, "But oh, Irma, you were simply wonderful!"

Mother had good reason to be proud of me, for only a year ago I had lived at home inconspicuous as a blade of grass; then events in my young life moved so fast that here I was returning to my home town dancing at the same theatre Isadora Duncan had appeared in that memorable week of our first encounter. In the interim I had not only made my dance debut and gone on tour, but I was already featured in two solo numbers of my own choreography. Enough to encourage any talented youngster, no matter what restrictions were necessary to achieve success.

Mother must have realized this when, after once more requesting permission to take me home and being refused by Tante Miss, she did not insist on her inviolable parental rights. Since I was a scholarship pupil, Tante Miss considered me school property, and there was nothing mother could do but take me away for good. Knowing how much I loved dancing and being Isadora's pupil, she naturally did not wish to hurt my chances.

Actually, however, none of us really knew what our future was to be at that extraordinary institution dedicated to an untried, idealistic experiment. Doubts of any sort were hardly ever raised by those who saw us dance, but there happened to be someone among the spectators that day in Hamburg who did voice them. His article was signed only with the initials V.M.:

> The house was well attended, everyone was delighted and enthusiastic. The contrast was immense. In the middle of a snowy winter's day this charming idyll of spring, these tender human buds who devote themselves with such earnestness and understanding, and at the same time with all the grace and ease of youth, to this art although they can't possibly know what it will later offer them in return for all this devotion.
>
> This thought must occur immediately to every philanthropist. And it is reassuring to learn from the school prospectus that the leaders of the Duncan Dance School have taken this point well into consideration, that they are preparing their pupils adequately for the struggle of existence.
>
> There also arises another concern as one views this performance for the second time. Will this art be strong enough to continue to hold attention, or is it merely a beautiful dream, which one may dream only once? . . . But it can't be denied that it is a beautiful art, in its present form perhaps not yet an end in itself, but surely a good seed to which one may wish a favorable growth and fruitful ripening.

During the first year at school we developed a strong attachment to our pretty young nursemaids, a brunette and a blonde, Fräulein Lippach and Fräulein Konegen. The day they packed

their things and departed, what a wailing went up among the
smaller children! Tante Miss, however, was deaf to our laments
and remained adamant in dismissing them. What we needed,
she explained, was an English governess, so we could learn to
speak English. I had learned my first English words at Isadora's
knee when she taught her pupils to recite Keats' immortal lines:
"Beauty is Truth, Truth Beauty,—that is all/Ye know on earth,
and all ye need to know." "That is the motto of our school,"
she said, "and I want each and every one to learn these lines
by heart."

If she could only have remained with us, and continued to
instruct us in this way, what a difference it would have made in
our young lives! Instead of growing up directly under her benign influence, we were subjected to all kinds of indignities and
abuses under the regime of our new English governess, a veritable ogre if there ever was one. A woman of vague features,
completely colorless, with bad teeth and pale gums, she struck
terror in our hearts the moment we laid eyes on her. She had,
besides, the revolting habit of cracking her knuckles incessantly;
we were convinced she cracked them even in her sleep. And her
methods of teaching discipline were thoroughly antiquated. She
treated us as if we were hard metal and she a blacksmith ham-
mering us into shape.

I would not be living up to the maxim Isadora taught us if,
in this history of her school, I refrained from telling the whole
truth, the good and the bad. "The web of our life is of a mingled
yarn, good and ill together." In later years, when we were grown
up, we often would harp on this unhappy period in our childhood, much to Isadora's annoyance. Finally she was driven to
exclaim, "Why do you girls always talk about the bad things?
Why don't you sometimes also remember the beautiful things
that happened to you at school? I am sure there was more of that
in the long run."

And so it undoubtedly was. However, it is a queer quirk of
the human mind to recall the unhappy things of childhood more

vividly than the beautiful. The good things are taken for granted by children. Cruel treatment comes as a shock and is resented and has psychologically a traumatic effect, sometimes with bad results. I firmly believe that stupidity is the root of all evil. There were unhappy things that can definitely be traced to the stupidity of our English governess and the unenlightened attitude of Tante Miss when it came to cruel treatment. Their behavior was in direct contravention of the instructions of Isadora, who did not believe in punishment and personally used only logical reasoning to correct our misdeeds. Unfortunately, her prolonged absences made her completely unaware of what went on in the intimate lives of her charges. Insufficient control and superintendence is the only blame attached to her, since she sincerely believed that by placing us in the trusted care of her sister, she had left us in the best of hands.

With the arrival of our hated governess I, for one, developed a real propensity for what she called "being naughty," and the occasions when I was sent hungry to bed were innumerable. Often, when I disobeyed, the governess tied me to the foot of my bed, leaving me there for hours like a martyr at the stake. Her sadistic corporal punishments belonged to the dark ages, and after she had inflicted this hurt I would weep and look at the picture of my guardian angel. Where was Isadora? I could not understand why she was never there when we needed her in this beautiful house in the pine forest, which she had wanted to be a children's paradise. She herself found Grunewald to be "very melancholy" when she did return. No wonder!

No use complaining to Tante Miss; she knew very well what went on and punished us herself, only in subtler ways. Writing to mother was of no avail; all our mail had to be censored. I felt trapped. Then I thought of our kindly old Norwegian cook. Frequently, out of pity, she would surreptitiously slip me a slice of dark, dry bread when I had been sent to bed without my supper. With her help, I managed to smuggle a letter out to mother.

Within a few days mother's short telegram, saying "I am coming to take Irma home," came as a great surprise to Tante Miss. That was the last thing she wanted to happen. In a state of considerable alarm for fear Isadora would hear of this, she called me to her study for a private interview, something she had never done before. By cajolery and flattery she finally persuaded me to change my mind, but not until she had promised to stop the more cruel kinds of punishment. When mother came, some blind, childish loyalty to my absent idol made me refrain from telling her everything. Her protests to Tante Miss did some good, for the harsher treatment ceased, but she could not persuade me to go home. "Just for a little while," she urged, "till Isadora returns and we can explain it all to her directly. I know she will understand. She was very nice to me and said such nice things about you the last time I saw her." But I heard an inner voice prompting me: "Don't go. Stay here. This is where you belong."

Usually, with the coming of spring, we could count on our idol's return. And, as anticipated, one fine morning in early May she breezed in, looking radiant in a brown and pink traveling costume. Her small brown cap had a pink chiffon veil becomingly draped around it. (She loved veils and wore them in various attractive ways.) All unhappiness was instantly erased from our minds; we gathered about her with happy smiles. Then she asked us to dance. That was always the first thing she wanted to see. Afterwards we were called into the library, the most elegant room in the house, where the two sisters were seated together on the couch below the big window. We knew something was in the wind or we would not have been asked to come there. Isadora said:

"You have danced so well I would like to take all of you to have tea at my apartment. But it is just a small place, so I can ask only four or five." With her sister's permission she invited three of the smaller ones and her niece. Then she said, "And

I would like Irma to come too." I glanced in agitation at Tante Miss, who of late had substituted deprivation of privileges for corporal punishment. She stared at me, wrinkled her brow, smacked her tooth, and said flatly, "Irma cannot go; she has been naughty."

I could not recall what sin I had committed; I never could. My trespasses consisted entirely of talking back, for I never did anything really bad. Nor, as far as I remember, did the other children ever commit any really offensive acts. I was close to tears and stood there shamefacedly with lowered eyelids, scraping my foot on the carpet. Isadora, who had just seen me dance my "Poor Orphan Child" for the first time and liked it, said placatingly to her sister, "Oh, Elizabeth, let's make an exception for once and let her go."

"No, that would be a bad example for the others. I am sorry, but I can't allow it."

Isadora was not in the habit of being contradicted by anyone. However, she did not say anything further, although she seemed annoyed. While the other invited children rushed upstairs to don their party clothes (the new swansdown-trimmed dresses Isadora had given us for Christmas), I lingered in the hall trying to hide my tears. Suddenly I felt a light touch on my shoulder. I turned around and there was Isadora whispering quickly, "Shh, keep quiet, darling! Go and get dressed and then wait in my carriage, but don't let anyone see you! Hurry!"

How we children giggled at the wonderful trick Isadora had played on old Tante Miss! When we arrived at the apartment in Hardenbergstrasse, we found Gordon Craig seated there on the sofa smoking a pipe. I had not seen him since that day in Hamburg over a year ago. After tea, Isadora took a stack of her photographs out of a drawer and threw them on the floor saying, "Here they are, children; pick any picture you like and I will autograph it for you!"

While we carefully made our individual choices, she and Craig sat together watching us with the affection of indulgent parents. It gave me such a comfortable, homey feeling. Children always crave affection and loving kindness, and parents try to give it to them. But children harbored in an institution, no matter how humane the treatment, are starved for that loving individual attention of caresses and endearments that a mother usually bestows on them. Most regrettably, Elizabeth Duncan, in whose charge we were left and to whom we instinctively turned for those signs of comfort and affection, never—in all the years we were in her care—offered an endearment or a gentle pat on the cheek to any of her pupils. That is why most of them did not feel any affection for her either.

With Isadora it was entirely different. Children know instinctively when they are loved. That afternoon in her apartment we were completely happy. She autographed all our photographs, inscribing mine "With love and kisses." I hugged the pretty picture to my breast and carried it back to school like a trophy.

As if she had sensed what troubled her little pupils and had seen into their hearts, she came next day to Grunewald to teach us an unforgettable lesson. Early in the morning, while we sat at our desks, she opened the door and entered the classroom. Our teacher and the entire class rose to their feet.

"Good morning!" Isadora said cheerfully. "Please be seated and don't let me interrupt." Turning to our schoolmarm, Frau Zschetzsching, who sat at her desk on a raised dais looking very prim in a white blouse with high boned collar and hair done up in a pompadour, Isadora said, "Please continue with whatever you were studying. I'll sit here quietly and listen."

Our schoolmarm was flustered in front of the famous personage whose acquaintance she had not made before, this being Isadora's first visit to her classroom. "We were doing arithmetic," she answered, "but I don't think that will interest you, Miss Duncan. Let us turn to another subject. Would you like to hear the children recite poetry?"

"Yes, I love poetry, that would be very nice."

Although we had no inhibitions about dancing before a public, we all were tongue-tied and embarrassed to stand up and recite. The stuttering and loss of memory were pitiful to hear. It was in turn painful for us to see our schoolmarm's angry discomfiture mounting by the minute and Isadora's puzzled look as she made a concentrated effort to understand our incoherent German. With an embarrassed smile, Frau Zschetzsching finally said, "Well, they don't seem to be in very good form today. I think, perhaps, with the *Gnädige Frau's* permission . . ."

"May I put a question to them?" Isadora interrupted her.

"Of course." Our schoolmarm looked relieved. Isadora stood up, assumed her familiar stance with head slightly inclined to one side and chin tilted upwards, while all eyes were riveted on her.

"Tell me, children," she said earnestly, "what is the greatest thing in life?"

A ray of intelligence flowed back into our dull minds. Instantly, a flurry of hands shot into the air, furiously wigwagging for attention. The answer to that one was obvious. We all knew it. So when she asked, we all shouted in unison, "To dance!" and sat back with an expression of triumph on our shining faces.

But Isadora sadly shook her head. We could not believe our ears when we heard her say, "No, dancing is not the greatest thing in life."

That sounded like heresy, coming from her—of all people— the greatest dancer in the world! What could it be? Music? Painting? Singing? Our choices showed the influence of our thorough artistic education. No, no, no, none of those, she told us. We gave up. Lifting one forefinger for emphasis, she announced in a clear, vibrant voice:

"The greatest thing in life is—LOVE!"

We stared at her dumbfounded. She turned for corroboration to our schoolmarm and asked, "Is it not true?" To our astonishment, the prim schoolteacher had turned crimson with confusion. Delighted with the dramatic effect she had created, Isadora waved a graceful farewell, said "Adieu!" and disappeared.

No sooner was the door closed than a chorus of eager voices questioned our schoolmarm. "What did she mean, Frau Zschetzsching? Why is love the greatest thing? Why, why, why?"

She rapped her desk for order and said, "Be quiet! Sit down, and I will explain."

Slowly she opened a drawer of the desk and drew forth a black book. We recognized it as the New Testament, from which she read us a lesson each day. With a solemn expression, she announced, "Let me read you a verse from First Corinthians." While we sat with hands folded in prayer and assumed the proper, pious mien expected of us, she intoned:

"Though I speak with the tongue of men and of angels, and have not love, I am become as sounding brass, or a tinkling cymbal" and she continued through the whole thirteenth chapter, which ends, "And now abideth faith, hope, love, these three; but the greatest of these is love."

Our teacher fixed us with a stern look. "This, my dear children, is what Miss Duncan meant when she said the greatest thing in life is love." She closed the book with a loud thud and said, "Class dismissed!"

It was entirely by chance (because printed material of that sort was carefully kept away from our hands) that a few weeks later we saw an item in an illustrated weekly telling of Isadora's marriage to Gordon Craig. Naturally Isadora's personal life was a closed book to her young disciples, so this piece of news aroused the wildest interest. There was one thing we could not comprehend—why had we not been told? Surely, if this story were true (we had no way of knowing then that it was not), we reasoned that we would have heard about it from Tante Miss. This fascinating news item remained an unsolved riddle as far as Isadora's pupils were concerned.

For a whole year thereafter we did not obtain as much as a glimpse of her. She was at that time expecting the birth of her first child at a secluded beach cottage in Nordwyck, Holland—fact of which her pupils were kept in strict ignorance. She had invited her niece to visit her and had included Erica and me too, but Tante Miss as usual said No. So that we would not feel too disappointed, Isadora in the kindness of her heart sent us some toys. I remember the penciled note she included saying: "Dear Irma, Here is a lamb for you and a pink kitten for little Erica. Love, Isadora." I treasured the note more than the toy lamb on wheels, for which I considered myself too old, as I had reached the ripe age of ten.

Years later, I found a thought she wrote in her diary while awaiting her first born. It said: "Yellow tulips, white hyacinths, great window spaces of sky, black steps leading to a balcony—four red pillars. Dearest Baby, if you can remember these things and always love them."

When at last we saw her again in Grunewald the following spring she appeared with a sweet blue-eyed baby in her arms. Her own contribution to "the greatest thing in life." She held the child up for all of us to see and admire and said, "Very soon, she will be the youngest pupil in the school."

4

European Tour

It was night and the train sped eastward. We always traveled third class. At night the smaller children, leaving the hard benches for the older girls to stretch out on, climbed up into the *Gepaecknetz*, a luggage rack that was shaped like a tiny hammock though it was not as comfortable. The iron braces hurt my back even though I tried to pad them with my coat or woolen shawl. However, it was better to lie down, no matter how uncomfortably, than to sit up all night.

Contrary to the policy of the school (that we were not to appear on the stage together with our famous teacher until we reached the age of seventeen), Isadora had decided to take us on tour with her. All agog over the big adventure, I could hardly sleep, knowing that at this moment, in the middle of winter, we were traveling at top speed to St. Petersburg in Russia. What a fantastic place the name alone conjured up in my lively imagination! I had read about that frozen land to the north where fierce animals, such as wild bears and wolves, roamed through the endless forests; and of the cities where men called tsars lived in courts of Oriental splendor, speaking a barbaric tongue no one could understand. Though I was not, as a rule, a very good student—lapsing too often into daydreams during which I listened to the long-drawn hoot of the suburban trains and imagined I was on the way to some far-off place—I always gave undivided attention to geography. It was my favorite subject. I did not have a good memory for verses, but the jingles Frau Zschetzsching taught us to remember geographical names,

I seldom forgot. There was, for instance: *"Ural Gebirge, Ural Fluss, Caspisches Meer und Caucasus."* Was this an omen of the future? How was I to know that a time would come when I would traverse the Urals, the Caspian Sea, and all of the Caucasus on many occasions with the pupils of my own school to dance for the Russian people. Now as a child of ten, the largest part of Europe had appeared merely as a colored blotch on my geographical map. It was most exciting to see it take on actual dimension and reality.

This was vividly brought home to me the instant we changed trains at the frontier to the wider-gauged Russian cars, with a Russian conductor, big brass samovars of hot water for *chai*, and candles that burned during the night instead of gaslight. I kept my eyes glued to the window, as did all the other children, on the lookout for wolves and wild bears when the gloomy woods, deep in snow, stretched out on either side. But we saw nothing. That did not prevent us from having goose pimples all over.

All would have been perfect but for one thing. Dining car meals being far too expensive, Tante Miss provisioned us with a hamper of the most outlandish food. A faddist by nature, she was currently addicted to a health-food diet. Throughout the three long days of our trip she fed us, three times a day, nothing but dried figs, dried bananas, and nuts. "Don't make a fuss," she admonished me when I refused to eat any more. I tried to explain that my stomach was upset. She wouldn't hear of it. "Nonsense, this is good for you," she insisted. "Just think of something else while you eat. The other girls seem to like it, why don't you?"

There was no use protesting. No one could be more tyrannical than Tante Miss, and it was health-food diet or go hungry. I knew something awful would happen, and it did. As we stood disheveled, unwashed, and travel-weary in the middle of the elegant lobby of the best hotel in St. Petersburg, I experienced an awful attack of biliousness. While waiting there for our rooms to be assigned I saw, as through a green miasma, the golden open-caged elevator ride up and down discharging passengers, who leisurely wended their way toward the restaurant hidden behind pots of tall palms. The odor of expensive food wafted my way, together with the sounds of dinner music, the usual selections from *The Gypsy Baron*. And then it happened! Like a contagious wave, my sickness started to spread among the other girls. A group of green-looking children was led upstairs and put to bed. Tante Miss shook her head in dismay. "Too much excitement, I'm afraid," she said. We knew better. Too many dried bananas, figs, and nuts!

Feeling fine the next day, after a good night's rest in real beds and some real food, we made the acquaintance of St. Petersburg. In those forever vanished times the city was lively and brilliant in its mantle of deep snow. The jolly sleighrides from the hotel to the theatre and back every day were our special delight. To children, there is nothing quite so much fun as a ride in an open sleigh. There was always a long string of them when we sallied forth, since each accommodated only two passengers. The bulky clothes of the *Isvostchik*, with his long beard covered with frost, reminded us of Santa Claus. Off we went at a fast clip, sliding down the broad Nevsky Prospect, a bear rug across the knees and the merry tinkling of little bells in our ears, sounding so festive and gay we could hardly refrain from shouting for joy.

Our first performance, on February 9, 1908, proved a gala event in the Russian capital. Presented as a benefit for a charitable organization under the august auspices of H.I.H. Grand Duchess Olga Alexandrovna, sister of the Tsar, it drew the elite and aristocracy of St. Petersburg society to the Maryinsky Theatre. Isadora danced her "Iphigenia" program, and we appeared at the very end in a "Werber Waltz" by Lanner, which she had choreographed and taught us in May of 1907, and which we had first performed in Mannheim that summer for the city's three-hundred-year jubilee. Isadora wrote of this dance:

I taught them to weave and entwine, to part and unite, in endless rounds and successions. Now resembling the Loves of a
Pompeian frieze, now the youthful Graces of Donatello, or again
the airy flights of Titania's following, the light of inspiration and
divine music shone in their youthful forms and faces. The sight
of these dancing children was so beautiful it awakened the admiration of all artists and poets.*

"How darling they are! Look at the one over there, isn't
she cute! My, what beautiful hair! You must simply love to
dance, you look so happy!" Such were the usual backstage
compliments we heard when people crowded into our dressing
room. But after that performance at the Maryinsky Theatre,
there was so much Russian spoken it made my head swim. We
all sighed with relief when the audience was gone.

Then there was a soft knock at the door, and a soft voice
said, "May I come in?" The moment she entered, we recognized
Anna Pavlova. We had seen her dance in an old-style ballet
the night before. She approached and kissed each one of us,
murmuring "Dooshinka, dooshinka." † Dressed in a white gown
with a long, glittering white shawl over her shoulders, she
looked as she had on the stage—tiny, dainty, and very pretty
with her dark hair tied back into a knot, ballerina-fashion. The
young man with her carried a large box of candy which she
offered us. Our hawk-eyed English governess stepped forward
and took it away saying, "Sorry, Madame, but the children are
not allowed to eat candy, except one a day." With these words
she disappeared, carrying the candy with her.

As soon as the door closed behind the ogress, Anna Pavlova
(who also had been brought up in an institution) whipped out
another box of candy from beneath her long shawl. With
gestures of her hands indicating for us to hide it quickly, quickly,
she helped us to stow it away in one of our wicker suitcases. We

* *Life,* p. 214.
† "Darling"

simply loved her for that clever trick. Lying in bed that night, under cover of darkness, we had a feast. Needless to say, we saw no more of the other box of candy, except the telltale wrappings scattered about our governess' room.

Summoned one morning to Isadora's suite, we found her seated on a chaise-longue surrounded by shoe boxes. "There is a pair of golden sandals for each of you," she said. "Try them on and see if they fit."

From a bolt of pink silk two lengths of material were cut and stitched up at the sides. With two small buttons, one for each shoulder, the material was caught up and fastened together to form armholes and "voilà, presto!" we soon each had a new pink silk tunic. A Russian embroidered belt completed the costume.

Our suspicion that this new getup signified that something special was afoot was verified when Isadora announced, "This afternoon we are going to have tea with a real grand duke. What do you think of that!" She explained that his name was André Vladimirovitch and he was a cousin of the Tsar. "He lives in that big white house on the other side of the river; you must have noticed it when you took a walk along the Neva. You must be on your very best behavior," she admonished.

We found the idea of meeting a royal personage quite overpowering, for in Germany everybody, from infancy on, was taught to look upon royalty as some kind of demigod. We did not look forward to the encounter with great pleasure.

When the time came, instead of going by the Troitsky Bridge we crossed the frozen river in sleighs and got out directly below the house. André Vladimirovitch, resplendent in uniform and decorations, greeted us jovially. A young man of twenty-seven, he was tall, blond, and good-looking, and he spoke to us children in German. Without formality, he proceeded to show Isadora and the rest of us his brand-new mansion, including the bathrooms with sunken marble bathtubs, which he had built for his mistress the prima ballerina Mathilde Kschessinska, who was seven years older than he. The latter, holding a little boy by the hand, followed the Grand Duke silently wherever he went. This tiny, mouselike woman dressed in black, with small features and dark frizzy hair, I took at first to be the boy's governess, but the child was their son Vova.* Next to the brilliant personality of the Grand Duke, she made no impression at all.

Soon many other guests arrived and crowded into the dining room, where we children were seated at a table laden with the most mouth-watering assortment of French pastries, towering layer cakes, fruit tarts, and candies—none of which we touched despite the repeated urging of our friendly regal host. We hated to be on display and reacted with chronic shyness. Finally the Grand Duke took a plate filled with chocolate candies and personally passed them around.

"Notice how polite they are," he said. "Each takes only one little piece. None of them would dare take two."

When he reached me with the silver platter, I took one like the others, but—being a child of spirit—I stopped him when he was about to withdraw and deliberately chose another.

"Ha, ha!" he threw back his head and laughed. "Good for you," he said, patting me on the head. That broke the ice, and the adults retired to the salon for their own refreshments, leaving us in peace to enjoy ours.

After tea, the Grand Duke wanted to know whether Isadora would favor them with a little dance. But she refused. How about the children? He and his guests would love to see them dance. Our music director, a young Viennese by the name of Max Merz, regretfully informed Isadora that he had not brought any music with him. However, he liked to improvise, and sitting down at the piano he started to play. Isadora conferred with Elizabeth about what to do when the latter surprised me by saying:

"Let Irma dance something, she knows how to improvise."

* Vova, short for Vladimir.

Isadora looked undecided. "Well, if you say so, Elizabeth," and she told me to try.

I had never improvised before so large a company and felt very timid. A command is a command, however. Trembling with nervousness, I hid behind one of the tall columns in the Greek-style hall to take off my pink socks and golden sandals. Unfortunately the hall had a marble floor not at all pleasant to dance on in winter. Concerned about this situation, Madame Kschessinska suggested spreading sheets on the floor. But they proved too great a hazard because they slipped. I much preferred the solid ground to dance on.

In her "Memoirs" Mathilde Kschessinska recalls this scene when she tells of our visit to her new palace. An old woman in her nineties, she now resides in France and still teaches ballet in her school in Paris. When I wrote to her a few years ago she very kindly responded, giving me news of herself and her work. After the Russian revolution she became the morganatic wife of the Grand Duke and goes now by the title of H.S.H. Princesse Mathilde Romanovsky-Krasinsky. Having always been a friend and genuine admirer of Isadora, she assured me that she had not forgotten her or her performances in St. Petersburg, which she always remembered with great pleasure.

On that freezing day in February, 1908, when I put my bare feet on that marble floor I felt as if standing on ice. So I moved about quickly and danced with great verve to keep my feet off the ground as much as possible. My spirited dance was much applauded, though no one guessed the reason why. I must have given a good account of myself, for Isadora hugged me warmly—more for my sportsmanship, I imagine, than for anything else. The Grand Duke shook my hand, saying, "That is something our ballerinas can't do—improvise." I felt very proud of myself and only wished mother could see me now. . . .

Having made the acquaintance of a Grand Duke, we now wondered whether by good luck we might not obtain just a glimpse of Tsar Nicholas II himself. Every time we passed the dark red façade of the Winter Palace, my childish curiosity was aroused. What did the ruler of this vast country look like? I soon discovered. Once, coming back from a walk near the river, we noticed a closed carriage accompanied by several outriders in uniform. A pale-faced man with a small goatee, wearing a peaked cap, glanced out the window. When he saw us, he smiled and waved his hand in greeting. Somebody shouted, "The Tsar! The Tsar!" We all stared after the retreating vehicle. Could that really have been the Tsar? Where was his crown, his ermine robe, his golden coach? Little did I suspect that the time was soon at hand when the last of the Tsars would be deprived forever of these imperial appurtenances, or that I would one day stand in that tragic cellar in the Urals where he and his family had been shot to death during the revolution that would topple his throne and cause all this brilliant life to collapse.

Our two weeks in St. Petersburg passed all too swiftly. Of the many interesting sights we had seen there, one other experience remained outstanding—our visit to the Imperial Ballet School. "I took my little pupils to witness the training of the children of the ballet school," Isadora said, "and they observed them with the view of swallows circling freely in the air looking at caged canary birds." *

Under the direction of Marius Petipa, who obstinately clung to the passé traditions, the ballet was not amenable to any change whatsoever. Only with the coming of the young, forward-looking ballet master Michael Fokine, who took over several years later, did a radical change take place. He adopted many of the new ideas Isadora Duncan had brought to the dance, and thus the Russian ballet underwent the transformation for which it is known today. These revolutionary ideas, which marked a new epoch in the art of dance, Fokine saw demonstrated for the first time in January 1905, when Isadora made her initial appearance in Russia.

* *Life*, p. 215.

Mathilde Kschessinska saw Isadora Duncan dance for the first time in Vienna in 1903. She frankly confesses to having been completely conquered by her art. She was so carried away, she says, by her "Blue Danube Waltz" that she climbed on her seat and cheered as loud as she could with the rest of the audience. As a professional dancer of the first order herself, she easily recognized the hard work that had produced such beautiful dancing and made Isadora the perfect mistress of her art.

I think that this above-mentioned earlier date is of special interest. Because of her position as prima ballerina assoluta of the Imperial Ballet in St. Petersburg, possessing enormous authority in that organization, she must surely have adopted and made use of some of the new ideas Isadora Duncan originated. Thus Isadora's influence undoubtedly made itself felt on a part of the Russian ballet as early as 1903, although she herself made her debut in that city only in January 1905.

Kschessinska, reminiscing about how the new changes came about that transformed the old-style ballet, stresses in her "Memoirs" the overwhelming impression the young American dancer made on Fokine. With a wild enthusiasm he immediately commenced to initiate the necessary reform. Hoping to obtain the same inspiration from the same source as Isadora did, for her new-found art, he went to the Hermitage Museum to study the Greek vases for dance movements. His first Greek-inspired production was a ballet called *Eunice*, in which Kschessinska danced the principal part. On that opening night performance the many old balletomanes criticized him severely for his obvious copying of what they termed "Duncanism." But being a staunch supporter of Fokine, M. Kschessinska always considered that first performance on December 10, 1906, a date of importance in the transformation of the old-style ballet to a freer expression. She and Fokine worked closely together toward that goal. In 1907–08, Kschessinska decided to take Vaslav Nijinsky, who had graduated from the Ballet School only the year before, for a new dancing partner, recognizing in him a great talent. After our performances in St. Petersburg in 1908, and having seen Isadora's Chopin program, they initially danced together at the Maryinsky Theatre to Chopin's "Nocturne," choreographed by Fokine. At the time of our visit, none of the famous dancers associated with the ballet school in St. Petersburg had yet been completely emancipated artistically. Nor were their names (with one or two exceptions) known outside of their own country. Not until five years after their first contact with Isadora's ideas did they form the great company known as the Diaghilev Ballets Russes, which brought that roster of world-renowned names, such as Nijinsky, Pavlova, Karsavina, Fokine, and others to the attention of foreign countries for the first time. While most of these ballet dancers freely admitted that Isadora Duncan's ideas gave new life to their once moribund art and helped to beautify it, they all maintained that neither Isadora herself nor her pupils could execute ballet movements, whereas any well-trained ballet dancer could easily assimilate and execute any Duncan movements.

This assumption to my mind has always seemed both illogical and absurd. They forget, or don't seem to comprehend, that Isadora Duncan's theory of the dance precludes any assimilation of movements based on ballet technique and therefore no ballet technique can produce the proper Duncan movement and expression. Although Isadora's art has incontestably helped to beautify the ballet and given it new life, the converse does not apply. The art of Isadora Duncan has never been either beautified or re-vitalized by the ballet.

That morning we watched for three hours while the ballet girls of different age-groups stood in rows on the tips of their toes going through torturing exercises in a bare room with a large portrait of the Tsar hanging on the wall. We were familiar with many of the exercises. We practiced barre work ourselves—though of course in a much more relaxed style, without distortions, and from natural positions of the feet.

What amazed us Duncan pupils was the way the ballet

students danced continuously in front of a mirror, closely watching every move they made. There were no wall mirrors in our school. Our teacher's philosophy of the dance forbade any such visual aids. Isadora taught us to close our eyes and listen to the music with our souls. Then we were to dance in accordance with this music heard inwardly and, while listening, feel an inner self awakening deep within us. Its strength would animate our bodies.

"This is the first step in dancing as I understand it," she used to say. "This is the truly creative dancer, natural but not imitative, speaking in movement out of himself and out of something greater than all selves. It is the mission of all art to express the highest and most beautiful ideals of man. What ideal does the ballet express? All ballet movements are sterile because they are unnatural; their purpose is to create the delusion that the law of gravitation does not exist for them." *

She pronounced an anathema on dancers who comprehended only with the brain, who loaded down their dances with empty gestures devoid of meaning, and on all those systems of dancing that are merely arranged gymnastics, too logically understood. In this connection, as far as physical education for children was concerned, she once said, "It seems to me criminal to entrust children, who cannot defend themselves, to this injurious training. In my opinion it is a crime to teach the child to guide his growing body by the stern power of the brain, while deadening impulse and inspiration."

To which I might add that ballet of the present period has not fundamentally changed its principles. Despite some liberation from old bonds, it still does not represent a true art of the dance, but only highly accomplished acrobatics. The male dancer, not going on toe, is not as hampered in the evolution of kinetics as the ballerina. But so long as the latter cannot make more than a few movements unaided, or is kept in a constant

* Cf. *Art*, pp. 52, 55–56.

state of levitation by her partner if not tossed about like a set of Indian clubs between several assistants, her physical activities can hardly be dignified by the term *dancing*.

I recall almost nothing of Helsingfors, Finland, the next stop on our itinerary, except the abnormal amount of butter we were urged to eat in order to keep from freezing, for the temperature was below zero. Then we gave performances in Warsaw and Lodsz in Poland. Warsaw, where we stayed for a week at the Hotel Bristol, stands out primarily because of the new coats Isadora designed and had made to order for us. Of coarse gray military material, they were edged off and embroidered each with a different color—blue, green, brown, wine red—and we also had those little pillbox caps that are now so much *en vogue* to match. We referred to them as our Polish coats and, although they scratched quite a bit, being unlined, we took inordinate pride in them and even insisted on wearing them in the summertime.

The tour continued through Holland and Belgium and, since each stop took up a week or more, it was spring by the time we returned to Germany to dance at the various southern watering places such as Wiesbaden. By this time the weather was warm enough for us to perform out of doors, as we did on the extensive lawn in front of the Kurhaus in Baden-Baden.

At the International Art and Landscaping Exhibition in Mannheim in the previous year, we danced in the middle of a rose garden, against the dramatic background of an illuminated fountain and its reflecting pool. For this occasion the water was turned off, and the fountain proper was boarded over to provide a stage. To reach it, we were paddled across the pool in flower-bedecked gondolas manned by costumed gondoliers. At night the scene was lit by floodlights; and the performance, seen as if suspended in mid-air, took on a most romantic aspect. A select but enthusiastic audience attended. An article in a local newspaper described the end of the performance:

The crowd swiftly passed by the brightly illuminated water tower and fountain so as not to dim the inner vision glowing with the beauty and grace they had just witnessed. For they were all very much moved by the wonder of the dances a small group of children had presented there. Repeatedly one hears men both old and young exclaim: "How delightful! That was really quite enchanting!"—not to mention the enthusiastic remarks of the women! While Isadora danced alone, her reform movement in the art of the dance did not carry quite the conviction it has when she shows us her graceful dancing children. What appears to our present doubting generation only as a dream will become a reality for the children of the next generation.

We children were apparently successfully putting our message across to the people, as Isadora had hoped we would, proving that her efforts had not been in vain. More and more people began to understand what Isadora's art was all about now that they saw it could be transmitted to others. She had wanted her pupils to set a good example to all the other children in the world. With what fine result we fulfilled this wish can be gleaned from the following article, which appeared in a Swiss paper after a performance we had given in Zurich:

To begin with: the appearance of the Duncan Dancers was a complete victory! We noticed with the greatest pleasure the many children present in the audience and hope there will be an even greater number here tomorrow, because here they have an example of what the true dance should be, so different from the instruction they receive in their usual social or ballet dancing classes. One must see with one's own eyes with what clarity of expression these Duncan pupils perform in order truly to appreciate their unique art. . . . The magnificent free strides of their simple walk, which one has already much admired in Isadora Duncan, has also become a salient characteristic of her young pupils. The arms, the hands, the entire body is here awakened into graceful motion and rhythmic life.

For instance, with what grace did a group of three slender girls raise their arms and close into a small circle . . . or, as in

the Lanner Waltz, when a fine silken fabric arched overhead
into a triumphal arch beneath which the dancing children passed
in pairs and then scattered to the four winds; or that supple backward thrust of the body and head with raised arms indicating a
delightful Dionysiac joy. . . .

To correctly evaluate what these children achieve with their
dancing one should immediately afterwards see some of the ster-
eotype movements of the ballet. Anyone endowed with a normal,
healthy perception would not be able to stand it by comparison;
for the latter is all artificiality while the former offers us, together with simplicity, a truly artistically styled naturalness.

Appearing on the same program with Isadora, as we were
now doing, did not imply that we actually danced with her; we
were still too young for that. The only exception to this rule
was the "Reigen" we did together at the very end of each performance by way of an encore. It was always a wonderful event
for us. Then the act of dancing invariably took on a special
meaning for me. Just to hold hands with Isadora, as I often did
in the circle, and to watch the radiant expression on her face
when she danced, was so inspiring that I carry the memory of
it with me to this day. Isadora herself derived unique pleasure
from this, for she said:

Whenever I felt their willing hands in mine, felt the pull and
swing of their little bodies as we danced our fast-paced rondos,
I always envisioned that orchestra of dancers I would one day
bring to life. The sight of these dancing children was so beautiful they strengthened my faith in the ultimate perfection of an
orchestra of dancers which would be to sight what the great
symphonies were to sound. A vast ensemble dancing the Ninth
Symphony of Beethoven.*

That artistic goal was still a long way off. In the meanwhile,
she presented her pupils to the European public, with the promise that in the future they would dance in a mighty array such as
the world had never seen.

* *Life*, p. 140.

So far, the tour had taken us in three months to six countries. At the end of our engagements in the south of Germany, we continued on to France. How thrilled I was to be going to Paris! At the Gare du Nord the porters dressed in blue smocks rushed into our compartments shouting, *"Porteur! porteur!"* and I had a hard time holding onto my now well-traveled wicker suitcase. Tante Miss, who had been reading a novel—Renard's *Poil de Carotte*—to brush up on her French while sitting up all night in the day coach, shushed the swarm of blue-smocked porters away. *"Allez-vous en, allez-vous en,"* she kept repeating until they had gone.

We finally managed to evade their grasping hands and reached the street safely through the noise and bustle of a busy terminal. We found an old-fashioned horse-drawn omnibus waiting for us. On the steps outside the French station I breathed in the soft, caressing night air, eagerly observing the sights and sounds of Paris. They immediately struck me as being, in some indefinable way, unlike those of any other country I had seen. No one who has been to Paris in the month of May will ever forget it.

Sitting on two banquettes facing each other, and attired in our Polish coats and pillbox caps, we were able to take in the sights at leisure. The stodgy omnibus lumbered down the Rue de la Fayette and then continued along the Boulevard Haussmann while the horses' hoofs clumped hard on the uneven pavement, making the windows rattle. Debouching onto the Place de l'Étoile, straddled by the massive Arch of Triumph, we saw the heart of the city suddenly open like a picture book before our enchanted eyes. Illuminated by garlands of lights strung along both sides of the magnificent Avenue des Champs-Élysées and reaching toward the Place de la Concorde where the fountains were playing, Paris was beautiful.

In the spring of 1908, the uncrowded traffic moved at a much slower pace than it does today. It did not obliterate the sense of calm spaciousness that was such a notable characteristic of the French capital, for vehicles then consisted mainly of elegantly accoutered phaetons and equipages. Every now and then a silent electric automobile, signaling its approach by delicately ringing a bell, would overtake our steadily plodding omnibus. Progressing at a slow pace, we finally entered the suburb of Neuilly.

The long passage from east to west across Paris had occupied the better part of an hour. During the last part of it we began to feel drowsy. I glanced over at Tante Miss sitting in one corner with her eyes closed; she seemed to be dozing. We had been very quiet, since her presence was enough to curb our speech. She frowned on any kind of chit-chat and always told us to keep quiet. But as soon as we entered the wide Avenue de Neuilly, with its broad center strip of grass and trees, we saw that a spring fair was in progress. Instantly we were wide awake.

"A carnival! A carnival!" we shouted in unison. In all the years at school we had seen plenty of museums, but not one fair. The sight of this one made us hop up and down on our seats with glee. At home in Hamburg mother had taken me to the Christmas fair. Everything was there just as I remembered it: the milling crowds; the double row of lighted booths filled with toys and gingerbread; the incessant shouts of the hawkers offering their wares; the spinning carrousels, each blaring forth another brassy tune; the pungent smell of steaming sausages. Above it all an acrid odor of magnesium flares floated like a cloud of incense offered to the spirit of King Carnival. We clapped our hands in childish rapture and laughed, wishing we could jump out and join in the fun; but the stern voice of Tante Miss spoiled our innocent enjoyment with, "Come down off those benches immediately and keep quiet!"

We obeyed reluctantly. Her attitude toward us was one of perpetual reproof. She never missed a chance of reminding us to behave with more dignity because we were pupils of the Isadora Duncan School—as if that should stop our normal urge for fun and mischief. Disgruntled grumblings and little grimaces behind her back were our ineffectual revenge. We were craning our necks to get another good look at the gay fair despite her reproof, when the lumbering omnibus suddenly veered sharply to the right, jumbling us together.

We had turned into a quiet side street of the residential section. By comparison with the broad and lively main thoroughfare, it seemed as deserted as a cemetery. The strident music of the calliopes and hurdy-gurdies grew fainter and fainter until only the monotonous clop, clop of the horses remained. The street was dark, with only a gaslight flickering here and there. After a while the brakes screeched, and the omnibus came to a sudden halt.

"This is where we get out," Tante Miss said wearily. The omnibus did not deposit us in front of a hotel or pension as we had expected, but had stopped in front of a church with a tall, slender steeple. A churchyard on one side and a small house on the other presented an eerie picture. All was silent and dark except for a light burning in the window of the house. We did not know what to make of this. My curiosity got the better of me. I timidly asked Tante Miss where we were, not really expecting an answer because she never told us anything. She surprised me by explaining wearily but patiently, "This is our new home, we are going to remain here for as long as we stay in Paris."

"In this church?"

"No, silly, of course not. In the little house beside it. Just follow me." And she added, while we trouped up to the house together, "This used to be the rectory of the American church, but it isn't any longer. Now, no further questions. Take your suitcases and go inside; supper is waiting."

There was something important that she did not explain. None of us had any inkling when we went to bed that night that we would never return to Grunewald. Isadora considered Germany (mainly for personal reasons but also because of the Kaiserin's puritanical views) no longer the proper place for her school. With the closing of the house in Grunewald, she now had just twelve of her most talented pupils left.

We appeared with her for a month or more at the Théâtre de la Gaieté Lyrique in Paris that spring. Gordon Craig, who was then living in Paris and came to our performances, wrote in his notebook:

> It was here that she first used the great blue curtains some twenty or twenty-five feet high, which followed my designs as may be seen in my *The Arts of the Theatre*, published in 1905 and which I had made in 1901–2–3. She pretends that she used them in 1904 in Berlin where I saw her dance for the first time in December. She did not use them then. She used a few curtains six feet in height.

Performing every night, practicing, and rehearsing, we were kept busy. During the day, out for a stroll and some fresh air— always walking in orderly pairs—we often stopped in the Bois where the acacia trees were in bloom to watch the Parisian children at play. They rolled hoops or tossed diabolos into the air or played *cache-cache*, hiding from their nurses behind the big trees. We sometimes envied them, for our toys were left in Grunewald and we had nothing to play with. But at night, when the little Parisians slept, we envied them no longer. For then came our turn to play. Dancing on the stage to our hearts' content in harmony with beautiful music played by a fine orchestra under the baton of the great Colonne—what could be a more stirring game! We never tired of it and eagerly looked forward to our nightly gambols.

Not that our academic studies were neglected. Frau Zschetzsching came from Germany to resume them after a three-month vacation. She also taught us French, a language she pronounced with a strong Germanic accent, which bore no resemblance to the way the natives spoke. We learned to pronounce it better from singing the old folk songs "Sur le pont d'Avignon" and "Le Chevalier de la Marjolaine."

Although we had contributed to our upkeep by giving paid performances ever since our stage debut, the expenses of the school mounted and became more and more difficult to meet. Away on tour, Isadora would be constantly bombarded by telegrams from her sister or mother asking for funds—a thousand marks here, two thousand marks there, until she felt like saying, "To heck with it all!" She always remembered this effort of sustaining the school's expenses as uphill work, like straining forward against the rapids of a river. She had no sooner returned from Russia at the end of June than Charles Frohman proposed an extended engagement in London, together with her pupils. This was all so quickly organized that she had no time to rest from her strenuous tour. It seemed that the Duchess of Manchester, who was a dollar princess, was ready to sponsor the Duncan School in England, and so we all went there to dance at the Duke of York's Theatre, beginning July 6, 1908.

It rained almost the whole time, and we took melancholy walks into Hyde Park from our nearby lodgings in Half Moon Street, finding no gay children at play but only placid sheep grazing on the common. Frohman had advertised us somewhat sensationally as "Twenty Parisian Dancers." That this statement was misleading and inaccurate on both counts did not bother this seasoned showman one bit. However, he gave us the thrill of our young lives when he presented each of us with a little gold watch. We simply squealed with delight. To be in possession of a real gold watch was the height of our ambition. We were seldom given presents. No longer were our daily outings in Hyde Park melancholy; we positively beamed with pride as we walked about in the rain with our watches pinned to the outside of our coats. After a week of this, alas, our golden watches turned a nasty green.

Ellen Terry, the mother of Gordon Craig, tried to make up for this disappointment by taking us to the zoo; then to see *Peter Pan* and *The Pirates of Penzance*. She loved children and we loved her. She was the second celebrated actress we had met.

The first one had been Eleonora Duse, who did not take us to a zoo. Instead, reclining on a couch à la Dame aux Camelias, she had placed her long, slender hands on our heads in benediction and murmured, *"Que dieu vous garde!"*

The highlight of our month's stay in London turned out to be a command performance for their majesties King Edward VII and Queen Alexandra. The day before this important occasion we lunched with the Duchess of Manchester at her lovely estate on the Thames. For a change we enjoyed a spell of beautiful weather, and the command performance was planned to be given outdoors.

When we went in to luncheon, Isadora sat next to the Duchess and then asked me to sit beside her. This honor, pleasant as it was, made me nervous. Luncheon was served in grand style, with a uniformed footman in the ducal colors standing behind each chair. For a main course we had scrambled eggs and string beans. The latter happened to be my great aversion. I didn't think anyone would notice if I left them untouched, though I had been taught that leaving food constituted a grave social error. Just as the white-gloved footman was about to remove my plate, Isadora—who had been engaged in conversation with the Duchess—glanced my way and said, "Irma, eat your string beans."

What to do? Both she and the Duchess were giving me their undivided attention. Luckily the situation was saved when the Duchess, taking pity, said, "I know how she feels. I have a little niece who can't stand them either," and motioned to the footman to remove my plate. Then I heard her say to Isadora, "Their majesties are definitely coming tomorrow night, so why don't we have our coffee in the drawing room and talk about the arrangements, while the children go outside to play? It's such a lovely day."

We breathed a sigh of relief. Amid heavy tapestries and embossed silver, the ducal luncheon had been a bit too formal and skimpy. Once out in the sunshine, the velvety lawns and the carefully tended flowerbeds restored our normal spirits. We roamed unattended through the park. At one point we came upon a charming sunken garden surrounded by a high wall, which—we noticed with delight—was covered with luscious peaches growing in espalier fashion. They hung there, well spaced, in glowing colors, like nature's miniature masterpieces, ripe for the picking. In the twinkling of an eye, two of the older girls had jumped into the garden whence they threw the golden fruit, flushed with pink, up to us. The first peaches we had ever eaten (they are considered a great luxury in Europe and are very scarce in the northern countries), they tasted as delicious and sweet as stolen fruit is supposed to.

But suddenly we heard someone call from a distance, "Children! Children! Where are you?"

Hastily we wiped the telltale juice from our hands and lips, and walked sedately back, putting on an innocent air. We kept our fingers crossed that Isadora would not discover our misdeed.

After the dance the next day, their majesties graciously shook hands with us, and the King wanted to know what everybody else in that overdressed era was always asking: "Are you not cold with so little on?" Bored with the same old question, we simply shook our heads and smiled. Queen Alexandra, elegantly gowned in the Victorian style with trailing skirt, feathered hat, and long feathered boa, enjoyed our dancing so much that she attended several of our matinees when we children presented our own program. She particularly liked the old German folk songs we sang and danced, such as *"Haenslein sass im Schornstein und flickte seine Schuh,"* in which I had the solo part, or the one where little Isabelle with the bushy hair was so amusing, which was called, *"Hexlein, willst du tanzen."* They probably recalled to the Queen her own childhood in Denmark.

I must mention here that despite the frequent paid performances we children gave, none of us ever received any weekly allowance or pocket money. We got not even a penny's worth to buy an occasional lollipop or a ribbon for our hair. Naturally,

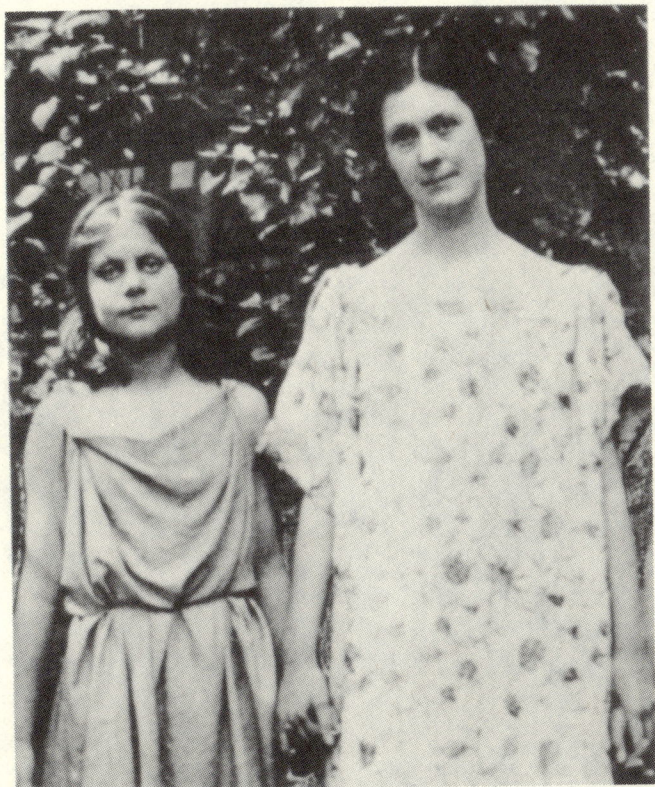

Irma and Isadora, Neuilly, 1908.

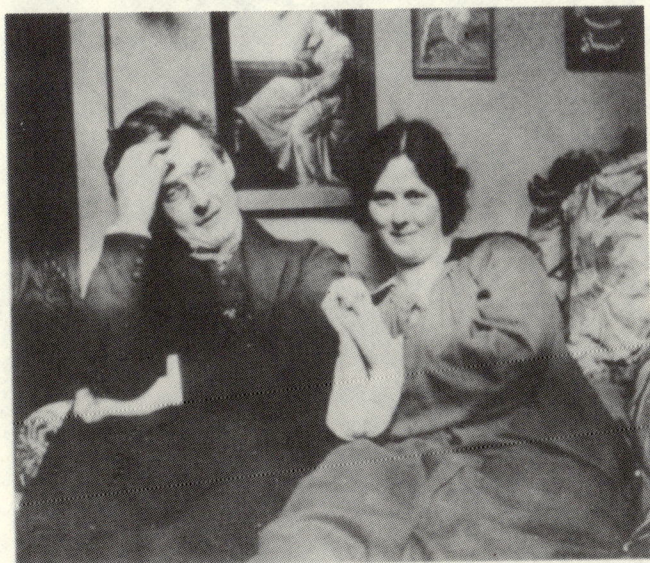

Gordon Craig and Isadora, Berlin, 1904.

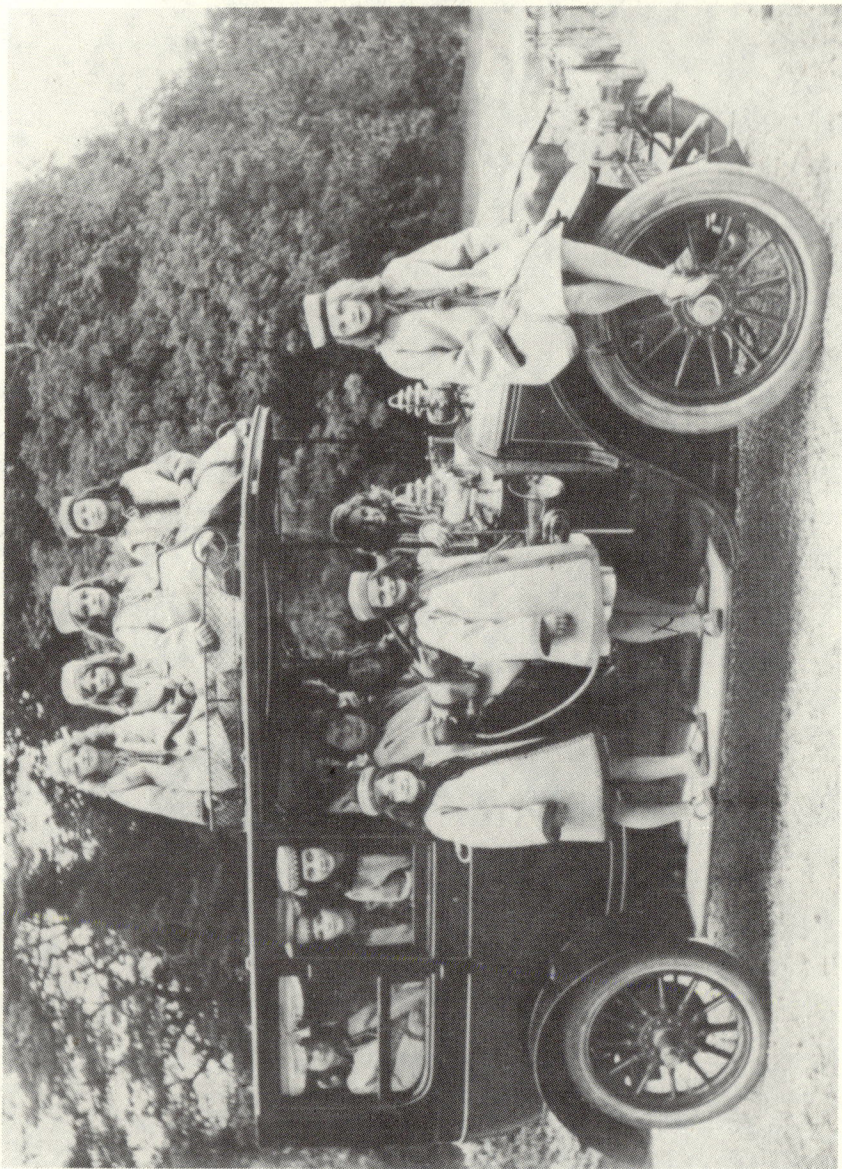

Pillbox hats and Polish coats, Château Villegenis, October 1908. Irma on running board, center; Preston Sturges behind shoulder of girl at wheel.

with our strict upbringing, we dared not ask for any. Even small sums sent from home by our parents were frowned upon. Thoughts of filthy lucre had no place in our spiritual education dedicated to the true dance. So one can imagine the thrill I experienced when one day, in a restaurant in Piccadilly, I found a golden sovereign lying on the stair carpet. My exclamations of glee drew the governess' attention, and she grabbed it away from me. Like all children I believed in the rule "finders, keepers," but she said with a righteous air, "This must be returned to the management, immediately." Then the old hypocrite put it in her black leather bag and kept it. She happened to leave us that season for good. We children were so overjoyed to be rid of our dragon that I did not begrudge her my lucky find. To be rid of her was well worth the loss of a gold sovereign.

The noted English novelist John Galsworthy saw us that June and wrote an article about the Duncan dancers:

DELIGHT

I was taken by a friend one afternoon to a theatre. When the curtain was raised, the stage was perfectly empty save for tall grey curtains which enclosed it on all sides, and presently through the thick folds of those curtains children came dancing in, singly, or in pairs, till a whole troop of ten or twelve were assembled. They were all girls; none, I think, more than fourteen years old, one or two certainly not more than eight. They wore but little clothing, their legs, feet and arms being quite bare. Their hair, too, was unbound; and their faces, grave and smiling, were so utterly dear and joyful, that in looking on them one felt transported to some Garden of Hesperides, where self was not, and the spirit floated in pure ether. Some of these children were fair and rounded, others dark and elf-like; but one and all looked entirely happy, and quite unself-conscious, giving no impression of artifice, though they evidently had the highest and most careful training. Each flight and whirling movement seemed conceived there and then out of the joy of being—dancing had surely never been a labour to them, either in rehearsal or performance.

There was no tiptoeing and posturing, no hopeless muscular achievement; all was rhythm, music, light, air, and above all things, happiness. Smiles and love had gone to the fashioning of their performance; and smiles and love shone from every one of their faces and from the clever white turnings of their limbs.

Amongst them—though all were delightful—there were two who especially riveted my attention. The first of these two was the tallest of all the children, a dark thin girl, in whose every expression and movement there was a kind of grave, fiery love.

During one of the many dances, it fell to her to be the pursuer of a fair child, whose movements had a very strange soft charm; and this chase, which was like the hovering of a dragon-fly round some water-lily, or the wooing of a moonbeam by the June night, had in it a most magical sweet passion. That dark, tender huntress, so full of fire and yearning, had the queerest power of symbolising all longing, and moving one's heart. In her, pursuing her white love with such wistful fervour, and ever arrested at the very moment of conquest, one seemed to see the great secret force that hunts through the world, on and on, tragically unresting, immortally sweet.

The other child who particularly enchanted me was the smallest but one, a brown-haired fairy crowned with a half-moon of white flowers, who wore a scanty little rose-petal-coloured shift that floated about her in the most delightful fashion. She danced as never child danced. Every inch of her small head and body was full of the sacred fire of motion; and in her little *pas seul* she seemed to be the very spirit of movement. One felt that Joy had flown down, and was inhabiting there; one heard the rippling of Joy's laughter. And, indeed, through all the theatre had risen a rustling and whispering; and sudden bursts of laughing rapture.

I looked at my friend; he was trying stealthily to remove something from his eyes with a finger. And to myself the stage seemed very misty, and all things in the world lovable; as though that dancing fairy had touched them with tender fire, and made them golden.

God knows where she got that power of bringing joy to our dry hearts: God knows how long she will keep it! But that little flying Love had in her the quality that lies in deep colour, in music, in the wind, and the sun, and in certain great works of art—the power to set the heart free from every barrier, and flood it with delight.

John Galsworthy remembered our dancing years later. Lecturing at Princeton University, he spoke of losing oneself in the contemplation of beauty. He said, "How lost was I when I first looked on the Grand Canyon of Arizona; when I first saw Isadora Duncan's child dancers . . . or the Egyptian desert under the moon."

This tribute by the English writer fittingly closes a chapter in the lives of Isadora's little pupils from the Grunewald school. The innocent years of childhood were rapidly drawing to an end. This long voyage to foreign lands had broadened my outlook and perceptions and had made me more aware of the outside world. With it, too, had vanished many of my childhood illusions.

❧5❧

Sojourn at Château Villegenis

EVERY life has its ups and its downs, its prosperous periods and its meagre ones. The same was true of Isadora's school. Ever since she founded her philanthropical institution, she had tried to keep it going despite financial difficulties. This meant an endless succession of dance tours with no time out to put down roots for the establishment of her private life. Once more, no sooner had the London season ended than she was off again. This time her destination was America. And once more she entrusted the school to the management of Elizabeth. She had no other alternative and no reason for not trusting her sister.

It had not been easy for Isadora to decide on this trip, putting the whole expanse of an ocean between herself and her loved ones for who knew how long. She said, "It cost me many pangs to part from my little baby Deirdre, who was now almost a year old, and from that other child—my School."

Although the number of her original pupils had dwindled to a mere dozen, she continued to pretend they still numbered twenty. Constantly on the lookout for people who might be persuaded to become patrons of her school, she was delighted upon her arrival in America when she met Mrs. W. E. Corey, a wealthy American lady who took an interest in furthering the arts. Before her marriage to a steel magnate, the former Mabel Gilman had been on the stage in musical comedy. An article appearing in a New York newspaper on September 20, 1908, said in part:

> It is owing to Mrs. W. E. Corey's desire to devote some of her present fortune to encouraging artists who need it that the twenty little members of Isadora Duncan's school for dancing are just

now enjoying the delights of residence in a chateau, about forty miles from Paris.

Mrs. Corey, who wants to help not only young dramatists but artists of all kinds as well, heard from Miss Duncan of her plans and the struggle that it was for her to maintain the school by her dancing. Even in France to clothe, feed and educate twenty children is not a slight financial undertaking, especially when they are reared carefully. . . .

"To think that you should be paying to house your school in Paris," said Mrs. Corey when she heard of the work that the children are doing, "when I have a chateau standing empty which they might as well occupy! There is a farm there, too, with all that they could want to eat, and there are servants with nothing to do but wait on them."

Unfortunately, our unknown but very generous American hostess was not there to extend a welcome when we arrived late in September at her beautiful château. Instead we were met by her Irish mother, Mrs. Gilman, a short, square-shaped woman in her fifties, who displayed none of her daughter's generous traits. With Tante Miss and our French governess we had come on foot from the small station at Massy-Palaiseau two miles away, when we saw her standing by the front door. Her daughter's sudden affluence through a rich alliance did not change Mrs. Gilman's manner or outlook from the skimpy days when Mabel had worked in the chorus line to earn a living. Dressed in a gray suit and wearing shiny black low-heeled shoes, she stood with feet apart and firmly planted in the graveled driveway. Like a watchdog, she was grimly determined to bar all comers from entering the house. Without offering a greeting she exclaimed, "Well, bless my soul! If they aren't here, the whole lot of them!" Pointing at some buildings across the driveway enclosing a large courtyard where the stables were, she said to Elizabeth, "Their quarters are over there. I'm afraid your kids will only scuff up the parquet floors and scratch our nice furniture if I let them in here." She jerked a thumb behind her at the château. "Those rooms over there are plenty good enough for them. Come on and let me show you."

With that remark, not very flattering to our general upbringing (especially since the Grunewald school prided itself on an immaculate cleanliness and neatness), she stepped out energetically and conducted us to an apartment near the stables, probably originally occupied by the grooms. To my amazement I saw that, except for a large table and some chairs occupying the entire space in the small dining room, the rest of the rooms were completely devoid of furniture. There was not even a single chair. Furthermore, we children were obliged to sleep— not, as Isadora and her generous art patron in far-off America imagined, in the comfortable beds of the château—but on simple pallets spread on the hard floor. These primitive living quarters provided neither electricity nor sanitary facilities of any sort. Moreover, we later discovered, the whole place was infested with mice. At night, after blowing out the solitary candle serving as light, we could hear them hungrily gnawing at the woodwork.

Quite patently Mrs. Gilman had seen to it that her daughter Mabel's little guests would not enjoy "the delights of residence in a château." Nor, if she had any say about it, would they have "servants with nothing to do but wait on them." Her daughter's decision to place the château and everything in it at the disposal of Isadora's dance school obviously met with her complete disapproval. It must have been a real disappointment to her when Elizabeth left us there.

Tante Miss made no visible protest nor, for that matter, did she inform Isadora of the true conditions concerning our reception and accommodation at Mrs. Corey's château. She told us, "I am going to leave you here with Mademoiselle and a woman to do the cooking. I want you to be good children and obey Mademoiselle because I will be able to come out and see what you are doing only once in a while. I am staying in Paris at Isadora's apartment to take care of Deirdre."

Château Villegenis, where Elizabeth apparently was satisfied
to leave us, was situated in the lovely Bièvre valley, a few kilo-
meters south of Paris and not far from Versailles to the west.
It had once belonged to Napoleon's brother Jerôme Bonaparte,
the sometime King of Westphalia, who died there in 1860. To
the north it was dominated by the imposing mass of the wood
of Verrières, a heavy stand of pine, oak, beech, and chestnut
trees; and a river ran through the extensive property.

The château itself stood in the center of a wooded park,
reached by a half-mile driveway from the main gate in the
surrounding wall. The white house, with two wings in typical
French style, mirrored its façade in a small lake, with a parterre
of flowers extending to each side. The estate contained tennis
courts, orchards, hot houses, a little ivy-covered chapel, and even
a medieval donjon hidden deep in the woods. The house was
beautifully appointed, with all the conveniences and servants
galore; but Mrs. Gilman, together with a little girl called
Françoise (a distant relative by marriage), lived there in solitary
splendor. We were not invited to set foot in it, not even to take
an occasional hot bath. For our daily ablutions we used a large
tin pan and cold water drawn from the pump in the courtyard.
The French governess pleaded in our behalf for the use of a
bathroom, but to no effect. "I don't know why I should let you
kids run all over my house," was Mrs. Gilman's only answer.

And so, in the midst of these beautiful surroundings we
children were destined to live in squalor, which made our stay
at the château completely miserable. At first, in balmy October
when we could spend all our time outdoors, it wasn't so bad.
But we knew that October could not last forever.

At one point we even had hopes of leaving. Late one night
we were told to pack our things quickly, and we were whisked
off to Paris—only to be returned the next day. As usual, no one
told us where we were going. But when I peevishly remarked
at being kept in the dark that "we might be on our way to

America; even then no one would tell us so," the response was that I had guessed correctly.

It seemed that Isadora's American tour had had an inauspicious beginning. To help drum up more interest, Mr. Frohman —remembering how our dancing had captivated even the sophisticated London audiences—may have had the idea of sending for us, and Isadora may have countermanded it because of the extra expense involved. In any case, we returned, greatly disappointed, to the château.

That one night and day in Paris, we stayed at the tiny three-room apartment of Mrs. Mary Sturges (later Mrs. Desti), at 10 Rue Octave Feullet. She was an old friend of Isadora, an American divorcee and expatriate who made her home in France. A few days later she motored out to see us, bringing her little son Preston and a photographer. "I want to send Isadora a picture of you children," she said, "so that she can see how well you look and how happy you are here."

A gay, rather frivolous woman, who liked to laugh at everything and was constitutionally unable to take anything seriously, she conceived the idea of posing us festooned all over her automobile. We put on our Polish coats and climbed aboard her 1908 model limousine, which had more polished brass trim than room to sit in. Preston (who later became the well-known playwright and movie director), climbed in too and had his picture taken with us. It must have reassured our absent guardian that all was indeed well with her pupils at Mrs. Corey's marvelous French château, where we were enjoying a delightful residence and being tended by the servants who had nothing to do but wait on us.

Mrs. Sturges only made matters worse by telling us in her gay, chatty manner, that she was taking Elizabeth and Mr. Merz, our music director, on a motor trip. "We are making a tour of the Rhineland," she informed us in her easygoing way. When we pressed her for further details, she chatted on, "Well, I'm not supposed to tell you, so don't tell anyone I told you, but it seems that the Grand Duke of Hesse"—she stopped and wagged a finger at us in mock-seriousness. "Remember now, this is a secret! Well, the Grand Duke has offered Elizabeth a piece of property near Darmstadt for the building of a school of her own."

When she saw that this piece of news left us gaping with utter astonishment, she hastily added, "Remember, not a word!" She waved gaily and grinned one last big grin as she got into her chauffeur-driven limousine, calling out, "Au revoir! See you again when I return!" The chauffeur tooted his brass horn, and we scattered like chickens. Then wheels crunched on the gravel and she was gone, leaving us shaken children trying to grasp fully this formidable piece of news.

Our first reaction was to wonder, "Does Isadora know of this?" and, "What will happen to us?" As usual, there was no one to enlighten us, and our future seemed as uncertain as our present. Abandoned here in France by our second guardian, who had been entrusted by Isadora to take good care of us, we couldn't help feeling that we were a group of lost waifs.

To cap it all, Mademoiselle packed up her things one day and left. Whether it was the bad food, or not getting paid, or that we were too much to cope with, we never knew. From that moment, left without any sort of supervision, we entered upon a state of total neglect.

The winter that year in France proved to be exceptionally severe. It was so cold that the pump froze and the older girls needed to hack the ice away to get water for our cold baths. By then our open sandals had worn thin and had such big holes in them that we were practically walking barefoot in the snow. Our clothing, too, was threadbare and provided little warmth. Fortunately, some coal fires in an open grate provided a little heat in the tiny rooms, otherwise we would surely have frozen to death. During the bad weather, confined indoors, we sat on the floor (there being no chairs) huddled close beside the hearth, and whiled the day away till bedtime. We had no books or games to keep us occupied. Apparently no one cared what happened to us. The *cuisinière*, a mute old peasant woman, concerned herself exclusively with cooking what meagre food there was. The provisions dwindled rapidly. Our daily fare during the winter months consisted entirely of either pumpkin soup or a dish of plain boiled potatoes. Forks not being available, even though we were guests of a millionairess, we ate with spoons, the only eating utensils provided by Mrs. Gilman.

Time seemed to stand still, with nothing to look forward to, not even the approach of Christmas. The usual Christmas packages from home failed to arrive. Our parents had no idea of our exact whereabouts in France, and mail from Grunewald could not be forwarded. Not that we children were remiss in wanting to correspond; we simply lacked the money to buy stamps, and in our ignorance we had no inkling that letters could be sent without them. The prospect of having to celebrate our beloved *Weihnachten* alone in a strange land caused a great deal of homesickness. Christmas Eve had dawned bleakly when Mrs. Gilman surprised us by calling us over to the château.

We tidied ourselves as best we could and eagerly approached our hostess, who stood waiting by a side door. With our bare toes sticking out of our sandals in the snow, we curtsied politely and said "Merry Christmas."

"Yes, that is what I want to see you about," she said, looking us over carefully without as much as a smile. She asked us into the glass-enclosed side entrance, but would not let us enter the house as if our presence might contaminate it. She opened the door and showed us the huge, decorated tree in the hall. With spontaneous exclamations at the beautiful sight of the tree and the many attractively wrapped presents beneath, we pressed forward for a closer view. But she restrained us. "No, don't go in," she said. "You will only scuff up the floors. I just thought you kids might like to see the tree since you haven't got one."

She stepped inside for a moment, returning with an open

box of candies. "Here, take one," she said in a more friendly tone, and offered each child a bonbon. Then she closed the box and replaced it on the table in the hall. We stood crowded together in the small entrance watching her, not knowing what to do or say, hoping for a little more friendly human contact.

"Well, run along now," she said, dismissing us. "I just wanted to show you the tree. You understand, don't you?" We nodded our heads and sadly trudged back to our bare rooms.

In Europe, the tree is lit and the presents are opened late on Christmas Eve. Glumly we sat on the floor close by the fire after our evening meal of pumpkin soup and waited for something to happen. But what? It was cold outside and snowing. We could hear the wind in the chimney. We talked, remembering other, happier Christmases. Presently, to get in the right mood, I started softly to sing: *"Stille Nacht, heilige Nacht; alles schlaeft einsam wacht."* The others joined in, and we sang on bravely till the end. With the last notes, our voices quavered and then failed. We all burst into tears. Through our tears, hungry as the mice in the wainscotting, we gnawed on raw acorns and chestnuts that we had gathered in the woods for Christmas presents—the only ones we had. We cried ourselves to sleep, lying on the miserable pallets on the floor.

The following day, we looked through the frosty windows and watched the fine little friends of Françoise arriving for a party at the château. We were not invited, Mrs. Gilman's excuse being that we did not speak French. But Christmas is a day for children the world over and needs no special language for their understanding.

It was a hopeless situation. With Isadora in America, Elizabeth in Germany—none of us knowing their exact whereabouts—and Mrs. Gilman ignoring our existence, we found ourselves helplessly trapped. In an effort to find a solution, I realized that outside help in our predicament could be obtained only by notifying mother. Not aware that an unfranked letter would actually reach her, this escape seemed closed too. As a result, a frightening sense of insecurity enveloped us all.

Because of the bad weather and for lack of proper clothing, our outdoor exercises had to be curtailed. The cramped rooms made indoor exercise equally impossible. We had no means of letting off excess energy, and so it was not surprising—cooped up as we were in four tiny rooms, like dumb animals in a cage— that the older girls should gang up on us younger ones for something amusing to do. The six older girls, all teen-agers, tyrannized the younger to such an extent that we lived in constant terror. Children can be very cruel. As the oldest of the younger group, and possessed of a latent fiery temperament that needed only strong fanning to erupt like a volcano, I did not suffer from their machinations. They knew me and my temper too well. But one day, after a fierce quarrel when I tried to remonstrate with them and their unspeakable behavior, they held a court and sentenced me to Coventry.

Now being sent to Coventry is not a pleasant experience, as most children in boarding school well know. In my case, where it lasted for weeks, it amounted to solitary confinement. If the youngest girls with whom I roomed even so much as glanced my way, they were severely punished. I became embittered, secretly vowing some kind of vengeance on the three ringleaders. At one point I became so morose I decided to run away. I had no money, and it meant walking all the way home to Hamburg. In desperation I packed my few belongings in a small satchel and sneaked out of the house before dawn. I got past the main gate without being seen by the gatekeeper and wandered determinedly along the highway to Paris. But after a few miles of walking in my torn sandals, I got footsore and so frightened at the enormity of my rash undertaking that I succumbed to my misgivings and returned to the chateau as the lesser of two evils.

I don't know how long this ostracism would have lasted (since I was too proud to ask the girls to forgive me) if a frightening incident had not occurred and changed their minds. As I have mentioned, coal fires burned in open grates in our bed-rooms. One day I happened to be sitting in the farthest corner of the room while two little girls played close to the open fire. I was supposed to be in solitary confinement, but I knew that both Erica and Temple secretly sympathized with me, having themselves been badly treated by the big ones. I sensed that they played in this room on purpose, despite the risk they took, to keep me company after my month-long loneliness.

I was drawing pictures and paying them no heed when suddenly I heard a terrified scream. Erica's dress had caught fire, and the flames rapidly spread to her face. Temple stood petrified beside her, screaming. I rushed over and was trying to extinguish the flames with my bare hands when the older girls came running in. Seeing me struggle with Erica in an effort to subdue the flames, they recoiled in panic, thinking I meant to throw her in the fire. For the first time I saw fear written on their own nasty faces—fear of what I might be capable of doing to them in revenge. Their cowardly expressions gave me inner satisfaction, for I realized I now had the upper hand.

"Don't stand there like idiots!" I shouted at them. "Go fetch the water cans quickly!"

They obeyed my command with alacrity, relieved that I was not going to destroy them after all. When they brought the water, I poured it over Erica till the flames were extinguished.

"Poor little Erica," I consoled her, rubbing her dry with a towel. "You'll be all right now."

She threw her arms about me, and we kissed. Temple came up and whispered, "Irma, dear, none of us little ones are sore at you. THEY forced us to ignore you. Both Erica and I are so sorry for you."

"I know, don't worry. You'll see, I'll get even with them yet."

That night, when I was about to drop off to sleep, one of the ringleaders bent down low over my pallet. I sat bolt upright in a combative mood.

"What do you want?"

"Sh, sh, don't be alarmed," she whispered. "Susanna wants to see you. She is ready to forgive you because of what you did to save Erica."

Susanna, the eldest of our group, asked me to apologize. "Never!" was my defiant retort. She came from the same city I did and did not in the least impress me with her absurd airs. The other girls looked on her as a queen, she had them so hypnotized. To me she was just a stupid, stuck-up kid, and I told her so. At this *lèse majesté,* the others acted stunned. When they had recovered sufficiently and saw that I was not going to kowtow to their silly queen, two of them crept up behind me. I stood there unaware in front of Susanna, who was propped up on pillows as if on a make-believe throne, when they suddenly doused me with a pitcher of ice-cold water. My fury aroused, I threatened them with dire destruction and rushed out of the room, bolting the connecting door. It was their only exit, and now I had them under complete control. I intended to keep them locked up in there for good. Now it was their turn to beg me to unbolt the door, and when they promised to behave and cause no more mischief, I set them free.

This life would have continued indefinitely but for the fortuitous arrival of a new governess. Fräulein Harting turned out to be a young, sympathetic Alsatian woman, who spoke both French and German. Overjoyed to have at long last someone who spoke our own language, I told her all that weighed on my mind and made me unhappy. When I confessed my big sin, my attempt to run away, I was ready for her to scold me. Instead, she asked earnestly, "Why didn't you? I would have done the same thing." I told her that I had no money to buy a ticket. "You need only go to the nearest station and ask for Travelers' Aid," she explained—and she told me how that society would always furnish a ticket home for anyone stranded in a foreign land.

She told me also that it was possible to send a letter without stamps, postage due. I immediately decided to put her advice to the test. Not having written home for four months, I tore a page out of my copybook and poured out my heart to mother, telling her that Elizabeth Duncan had a plan for establishing a school in Germany, but that Isadora had decided to have hers in France. And to make no mistake about my preference!

Fräulein Harting's advice had been correct. Mother received the letter and instantly sent me money and a large package with all the necessities I had had to do without for so long, such as a brush and comb, soap, tooth powder, and writing paper. From Tante Miss and Isadora, we had not a word; they seemed to have forgotten us.

Life in the rooms near the stables at Château Villegenis continued as before except that now we had a governess. We complained bitterly. For days we were fed only pumpkin soup, which I loathed. Once, rebelling, we refused to eat it. But our governess said, "I'm sorry. Pumpkin soup is all there is to eat. You will only have it again tomorrow for breakfast if you don't eat it tonight."

"Oh, no I *won't!*" I suddenly shouted. Disgusted with the whole business, not only the horrible food, I seized the bowl of soup and flung it across the table at the wall. It landed directly above a photograph of Mabel Gilman in musical comedy costume, dripping all over the picture. There was a shocked pause. Everyone present stared at me while I stared defiantly at the big stain on the wall. Then Fräulein Harting found her voice. She pulled me by the ear, saying, "I'll teach you to throw food around! Come with me!"

She dragged me to the upper floor, locking me into a dark, unused room. "You can spend the night here and cool off!" she shouted, and left. I threw myself against the door and rattled the knob, screaming, "Let me out! Let me out!" Suffering a fearful attack of claustrophobia, I was frantic. When my eyes became accustomed to the dark, I saw that the room was crowded with furniture—all the furniture Mrs. Gilman had begrudged

our using. In an access of fury, I climbed over the stuff, opened
the window, and proceeded to throw out the furniture. Out it
went, piece by piece: chairs, tables, mirrors, everything I could
lift. The crashing on the hard ground outside made a big noise
in the still night.

It wasn't long before Fräulein Harting came rushing back.
She unlocked the door, screaming at me, "Are you crazy? Stop
that immediately!" But I paid no heed and kept flinging furniture out the window with enormous gusto. It was a marvelous
relief for my long-pent-up resentment.

All this shouting and excitement brought old Mrs. Gilman
on the run. "What on earth is going on?" she wanted to know.
By this time the governess had gotten hold of me and dragged
me outside to the heap of broken furniture.

"Look what you have done!" Fräulein Harting pointed out
unnecessarily. I knew what I had done, and I was secretly glad
of it the moment I saw Mrs. Gilman. For a while, the latter
stood absolutely speechless. Finally she gave me a look of hate
and said, "Aren't you ashamed of yourself?"

With my heart still pounding wildly from the exertion and
the fury and the fear, I looked her straight in the eye and said
nothing. On seeing this woman—who had shown so little com-
passion for the starving, freezing children who were guests under her roof—now reproaching me, I felt only bitterness well up
in my heart. And although I cried hot tears of shame, I could
not bring myself to say to her, "I'm sorry."

She started to upbraid me in the angry tones of an outraged
woman, and I expected the worst in retaliation. But to my great
surprise and relief, Fräulein Harting simply took me by the
hand and led me straight to bed. She covered me up warmly
and brought me a bowl of hot milk with bread in it. "There,
calm yourself," she said. "Eat this and then go to sleep. We'll
talk tomorrow."

But we never did. I suppose she too had seen the mask fall
from Mrs. Gilman's face and suddenly realized where the guilt

of my rebellion really lay. Her sympathy was all for the neglected motherless children in her care, with no further concern about Mrs. Gilman's broken furniture. She told us she would go to Paris and bring us help.

It was the end of March. Spring comes early in this part of France, and the flowers and trees were budding with fresh, new life. Instead of our governess, Mrs. Sturges showed up again on a Sunday. She carried a bolt of gray cloth under her arm and brought scissors and sewing material. Greeting us with squeals of laughter, she said pleasantly, "I brought you girls some material to make new dresses. I wanted to buy a pretty blue, but Elizabeth said gray was more practical. So here is some blue embroidery yarn for decorating. I also brought you some new sandals."

With several more delighted squeals, she told us the wonderful news that Isadora was expected to return from America any day. We happily set to work on making new dresses for her arrival. And then, one marvelous sunny day in the first week of April, there she was! She actually stood before us, our idol, our goddess, our longed-for Isadora. The spell she cast with her very presence made everything seem rosy, all cares forgotten. She embraced us all tenderly and remarked how we had grown! She herself looked pale and worried. "Poor children," she said gently, hugging us, "poor children. Miss Harting told me everything. You must pack your things and come with me at once."

But there was nothing to pack. Our old clothes were torn to tatters. We had thrown them away for rags the day before and left them in an empty storeroom beside the stables, where we had discovered an abandoned marble tub that once belonged to Jêrome Bonaparte. With whoops of joy we had heated water in the kitchen and had taken our first hot bath in six months in the Napoleonic tub. No hot bath had ever felt so good!

Cleaned up now, our hair washed, wearing our new dresses and sandals, we were ready and oh! how willing to go and leave this place forever. At that moment Mrs. Gilman appeared to greet her distinguished visitor. When Isadora saw the squat figure in a gray suit and black low-heeled shoes, she cut her dead by turning her back and walking away without saying a word.

"Come on, children, get in the cars and let's go," Isadora called out. She took my hand, saying, "You come and sit with me in my car." I hopped in beside her, smiling happily. As we passed through the gate in the great wall surrounding Château Villegenis, I did not once look back at the place where I had been so unhappy. With my hand in Isadora's I felt safe once more and happy. I leaned back blissfully against the soft cushions of the limousine and sighed contentedly. Everything seemed well again with me and my small world as we sped along the sunny highway to Paris.

6

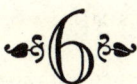

Elizabeth Takes Over

Upon Isadora's return from America, two events occurred that had a decisive bearing on our future as well as hers. One was the fateful meeting with the millionaire she had hoped would help to establish her school on a solid financial basis. This was Paris Singer. The other was her sister Elizabeth's quite unexpected competition.

After a short engagement at the Gaieté-Lyrique Théâtre in Paris there followed a month's vacation on the Riviera, for which Isadora provided us with a new, much more elaborate wardrobe. Then she resettled her pupils at Neuilly in a comfortable pension not far from the house she had bought with the dollars earned on her American tour. She once again devoted herself to the reorganization of her school in France. Starting with the nucleus from the Grunewald school, she found she had first to obtain the consent of the parents for our permanent residence in France. To this effect she sent them each a letter dated June 7, 1909:

My dance school no longer exists in Germany because of insufficient support. My own resources are no longer adequate to enable me to carry the expense alone. A group of influential friends, here in France, is now engaged in organizing a dance school under my sole direction, but supported by other funds.

In this new establishment the pupils will continue as hitherto, to receive an academic, as well as an artistic education. The parents are requested to agree by contract to leave the children at the school till they have reached the age of eighteen. Having finished their education, the graduated pupils will then be able to obtain dance engagements through the school organization. Half of their fee will then be deducted for repayment of the expenses incurred for their education.

If you should consider leaving your daughter with me under the above stipulated conditions, I beg you to let me know immediately. If otherwise, I shall find myself constrained to return your daughter to you. My address is: 68 Rue Chauveau, Neuilly près Paris. Teleg. "Duncanides."

At the same time, unbeknownst to all of those most intimately concerned with her project, Elizabeth Duncan had perfected and put into operation her secretly hatched plan of establishing a school under her own name in Germany. In order to start her enterprise with a trained group of pupils acting as her assistants, she caused a similar request to be sent to our parents. Hoping she would surely come out the winner in this contest for the possession of the original pupils, she placed enormous faith in the fact that the German parents were bound to prefer keeping their offspring in their homeland. She then made her intentions public by placing the following notice in the German press:

With reference to the sojourn of my sister Isadora Duncan and her school in Paris, I beg to state that I have been associated with this school since its foundation in the capacity of both teacher and director. My own activities have been widely recognized in Germany. I therefore declare that I am not taking any part in the re-establishing of a new school in Paris, France. As repeatedly stated, I shall continue my activities in Germany, specifically in Darmstadt, where my own school is now in the process of being built. I beg you not to construe this as going against my sister. I merely continue to pursue my long and successful—if at times difficult—activities in Germany. I shall proceed on my chosen path with the guarantee of the fine support I have received so far for my undertaking.

In the meanwhile, fearing that most of the pupils would prefer to remain with Isadora if given a choice, and egged on by

Max Merz, her friend and adviser who master-minded the whole scheme, she resorted to some audacious tactics.

We had not seen her for ages when she appeared one afternoon at our pension all smiles and innocence. Although most of us instinctively scattered like birds, *sauve qui peut*, at her approach, she managed to catch a few of the more trusting ones who had lingered behind. She made an unusually friendly gesture without arousing any suspicion and invited them to have tea in town. The girls accepted with pleasure. The next thing they knew, instead of having tea and cakes at Rumpelmayer's, they were on a train bound for Germany! But of course the rest of us at the pension had no inkling of this forced abduction till later.

"What do you mean by saying my sister has stolen five girls?" Isadora seemed terribly shocked by this dreadful accusation. Standing in the midst of a group of wildly excited children, she listened with growing amazement as we told our tale of how, through a ruse, the five girls had been kidnaped. We explained how, when the girls failed to reappear and Tante Miss returned without them on the following day at exactly the same time to try this trick on the rest of us, we became suspicious; how, under the pretext of getting dressed for the bogus party, we locked ourselves in and refused to come out of our rooms. As soon as she was gone, we had sent for Isadora in a hurry.

"This is an outrage!" she exclaimed angrily. "How is it possible that my own sister should do a thing like that to me? It is incredible!"

But it was only too true. I had never seen Isadora so angry. Her sister's underhanded action had evidently come as a great shock to her. She contemplated us for a while in silence. Then she asked whether the rest of us wished to remain with her. We assured her that we did. Visibly moved by our sincere attachment, she said, "Very soon I'll have a beautiful new school organized here. Just have a little patience."

Then she turned to me. "Oh, by the way, Irma, I have a nice letter here from your mother. I received it this morning." And she showed me the letter in which mother asked her to send me home for a long-overdue vacation and a consultation.

"I think your mother made a good suggestion," she said. "None of you has been home for over four years, and it is time you went back. You may visit your people for the summer months and I shall send for you when the new school is ready." And she added, "That is perhaps the best plan for the present, as I shall myself be absent for a while." Neither she nor her adoring pupils could possibly foresee that "absent for a while" would encompass the space of not only several months, but years.

For my part, living at home with mother was very agreeable and a nice change from school routine. Only after two months of this, I became restless and, as time went by, longed more and more for a speedy return to Isadora and the company of my schoolmates. Life at the Duncan School, for better or worse, had become so much a part of me that I could not envision any other existence. At home, delimited by my mother's narrow horizon, I felt shut in. My initiation into the art of the dance had given me a need for beauty and a sense of higher aspirations that could no more be denied me than breathing. So when July, August, September, and most of October passed and I still had not heard from Isadora, I was seized with despair, believing I would never hear from her again. On the other hand, we had frequently received word from Mr. Merz, who in his capacity as director of the newly established Elizabeth Duncan School repeatedly begged me to join that organization. Loyal in my devotion to Isadora, I steadfastly refused.

I had been in contact once with the eldest pupil, Susanna, who also lived in Hamburg. She wanted to know if I had news from Isadora, because she too wondered at her silence. We exchanged opinions, and that was all. But a couple of days later I told mother for the first time about the feud I had had with

Susanna at the château when she and the other two older girls had tormented the younger ones. Mother appeared shocked. "To think that I received her here in my house and was nice to her!" she said. "Why didn't you tell me before? I would have refused to let you associate with such a nasty girl. She is a bad influence, and I'm surprised that they kept her at the school."

Then early one morning, when I happened to be still in bed, the doorbell rang. Mother went to answer. Who could it be so early? I sat up in bed to listen. Never was I so surprised as to hear the familiar Viennese accent of Max Merz inquiring whether I was at home? Mother conducted him into the front parlor.

During my stay with mother I had discarded my Duncan uniform so as not to appear conspicuous, and had worn the type of dresses and shoes used by other people. At the sound of Mr. Merz's voice, I jumped out of bed and reached for the suitcase that contained my school outfit. I put it on in a jiffy. When mother came to my room and said, "Guess who is here?" she was taken aback to see me standing there in sandals and tunic. I answered, "Yes, I know, and I am ready to go with him."

Mr. Merz, a pleasant man in his middle thirties, greeted me warmly. "I knew you would never make the trip alone," he said, smiling. "That is why I came to fetch you."

My resistance to joining Elizabeth's school weakened the moment I heard his voice. My deep yearning to be within my accustomed milieu again, where music and dancing were of the essence and nothing else really mattered, made me decide impulsively to go with him. But when mother heard that he intended to take Susanna back too, she strenuously objected to my going. "You must make a choice between my daughter and that other girl," she told him.

Before making a decision, Mr. Merz, who was pedantic and given to lecturing on sundry topics, wanted to consult with Professor Hohle, who was a member of the local committee for the support of our school. He and his family lived near us and knew me quite well. We went there, and Professor Hohle paid serious attention to what Merz had to say, but seemed surprised that he needed advice. He told him to take me.

So Mr. Merz and I on that same day took the train for Frankfurt-am-Main, where Tante Miss and the other five girls were temporarily located. They were living in the house of a Dr. Kling, on the Bockenheimer Landstrasse. It turned out to be a pleasant, old, musty-smelling house filled with books, for Dr. Kling, a bachelor and a learned man, had been a founder of the Germanic Museum in Nuremberg. His house, overgrown with climbing roses and set in a wooded plot where he maintained a bird sanctuary, had a mysterious, enchanted air.

We arrived there late at night and I did not see the other girls, who were already in bed. But when I awoke in the morning, with the sun pouring through a window framed in climbing roses in which birds nested and kept up a constant twitter, I thought I heard a different kind of twittering besides. Without turning around, I became aware of the other girls clustered near my bed. I heard them whisper excitedly:

"Oh, look! there is only one girl in here!"

"Which one is it, do you think? Irma or Susanna?"

"I don't know. I can't see—she has her head hidden in the pillow!"

"Gee, I hope it's Irma."

"Oh, so do I."

"Me too."

"Sh, sh. Suppose it is Susanna!"

"I don't care!"

That was all I needed to hear to get their honest reaction. Joyfully I cast away the bedclothes and jumped out of bed. The moment they recognized me, we had a gay reunion. Laughing and chatting at the same time, they told me how glad they were to see me instead of Susanna. "We all hate her so," Anna said, and Theresa eagerly nodded assent. Both Lisel and Gretel chimed in, one saying, "We were afraid of her"; the other asking apprehensively, "Is she coming later?"

I delightedly assured them that neither of the two older girls would ever be allowed to return. We had got even with our former tormentors at last. With Erica and Temple scheduled to join us at a later date, we all rejoiced to be reunited again. Pleased and happy to be forming a smaller but much more congenial group, we hoped to remain together to the end.

Two years elapsed before the Darmstadt building could be completed. In the interim, led by Tante Miss and Merz, we girls gave combination lecture-dance recitals to support ourselves. These also served to make propaganda and drum up trade in the form of paying pupils for their newly founded institute for *Körperkultur*. Here young German girls would receive an education based mainly on physical culture and racial hygiene—a chauvinistic ideology that had nothing in common with Isadora Duncan's theory of physical education for children, which was founded on her dance art.

The motivating force behind all this *Rassenkultur* business was Max Merz. A fanatic on the subject, ambitious and an opportunist, he managed to exert a kind of Svengali influence over Elizabeth. Born in Vienna of Czech parents, he had studied composition and conducting at the Vienna Conservatory, finishing at the Hochschule für Musik in Berlin. Seeing Isadora Duncan dance one day, he became so fired with the idea of composing music for her that he applied for a job at the Grunewald school toward the end of 1906. There he met not Isadora but her older sister, and from that moment on they became close friends and allies. He acted as music director and conductor for the school performances. When Isadora decided to transfer her establishment to Paris, Merz prevailed upon Elizabeth to remain in Germany—the country he admired more than any other—and to open her own school there. Being more than devoted to him, she agreed wholeheartedly.

A clever man, obsessed with a theory to propound, he developed a natural bent for lecturing. He would get up and lecture at the drop of a hat anywhere, any time. His ordinary conversations invariably turned into speeches and, once started, he would harangue people for hours. In promoting the Elizabeth Duncan School for Physical Culture, he had at last found his true métier. Affable in manner and attractive to women—with the well-known Viennese charm of *Küss-die-Hand* type of flattery—he encountered little difficulty in getting people to part with their money for his pet project. It was gradually taking form on a hill near Darmstadt, Merz having first cajoled the ruling grand duke to donate valuable property. As a doctrinaire preaching physical culture and racial hygiene on the one hand, and providing the musical accompaniment for our dance recitals on the other, he managed to confuse many of his listeners. As one alert Hamburg critic observed:

> The Elizabeth Duncan School for young girls of the privileged class purports to be an institution devoted to physical culture— and not the art of the dance. Then why, for heaven's sake, do they distort the picture of their intentions by giving dance performances?
>
> I am convinced that the majority of the public, despite the explanations of director Max Merz, left the theatre with the impression that this physical culture institution really represents a dance school.
>
> This is probably due to the name of Isadora Duncan, whose spirit presides over the whole show.

No matter how hard Elizabeth and Merz tried to wean us away from Isadora's artistic influence, they did not succeed in obliterating the spirit of the dance as instilled by Isadora in her former pupils. To mold us into their concept of physical culture paragons, they even resorted to the desperate means of engaging an officer of the Swedish army to drill us in gymnastics. Isadora had expressly stated that "Swedish gymnastics is a false system of body culture because it takes no account of the imagination and regards the muscles as an end in themselves." *

When, after such rigorous physical training (resembling in every respect the stiff drill of soldiers on parade), month after month, year in and year out, we still kept the spark alive and continued to dance the way Isadora taught us, they continued to disparage our efforts. If people happened to praise our dancing, Elizabeth would tell them that we only "imitated" her sister. She was undoubtedly well aware of the fact that Isadora, as the creator and unique exponent of her art, was also our sole example, and that she, Elizabeth, had nothing whatsoever to contribute in this particular field. Her own pupils had to look elsewhere for inspiration and guidance if they wanted to qualify as genuine exponents of the dance as Isadora envisioned it. She knew that Isadora from the very beginning intended to train specially chosen disciples to carry on her art.

Her dancer's body being the instrument, Isadora represented in her own person two not necessarily related principles: both the creative and the interpretative. To interpret her choreography correctly, from both the physical and the spiritual points of view, we could not do otherwise than dance in her image. For reasons of her own, this was something Elizabeth wanted to prevent at all costs.

I for one, all the time I was a pupil of the Darmstadt school, could not reconcile Isadora's spiritual teachings with the materialistic ideologies expounded by Elizabeth or the racial theories advocated by Max Merz. Nor did I willingly submit to wearing their uncomfortable, unbecoming school uniform, consisting of scratchy gray woolen underwear, ditto clothes, and gray woolen stockings shaped like long opera gloves with a cot for each toe. The latter were meant to fit specially designed orthopedic footwear with a separate compartment accommodating the individual toes. The excruciating torture I sustained walking around in

* *Life*, p. 189.

these modern instruments of the Inquisition cannot be easily described. Tante Miss had a knack for making her pupils feel miserable. Not that she set a fine example by using them herself. Oh no, her implacable Spartan attitude excluded her own discomforts.

Thus my education, which had started as a dancer and follower of Isadora Duncan's lofty ideals, was persistently being perverted. I was, against my will and natural inclination, abruptly directed into channels alien to my artistic instincts. It all culminated at the Hygienic Exhibition in Dresden in 1911. In the great hall (where a giant replica of a transparent heart pumping red blood greeted the visitor) we had an exhibit consisting of white plaster casts of our torsos and limbs. My own contribution was a life-size replica of my arm from shoulder to fingertips. Models of our school uniform were also shown. Preceded by lectures from both Mr. Merz and Elizabeth, we girls daily gave free demonstrations of our physical prowess acquired under their guidance via Swedish gymnastics. They reached the high point of their endeavors in the field of physical culture in Germany with that exhibition. With the award of the gold medal, their greatest ambition was achieved.

One would have thought that Elizabeth Duncan possessed at least the intelligence, if not the generosity of heart, to acknowledge that we pupils of the original school had contributed largely to the success of hers; that as a group we represented a distinct asset to her and her work. More important, as far as our personal attitudes were concerned, she should have recognized that we could no longer be treated as children in constant need of correction and punishment. We were growing up (the eldest being seventeen) and desired her to establish a more amiable student-teacher relationship. But her unrealistic approach to her growing pupils made the relationship even more strained than before. And thus matters stood between us when, in the fall of 1912, the Darmstadt school was ready for our occupancy. Situated just outside the city on top of a hill, the new building commanded a sweeping view of the valley below, with the silver ribbon of the river Rhine winding away in the distance. Built along simple, functional, modern lines, the house had large airy rooms filled with the Grunewald furniture, which Elizabeth had appropriated. The large central hall was especially designed for such physical activities as the Elizabeth Duncan School had to offer. The day of inauguration was planned as a big event, with their highnesses the Duke and Duchess of Hessen-Darmstadt participating.

Some of us had met this ruler a few years earlier, when we had performed at the Hof Theatre. A grandson of Queen Victoria and a brother of the Tsarina, he was in his early forties. He was informal and democratic in manner, jovial of disposition, and somewhat given to practical jokes. He was also an enthusiastic patron of the theatre and often took part in amateur theatricals. He and his wife organized a dancing class at the palace so that their two little boys could learn to dance, and some of the older girls went there once a week to assist Tante Miss with the teaching. Under the benevolent patronage of the Duke and Duchess, the Darmstadt school was off to a good start. On the day of the inauguration they drove up in their horse-drawn carriage in grand style and, seated in the front row of the great crowd of spectators, graciously watched the ceremonies.

This was indeed the day of days for Max Merz. Triumphant, with coattails flying, he supervised and conducted the whole proceeding. He was reception committee, conductor of the choir singers, and main speaker all rolled into one. He even composed both the words and music for the pageant. It seemed to be entirely his show. His frenzied activity aroused my risibility, which gradually mounted to such a pitch that during the inaugural address I was suddenly seized with a terrible fit of the giggles. I stood directly behind him among all the other pupils, who were dressed in purest white to form a striking background for his slender figure attired in a dark frock coat.

When, inspired by the brilliant October sunshine and carried away by his own flamboyant oratory, he started to invoke his Teutonic gods, I could no longer control myself. Neither apparently could he, for without looking around he knew quite well whence these hysterical giggles originated. And so in the midst of his impassioned evocation of "Baldur! Oh, mighty sun god! I implore thee cast thy golden rays upon our work!" he suddenly stopped and startled not only me but the whole assembly by shouting, "Oh, Irma, shut up!"

That effectively took care of me, but not the Grand Duke. He pulled his silk handkerchief out of his pocket and blew his nose vigorously while his shoulders shook with hidden laughter. . . .

Following the official opening, the Elizabeth Duncan School settled down to its regular daily routine of academic studies in the morning and dance, music, or gymnastics in the afternoon. Many new pupils were enrolled, on both a paying and a scholarship basis.

In this school, once I had shown an aptitude for teaching, I was formally entrusted with all the dance classes for children. Thus, at the youthful age of fifteen, I became a full-fledged teacher without pay. But what I gained was immense practical experience (by developing my own method of teaching) in instructing others, not only in the fundamentals, but also in the finer expressions of the true dance as taught to me by Isadora Duncan. But I am getting ahead of my story.

7

Lesson in the Temple

I HAD not heard from Isadora for two years when, quite unexpectedly, she came to see us. This occurred in Dresden, where we were attending a hygienic exhibition; and Isadora, on a motor trip with Paris Singer, happened to be passing through. When she arrived to have lunch with her sister, we hardly recognized her. Her outward appearance had undergone a complete transformation. Gone were the simple tunic and sandals she always used to wear, as well as the flowing cape and skullcap that were almost a trademark of hers. Instead, she appeared in a very smart outfit that Paul Poirêt, the famous French couturier, had designed especially for her in accordance with her taste for simple lines. It was quite a departure for him, who had just launched the eccentric fashion of the hobble skirt and cartwheel hat bedecked with ostrich plumes. And here we have proof of how Isadora Duncan influenced modern dress reform, for it was directly through Paul Poirêt's designs copied from her ideas that the simple line of today's clothes evolved.

"How the girls have grown!" she exclaimed when she saw us. She held my hand in hers for a moment and regarded me fondly and then said to her sister, "Be sure to bring this one along when you visit me in July."

Back at school I lived as in a dream, counting the days from then on till Tante Miss would get ready to leave. The middle of July came and went, and still I had not received the impatiently awaited sign from her. Had she forgotten? I was secretly elated that Isadora had singled me out, and having missed her for so long I was naturally eager to be with my idol again. But

I also knew that Elizabeth suppressed favoritism, and judging by her former actions I did not count much on my chances.

Then suddenly, late one afternoon, the governess came to me, saying, "Can you get packed in five minutes? Miss Duncan is going to take you along. But only if you hurry!"

I got downstairs with my hastily packed wicker suitcase just as Tante Miss stepped into the waiting cab. I had no time to say goodbye to the girls. My heart was beating fast with excitement in my joy to be with Isadora again.

We arrived late at night in Ostend, and Isadora met us at the station. At the hotel she softly opened the door to the room where her two children were fast asleep with their English nanny. "You go and sleep in that bed over there beside the nurse, darling, and I'll see you in the morning. Goodnight!"

Getting into bed beside her sleeping children, I had the sweet sensation of actually being one of her children too. With this thought I went to sleep, feeling happier than I had for a long time.

I awoke the next morning in a daze, not realizing immediately where I was. Bright sunlight filtered through the shutters, and I could get a whiff of tangy salt air and hear the waves thundering on the beach. Then I remembered we had come to Ostend on the North Sea, and I jumped out of bed and stepped onto the balcony to have a good look. My movements must have awakened Deirdre, for when I returned she was sitting up in bed. The last time I saw her she had been a mere infant. Now five years old, she looked me over carefully before asking timidly, "Who are you?"

"I am your new playmate," I said. "I hope we shall be friends."

"Have you seen my little brother?" she asked and pulled me over to his crib. "His name is Patrick and he is twelve months old." The baby, who was the son of Paris Singer, had blond curly hair. He looked very delicate and spent most of the time sleeping.

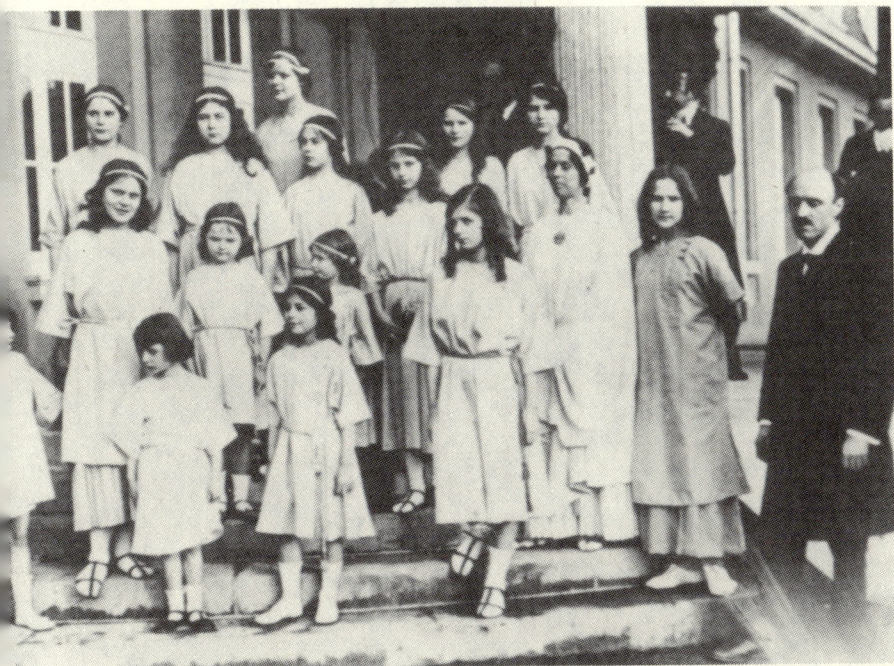

Elizabeth Duncan's school, Darmstadt. Irma at left among her little pupils; Elizabeth and Max Merz at right.

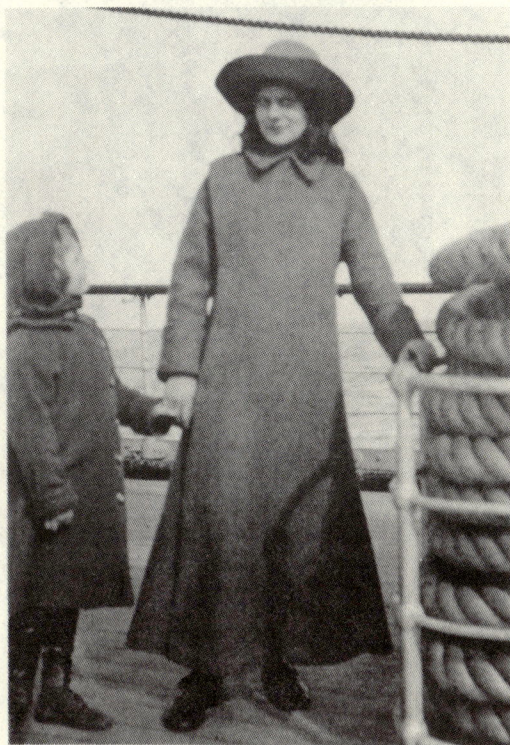

Deirdre and Irma aboard ship to Egypt, 1912: snapshot by Isadora Duncan.

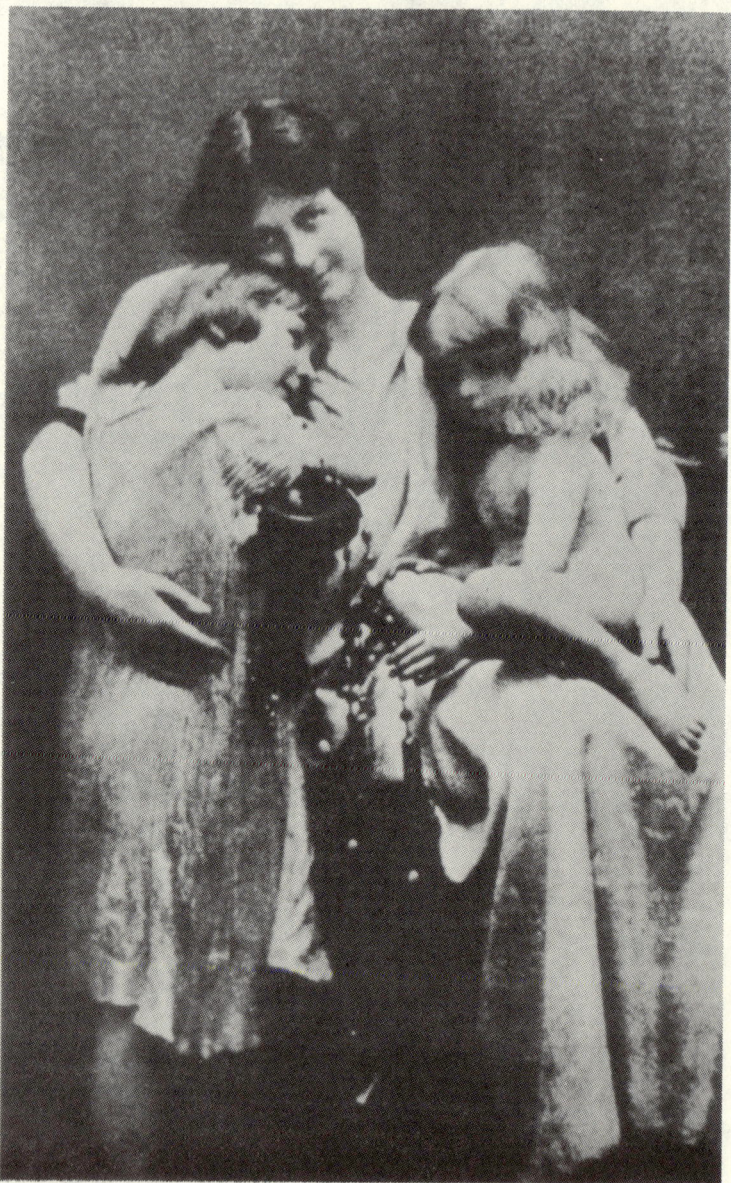

Isadora with Deirdre and Patrick.

"It would be a good idea if you taught Deirdre a few exercises," her mother told me one day. At that time I had never taught anyone, and so Deirdre, Isadora's little daughter, became my first pupil. She also suggested I teach her some simple piece of poetry like William Blake's "Little Lamb, who made thee?/Dost thou know who made thee,/Gave thee life, and bade thee feed/By the stream and o'er the mead?" Whenever her mother asked her to recite the poem, the poor child—timid and confused—could remember only the first line. Her mother would frown and scold, gently urging her to make more of an effort. Being a sensitive child, Deirdre would blush, hang her head, and start to cry.

To make her smile again, I dressed her in a pink candy-striped dress with a red sash, gave her a red pail and shovel, and took her down to the beach. There all the grownups sat in tall wicker chairs, which sheltered them from the stiff breeze that made the water too cold for bathing. The children, fully dressed, built sand castles at their feet. The band played in the pavilion on the boardwalk. And the fashionably dressed summer visitors—the women in hobble skirts with parasols, the men in white flannel trousers and blue jackets—paraded up and down. Few people ventured into the water. When they did, they entered a bathhouse on wheels, where they donned bathing suits that fully covered the body. Then a team of horses pulled the bathhouse out to sea. I found it a frightening experience and refused to do it more than once.

A most embarrassing thing happened to me at Ostend the day we boarded Singer's yacht, the *Lady Evelyn*. We were about to take a channel cruise. "If the weather is good," our host had told us, "we'll sail tomorrow for the Isle of Wight to see the regatta at Cowes."

There was a crew of fifty on the luxurious yacht, which had a festive air with all its pennants whipping gaily in the wind. She seemed to have more of them than any other boat lying in the harbor, especially on the afterdeck.

The instant I stepped aboard, Paris Singer came to me. "I am so sorry this unfortunate thing has happened," he said. "Please don't be too upset. It was an accident—it couldn't be helped. You see, the handle of your suitcase broke when it was carried across the gangplank, and it fell into the sea. The sailor who was carrying the suitcase jumped in and fished it out. But I'm afraid your clothes are ruined. I'm so sorry."

I gazed in horror at all my things hanging on a clothesline on the afterdeck, whipping madly in the breeze. It wasn't so much that they were wet as the dreadful fact that—since I had packed my new red diary with them—they were all hopelessly stained. Uncle Paris, as we children called him, gently placed his arm about me when he saw my consternation. "I'm afraid there isn't anything I can do," he said apologetically. "I wanted to telegraph Liberty's in London to send down some new clothes for you, but Elizabeth said not to do that. She said you could make out all right with what you have."

That was typical of Tante Miss. I was not surprised. It did not, however, increase my affection for her. On the entire cruise I wore the same dress I had on when I came aboard, thanks to her. Finally, when we reached Plymouth, Isadora took pity on me. She bought me the few new things I desperately needed, and everything took on a more cheerful aspect.

On that cruise we visited the Channel Islands and Mont-Saint-Michel, then motored through a part of Devonshire where Paris Singer had an estate near Paignton. All too soon the summer holiday was over. The trip had to be cut short because of Patrick's illness. The baby contracted a fever, and his mother was in a rush to get to her own doctor in Paris.

A week later I reluctantly had to say goodbye to Isadora. She came to see us off at the Gare du Nord where we boarded the train back to Germany. It was then she took me completely by surprise by saying quite casually, "Goodbye, dear. I'll see you next winter in Egypt."

EGYPT! I caught my breath. Had I heard correctly? I was

dying to ask Elizabeth a thousand questions but refrained out of fear of how she might react. She was often so peculiar in my regard that I thought it wiser to keep my fingers crossed just in case and say nothing. From then on, the fall and winter months seemed to drag along endlessly. Christmas came and went without a word from Elizabeth about our coming trip.

And then one day right after the New Year, word got around that she was getting ready to leave. I heard her hobble down the stairs from her top-floor bedroom, and anxiously I asked "Froecken," our Swedish governess, "Has Tante Miss said anything about my going with her?"

"No, she hasn't. Are you ready to go?"

I assured her that this time I was fully prepared. My bag was packed and all I needed was to hear my name called. At that instant from down in the front hall I heard Elizabeth's voice inquire impatiently, "Where is Irma? Why isn't she down here? If she isn't ready I shall have to leave without her."

"I'm coming! I'm coming!" I shouted exuberantly and flew downstairs.

"You lucky girl!" Theresa, my roommate, called after me. "Give my love to Isadora, and don't forget to write!"

I had only time to wave to the other girls from the taxi that waited at the side door. As usual, we were off in a rush. But I thought of my schoolmates left behind in the winter snow when the Simplon Express crossed the Alps into Italy, and how lucky I was indeed. For at Trieste we were to meet our host, Paris Singer, and the rest of the party that sailed with us to Alexandria and the fabled land of the pharaohs.

Ancient Egypt has a fascination all its own. To a young girl of my age, it was something straight out of the Arabian Nights. As in the days of Cleopatra, we sailed leisurely up the legendary river in comfortable houseboats. Arab servants in white caftan and red fez waited on us, bowing down to the ground exclaiming, "Allah be with you!"

During the day we watched mud huts and ruined temples

glide by. At night, when the stars shone so brightly they looked like small moons, the air was filled with the curious native chanting of the crew. Dark shadows danced to the rhythmic beat of drums around a campfire. Most of our days under the hot Egyptian sun were spent in sightseeing. On donkeys or camels, our party often started out before sunrise to visit the ancient temples buried in the desert; each one different, each one remarkable.

In Egypt, everything I saw took on the aspect of a fata morgana. Nothing seemed quite real. When, for example, after hours of sightseeing, one is tired and longs for a cool drink and a light collation—none of which can be obtained in the middle of the Libyan desert—then, lo and behold, a camel caravan appears like a mirage from out of nowhere. In a twinkling, like rubbing Aladdin's lamp, the camel drivers unload chairs and tables laden with sparkling cloths, and glass and silver are set up in the shade of a colonnade. A succulent meal of cold chicken, cold champagne, ripe dates, *rachat lukoum* (a Turkish delight), and Arabian coffee is served. After this repast fit for a pharaoh, all is removed and the caravan, with the swinging gait peculiar to camels, silently vanishes over the horizon.

One day, while visiting the Osiris temple near Abydos, I had another eerie experience. The temple was then still half-buried in sand, being explored by Professor Whittimore, the famous archaeologist. I walked along a raised boulder to get a better view of the desert and suddenly discovered that I was walking along one of the stone beams that was part of the roof, with a drop of fifty feet on either side. I cried out in alarm and was about to turn around in a state of panic, when I heard a quiet voice from way down below in the temple, saying, "Don't turn! Keep steady; look straight ahead and walk to the end. You can get off there."

It was Isadora's voice guiding me to safety as, dizzy from the height, I tried to step forward as firmly as I could. I felt like a tightrope walker in some kind of nightmare, scared to death, never thinking I could make it. I did so, but only because of Isadora.

The temple that was destined to have special significance for me was called Kom Ombo. Between Luxor and Aswan, our most southern stop before turning back, we passed through the narrow gorge of Silsileh, reaching Kom Ombo after dark. A full moon illuminated the temple, splendidly situated on a bluff directly above the river. It stood so close to the river that the propylaea had been washed away, but the building was protected by a high wall, and was the only ancient edifice erected directly on the banks of the Nile. Its other peculiarity was that it was dedicated to twin deities—Horus and Sobk—spirits of good and evil.

After dinner that night, I leaned against the railing on deck and gazed long and thoughtfully at the mysterious temple. All life and purpose gone, for how long had it brooded there in calm grandeur throughout the forgotten centuries? As I stood gazing, the silence was suddenly broken by strains of soft music. Beethoven's "Moonlight Sonata" came floating through the warm air; perfect music for a perfect setting. As if the great composer had written it especially for this scene, the beauty of the music blended with the radiant night and the mysterious temple bathed in white moonlight. Lost in my reverie, I was startled when someone suddenly whispered in my ear, "Quickly, come along with me."

I had not heard anyone approach. Elizabeth motioned me to join her. She conducted me to her cabin while Hener Skene, Isadora's pianist, continued to play on the grand piano that had been especially installed on the open deck for this journey on the Nile.

She asked if I had brought my dance tunic along. Then I knew. The last thing I wanted to do was to dance for the company. As for dancing in front of Isadora, the very thought made me tremble. She had not seen me dance for three years. In my secret heart I did not wish to show her the result of three years of Body Culture à la Elizabeth Duncan. I dreaded the outcome; and, hoping I would be let off, I said quite truthfully that I had not brought my tunic.

"Well, that doesn't matter," Elizabeth said. She took her silk nightgown off a hook. "Here, wear that," she said. When she had arranged the gown to look like a short tunic, she said, "There, that's not too bad. No one will notice. Isadora wants you to dance."

Imagining that I would dance on the open deck, which was luxuriously covered with deep-piled Oriental rugs, I asked, "Is Mr. Skene going to play for me?"

Elizabeth shook her head. "No," she said, "Isadora wants you to dance in the temple."

Quickly grasping at another excuse to get out of it, I asked, "How can I dance barefoot in the temple when the floor is covered with stone and rubble?"

"Wear your sandals. No, they make too much noise scraping the stone floor; wear your sneakers."

Again I grasped at a straw and told her I hadn't a pair with me, only to be disappointed when she said, "Here, take mine; they'll do."

When she said, "All right, let's go," I cried in alarm, holding back, "Oh, no! Tante Miss, I really cannot go!"

"Why not?" She gave me a sharp glance and clicked her tongue, a trick that always irritated me.

"Because," I wailed unhappily, "I really don't know how to dance any more—that's why!"

"Nonsense! Who ever heard of such a thing! Just do as I tell you to and let's have no more fuss."

With these words she led me by the hand into the temple, like a lamb to the sacrifice. The ancient shrine with its two altars dedicated to the deities of good and evil, which only a moment ago I had found so beautiful, now looked frightening. I was forced to dance here against my will and better instinct by the twin personalities who so far had shaped my life. What would the outcome be?

"Ah, here she is," I heard Isadora say as I entered the forecourt where the whole party sat on broken columns and other bits of ruins strewn about. "Are you going to dance for us, my dear?"

"I don't know what to dance," I murmured sullenly, "without music and everything. . . ."

"On such a wonderful moonlight night," Isadora enthused, "in this beautiful temple surely inspiration should not be lacking. Dance anything you fancy, whatever comes to mind."

Only one thought came to my mind and that was to run away as fast as I could. But my training as a Duncan pupil prevailed, and I automatically reacted to the old belief that the performance must go on. With a feeling of "Well, let's have it over with as quickly as possible," I started to move as gracefully as I could without stumbling in my too large sneakers over the broken masonry and rubble littering the floor. To keep some kind of rhythm, I silently hummed a familiar waltz melody to myself. To this unheard tune, I turned and swayed and leaped around in front of my audience for a few seconds in a perfunctory mood, simply to comply with Isadora's request until my sense of the utter inadequacy of the whole performance struck me dead in my tracks. That it must have seemed even worse to Isadora I could guess without being told.

The instant I stopped, the immemorial silence my scraping feet had disturbed settled once again over the ruined temple. No one had moved or clapped their hands or made any comment. Embarrassed, I sat there waiting for the verdict that was inevitably to come from my idol.

Slowly rising from her seat, Isadora spoke in gentle tones, but deliberately and distinctly:

"Have you noticed how entirely unrelated her dance movements were to these extraordinary surroundings? She seemed to be completely unaware of them. What she just did consisted of some pretty little dance gestures she has learned—very nice, very light-hearted, but not in the slightest degree in harmony with the almost awesome sense of mystery that pervades this place and of which you are all, I am sure, deeply aware."

In the pause that followed I felt like sinking into the ground. I realized how true her criticism was. But why did she have to make it in front of all these people? My pride was hurt, and in stupid, girlish fashion I resented this action, especially since I had been made to dance against my better judgment. I was about to get up and rush from the temple when Isadora resumed her impromptu lecture.

"Any dance movement executed in a place like this"—and she swept the vast enclosure with a majestic gesture of her right arm—"must be in close rapport with the mystical vibrations these temple ruins generate. Let me show you what I mean."

Adjusting her flowing white shawl, she strode across the court and disappeared into the shadows in the background. The members of our party regrouped themselves, seating themselves closer to watch what was going to happen. Among Isadora's and Singer's guests were the French artist Grandjouan * and the composer Dupin. There was also an elderly French couple, the Count and Countess de Bérault, whose given names were Tristan and Isolde. All of them were great admirers of Isadora's art.

Presently, as we peered into the background, we saw her emerge from the deep shadows cast by a peristyle of such massive proportions that it dwarfed her white-clad figure. But as soon as she started to move in and out of the tall lotus columns she seemed to grow in stature. The long shadows cast by the columns on the floor of the court formed a symmetrical pattern. And each time she stepped in her stately dance from the

---

* Grandjouan's sketches of Isadora were all made from life and give a true impression of her movements—which is not the case with those artists who depicted her from memory, in some instances even after her death.

shadows into the strip of bright moonlight in between, there was a sudden flash created by her appearance. Alternating in this manner the entire length of the colonnade, slowly in one direction and faster coming back, she created a striking rhythm of brilliant flashes, which in a strange way suggested the beat of music. It was a piece of magic that held her onlookers spellbound.

When Isadora returned to her friends, they voiced their admiration. The French countess embraced her crying, *"C'était magnifique, magnifique!"*

Chatting animatedly about the phenomenon they had just witnessed—one that only an artist of genius could produce—the company slowly wended their way down the narrow path to the houseboats below. I remained alone in the temple. I, her pupil, had not seen Isadora dance for years. For me, this demonstration of her great powers was like manna from heaven. Once more I wished, as I did when I first saw her, that I could dance like that. To my now more adult eyes, this was a revelation of what the true art of the dance should be. I had been taught a great lesson, one I would never forget, this moonlight night in the temple of Kom Ombo.

❦ 8 ❦

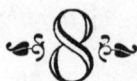

You Must Be My Children

My holiday with Isadora in Egypt came to an end on my fifteenth birthday. The next day Elizabeth and I started on our long trip back to Darmstadt. We would have continued on to the Holy Land with the others had we not received an urgent message from Max Merz to return immediately. He had arranged a command performance to be given for the Grand Duke and Duchess of Weimar.

Coming from ancient Egypt, where I had danced like some pagan priestess on the rough stones in a temple by the Nile, I was now to dance on the polished parquet floor of an eighteenth-century palace. We performed for the Duke and his court in a lovely music room in the old Amalienpalast, illuminated by hundreds of candles burning in golden chandeliers. Here we went through the same dance exercises Elizabeth had taught us. But the memory of Kom Ombo, still fresh in my mind, made her unimaginative physical culture drill even harder to bear. Oh, how I longed for just one more lesson from Isadora! Little did I realize then how soon my ardent wish would be fulfilled.

Ever since her liaison with the man who could provide her with luxury and every mundane distraction money could buy, Isadora's career had been neglected. But suddenly, upon her return from Egypt, she experienced an upsurge of her creative impulse. She once said of her constant struggle between her physical and her spiritual natures, "The woman in me and the artist are always fighting for the upper hand. But the artist always wins in the end."

She retired to her house in Neuilly and set herself to work

with renewed vigor, composing a whole program of new dances. She remarked at the time:

> There was a time when I filled my copybooks with notes and observations when I, myself, was filled with an apostolic sentiment for my art. When all kinds of naive audacities were mine. In those times I wanted to reform human life in its smallest details of costume, morals or nourishment.
>
> But ten years have passed since then and I have since had the leisure to prove the vanity of my noble ambitions. I now occupy myself entirely with the joys of my work and the preoccupation of my art. One can speak better of the dance by dancing than by the publication of commentaries and explanations. True art has no need for them, it speaks for itself.*

Entering her beautiful three-story studio in Neuilly was like entering a cathedral. The long blue drapes covering the walls and hanging down from the ceiling in heavy folds suggested a Gothic interior. The soft light filtering through alabaster lamps overhead lent a mystic atmosphere. An open stairway at one end led to her private apartment upstairs, which was lavishly decorated by Paul Poirêt. In this Parisian retreat the American dancer lived and worked alone. Her two children, with the nurse and servants, lived in a separate adjoining dwelling.

She took her work very seriously. Like other great creative artists, she craved solitude to work out her ideas. Nobody ever watched her doing it. Aside from the indispensable musician who acted as her accompanist and usually played in a corner with his back to her, no one was present. Not even her pupils were there unless she was choreographing special dances for them. That was the only time I ever saw her at work creatively. Otherwise, her studio was sacrosanct, and not even members of her family could enter. "My dance is my religion," she had often said; and she meant it. Of course, occasionally when she

---

* From a program note, Teatro Costanzi, Rome; cf. *Art*, p. 100.

gave some of her gay parties in the studio, she would improvise on the spur of the moment if her guests asked her to dance. But then it would be something light and frivolous; never anything serious.

Another detail connected with her method of work I want to explain: she never practiced her dances before a mirror. She used the large wall mirror hidden behind the curtains only to check on her gymnastics and exercises at the barre, which she vigorously engaged in every morning. But when it came to dancing, she rejected this method of self-observation, claiming it only interfered with her inner concentration and expression. None of her pupils used a mirror in her work. Her credo when it come to expressing music, as she often told her pupils, was "to look within and dance in accordance with a music heard inwardly."

She claimed that there were three kinds of dancers: first, those who consider dancing as a sort of gymnastic drill, made up of impersonal and graceful arabesques; second, those who, by concentrating their minds, lead the body into the rhythm of a desired emotion, expressing a remembered feeling or experience; and finally, those who "convert the body into a luminous fluidity, surrendering it to the inspiration of the soul." This last she saw as the truly creative dancer.*

In the spring of 1913 Isadora asked her sister to bring the older girls, her original pupils, to Paris to appear with her in a series of performances at the Châtelet Theatre. The last time we had entered her beautiful studio on the Rue Chauveau was in 1909, as children. We now returned as young girls, eager to resume our studies with the only person in the world who could teach us to progress in our art.

Our happy anticipation was dashed to the ground the day of our first lesson. It was only natural that Isadora (whose brain-children we represented) should be disappointed with our

* Cf. *Art*, pp. 51–52.

manner of dancing. Four years of regimented training under the tutelage of her sister had left their mark on us.

"They are terrible, simply terrible! Impossible! Whatever shall I do with them?" she wailed disconsolately, addressing her pianist Hener Skene.

Her reaction, though not quite unexpected, was nevertheless a shock to her doting pupils, who stood there speechless and with long faces, wishing they could crawl under a stone and hide. Her words cut deep. "What has happened to them? They dance without animation, stiff, without expression, without inner feeling—like automations!"

With these words she pronounced her verdict on the Elizabeth Duncan School of which we were only the pitiful products. But we girls, or rather victims of Max Merz and his obsession with his *Körperkultur* and racial hygiene, had to bear the brunt of Isadora's condemnation in silence. We swallowed hard, choked back our tears, and tried with all our might to do better, hoping that under her inspired guidance we would soon recapture her spirit and come closer to her ideal.

Unfortunately, she turned out to be a very impatient teacher. Her method consisted in demonstrating the sequence of a dance perfectly executed by herself. Then, without demonstrating it step by step, she expected her pupils to understand immediately and repeat it. Impossible, of course. She danced the sequence again and again without obtaining any result and then gave up in disgust. When her pianist politely suggested she repeat the fast dance movement at a slower tempo so we could get the steps, she readily consented.

And then a curious thing happened. She floundered and found herself incapable of demonstrating the movement step by step. She looked surprised and then annoyed at several unsuccessful attempts to come to grips with the situation. Wearily, she leaned against the piano and said to Skene, "How perfectly extraordinary! This is quite a revelation to me. I am apparently unable to dissect my own dance in order to teach it to others. I had no idea how difficult this would be for me. I can dance my own choreography, but am unable to analyse any part of it for the benefit of others."

"That often happens to creative artists," Skene interposed. "The methodical approach is not a basis for inspiration. Teaching is an art in itself. Your own style of teaching is entirely by example and inspiration. There is nothing wrong with this method, only it is more difficult for the pupil, that's all."

Difficult was right. She continued to train us in this "catch as catch can" fashion, repeating the dance movement until at least one of us caught on. Then she would say, "You have got the movement correctly. Now teach the others and I expect everybody to have it right by tomorrow." And that was that.

Our dogged determination to master the advanced technique she had developed over the past years, while we were deprived of her teaching, paid off in the end. Seeing us work so hard every day, eager to make up for so much time lost, she took note of our progress and eventually devoted much of her time to teaching us a whole series of new dances, most of them set to the music of Schubert and Gluck. The audience, when they watched us perform in the theatre and admired our dancing because it seemed so effortless and spontaneous, imagined that all they needed was a few yards of chiffon and they could do the same. They had not the slightest conception of the amount of work and technique involved.

Finally came the day when we once more danced with Isadora on the same Châtelet stage where we had last performed together in 1909. The French writer Fernand Divoire, who first coined the expression "Isadorable," wrote at the time:

Six slender young girls appeared on the scene attired in rose-colored scarves and crowned with flowers. Bare-limbed and light-footed they throw themselves joyfully into the dance. They are the little Isadorables we used to see dance when they were children. They are grown up now. Tall, supple and graceful, they combine their erstwhile naive gaiety with all the charm of young girls. No painting of Botticelli or Angelico, no Greek fresco depicting the vernal season expresses as much beauty, chastity and artlessness as these youthful dancers.

Isadora dances with them and is part of them. And the delighted audience applauds and applauds, freed of all everyday worries and care, left with no other thoughts but those of grace and youth eternal.

Such a performance rarely happens where, the orchestra gone, the lights extinguished, the ushers waiting to close the doors, so many of the audience remain to applaud frantically and acclaim the artist they worship. They insist on recalling the Isadorable one again and again, unable to part from her. After masses of flowers have been presented she gives the enthusiastic audience one last dance.

Joining hands with her six young girls they dance silently, without music, around the flowers heaped in the center of the stage—a ring around the roses—such as children play. This charming improvisation as we watch it unfold is unforgettable. Oh, garden of happy spirits!

Later that spring season we also danced with Isadora at the Trocadéro, taking part in her Orpheus program. I still recall the thrill I experienced when she taught me the solo part in the dance depicting the scene of the Happy Spirit, a part she had always danced herself. To make matters even more exciting, she gave me the tunic of pale blue Liberty silk that she herself had always worn. I treasured it for many years.

During this particular period Isadora was at the zenith of her career. At the age of thirty-five she had everything any artist or young woman could wish: fame, success, money, two lovely children, and a man who was not only devoted to her but willing to put himself and his fortune to work for the cause of her art. He planned to build a theatre of the dance in Paris that would bear her name. It was to outshine the recently completed Théâtre des Champs-Élysées, which in its exterior architectural decoration—as well as in its interior, painted frescos—had been inspired by her dances. The two artists who executed the decorations, the sculptor Bourdelle and the painter Denis, both admired Isadora's art profoundly and admitted to being greatly influenced by her. Among the dance decorations done by Maurice Denis is a gilded bas-relief panel on the mezzanine floor representing the six girls who appeared with her at the time.

The future seemed bright for me and my schoolmates, too. Our dream had come true at last—to be studying once more with Isadora. This had been our secret wish all along, while marking time at the Darmstadt school. When all looked so promising for the future that lovely month of April in Paris, in that "garden of happy spirits" the poet spoke of, who could have foreseen the unspeakable calamity hovering menacingly in the background, ready to pounce on its innocent victims, destroying them in a flash, and with them, our innocent dreams.

The nineteenth of April, that tragic turning point in Isadora Duncan's life, dawned wet and cold. We girls went as usual from our pension around the corner from the Rue Chauveau for our morning workout at the studio. A pleasant surprise awaited us. We found Deirdre and her little brother Patrick there playing games. They had come in that morning from Versailles, where they had spent the winter months. At the age of three Patrick could not yet talk except for a few words, but he understood quite well when his nanny coaxed him to show us how his mama bowed to the audience at the end of a performance. Deirdre always acted bashful when asked to do something, but not Patrick. Like a real actor he gave a cunning imitation of his famous mother acknowledging the applause. As we laughed and asked him to do it again, Isadora came in. She joined in the laughter and told us that we would all have luncheon at an Italian restaurant in town as the guests of Paris Singer. It was the last time we would all be so happily together.

We girls returned to our pension after lunch for our daily music lesson. Professor Edlinger, our teacher, had a nice baritone voice and loved to sing entire scores of operas, doing all the parts. That particular afternoon, while the rain continued unabated, he chose the stirring music of Wagner's *Die Walküre* for our lesson. All devout music lovers, we could sit and listen to him for hours.

While he sang Sigmund's impassioned *"Winterstürme wichen dem Wonnemond,"* I watched the heavy rainstorm bending the budding trees outside on the lawn, tearing off the tender green shoots and scattering them about in its fury. With branches wildly waving, the trees seemed to be dancing grotesquely to Wagner's music.

The room felt cold and damp. I shivered and drew my woolen jacket closer about me. The hours passed. Twilight was descending when we reached that state of repleteness which beautiful music engenders and which is accompanied by a mild state of drowsiness. Then suddenly, like one of the great composer's own leitmotifs, we were all roused from our lethargy by a frantic knocking at the front door. We heard a door slam and rapid footsteps approached our room.

Temple's father appeared pale and haggard-looking like a phantom in the twilight. In a frantic state, his clothes dripping wet, he rushed to his daughter and held her tight. Frightened, she cried out in alarm, "What is the matter, father, what has happened?"

In a broken voice that sounded hollow in the gloom he announced the dreadful news: "Isadora's children are dead."

After a night of terror in which I for one found little sleep, we all welcomed the sight of Mary Sturges who came to see us early the next morning. She described in detail the automobile accident that had caused the drowning of the two dear little children and their nurse in the river Seine. She told us to pack our things, since we would leave for Darmstadt immediately. But first we must say goodbye to Isadora.

The storm had passed during the night. Walking the short distance to Isadora's house in the sunshine, listening to the chirping of the birds, my mind was filled with the saddest thoughts. At sixteen one believes death happens only to older people. It is quite incomprehensible to see innocent children struck down. I was frightened at the thought of having to look at them in death, while remembering their laughing faces of the day before.

We entered by a side door. The house was shrouded in silence, and only the blue alabaster lamps were lit, shedding an eerie light over everything. With fear in my heart I entered the downstairs library. There, on a couch covered by a black silk shawl embroidered with many small flowers, reposed the lifeless forms of the two children, lying close beside each other, their blond heads touching. Deirdre had her right arm curved lovingly about her baby brother as if to protect him even in sleep. How often had I seen them together like this. I could not believe that they were dead despite the tall flickering tapers and the flowers heaped all around them. Seeing them thus I was more shocked than sad, and unable to shed tears. A black velvet rope stretched across the room separating us from them, and we stood there in silent contemplation for a few minutes. Then I heard someone whisper, "Come along now, girls, and say goodbye to Isadora."

We parted the long blue curtains and entered the vast studio. This was the moment I dreaded most. In the semidarkness I could at first barely see her. Immobile, like a statue, her head thrown back and eyes closed, she sat in an armchair. Tears flowed down her face. Her usually smiling, engaging countenance had, through unbearable grief, been distorted into a tortured mask. The picture of martyrdom incarnate, she resembled a Gothic saint carved in wood.

The moment we beheld her silent agony we all started to cry. Standing close beside her, I could not control my wild sobbing when she looked at me and, taking me into her arms, held my head close to her breast. Through my sobs I heard her say in a gentle, pitiful voice, "You must be my children now."

I doubt if there are many women in the world, including

myself, who would be capable of expressing so humane and generous a thought at so tragic a moment. That she could find no bitterness in her heart toward a fate that left her foster children unharmed while these of her own flesh and blood lay dead beside her proves the greatness of her soul. If all human beings are ultimately judged by their acts on earth, I would say this was Isadora Duncan's finest hour.

PART II. 1913–1921

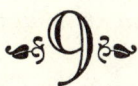

❧9❧

Dionysion

WOULD Isadora ever dance again? That was the question uppermost in our minds. It did not seem likely. She once confessed that in those dark moments she thought of committing suicide. She left her house in Neuilly after the funeral, never to return.

In her subsequent restless wanderings through Greece and Italy, all that summer, she found no peace. At the beginning of September she settled for a long stay in Viareggio, where her friend Eleonora Duse lived. Since Isadora did not have a telephone, Duse would leave little penciled notes for her at the hotel whenever she came to call and did not find her in.

These notes, written in French, expressed Duse's concern and devotion for a friend and fellow artist she so greatly admired. La Duse scrawled them in her large handwriting, three or four words covering a whole page. The first note, dated September 13 (1913), was delivered by hand to the hotel where Isadora was staying.

> *Chère*—My heart has been awaiting you for a long time—am here within two steps of you and shall come to you as soon as you desire—yours with all my heart.

> This morning at the Grand Hotel I left a letter and some flowers for you. *Chère* Isadora, *des roses de la campagne,* flowers from my garden. Tell me that you are not too sad to be in a hotel room. Dear, all day I hoped to be with you and tomorrow morning early I shall come and fetch you. But forgive my not coming this evening. It is raining too hard and I am not feeling well. I embrace you and thank you, *de tout âme,* for having

137

come and searched me out at this moment which is without life, without art for you.

Dear, I have called four times today at the Grand Hotel to see you. The last time they told me you had moved to the Regina. I would like to see you this evening but a headache and the thunderstorm prevented me from going out again. I hope the sojourn at the seashore, so lonesome for you, will not be too painful. Shelley will speak to you there. Dream, work, and be valiant in your beautiful strength.

Of seeking out Eleonora Duse to comfort her in this tragic moment of her life, Isadora has said, "If I had not been able to bear the society of other people it was because they all played the comedy of trying to cheer me with forgetfulness. But Eleonora said: 'Tell me of your children' and she made me repeat all their little sayings and ways."

In another note left at the hotel for her friend, Duse said:

Forgive my fatigue the other night. I could not speak to you, my heart pains me when I see you suffer. Be of good cheer tomorrow! I hope the view of the sea and the mountains will bring you peace. My thoughts watch over you and wish you courage, *Chère loyale amie.* To regain my own strength I must rest a little while longer by my doctor's orders. But I shall see you again soon and we will talk some more about the children— and art.

Isadora loved the sea, having been born near the Pacific Ocean, and she enjoyed swimming in salt water. She always used to go bathing wearing a black one-piece suit. Those were the days when women entered the water fully covered, even with stockings and shoes. In her simple, sensible attire, then considered outrageously scant, she naturally attracted much attention. Besides, she was a celebrity who only recently made tragic headlines the world over and photographers stuck to her heels and pestered her no matter how much she tried to evade them and other curiosity-seekers. When she complained of this to Duse, the latter said, "You cannot escape the crowds, they will always search you out."

Tired and annoyed by the curious throngs who trailed her wherever she went, Isadora rented a villa with a high wall around it, in a pine forest. Living there all alone, she had only the presence of Duse to comfort her. That great Italian actress was a devoted admirer of Isadora's art and encouraged her to find solace in her work. As the foremost tragedienne of her day, Eleonora Duse appreciated the noble sentiment of sorrow. They always spoke French together. Duse would say, *"Ne perdez pas la belle douleur."*

She advised Isadora to incorporate this ennobling experience into her art; to transfigure grief into a dance. And so Isadora wrote to her musician Skene:

> Life is nothing but chaos and terror; only music, beauty and art exist. Everything else is but a confused dream.
>
> Have you found a chorale or hymn by Bach or Palestrina on which I could work? I completely despair of life . . . but perhaps I could create something beautiful in movement grown in the midst of a requiem which might comfort some people on earth sad as myself. Please search for me.

In César Franck's *Redemption* she found the inspiration to translate her tragic experience into movement, guided by the Biblical words, "Thou hast turned for me my mourning into dancing."

Years later, after Isadora's death, I asked Mary Desti (who had been with her that tragic day in 1913) whether Isadora had actually danced at her children's funeral as some newspapers reported at the time. She said, "No, Isadora never even entered her studio where the funeral service was held. She only listened to the music (played by the Paris Symphony Orchestra) below while sitting upstairs in the narrow gallery fronting her private apartment. But everybody watched her intently, and every time she as much as raised her head or moved her arm—since all her movements were beautiful—they thought she was dancing! Only I could see that she was numb with grief."

Duse encouraged her with tender words to continue working as a form of salvation. Living in enforced retirement herself for lack of engagements, Eleonora knew from personal experience how it felt to be deprived of the exercise of one's art. Watching her dance one day and admiring Isadora's capacity to lose herself in the expression of music, feeling envious not to be able to do this herself, she told her friend:

"You, who can flee reality, *chère genereuse!* So courageous in life and gentle and submissive before death, how I wish I too could escape from reality! Without work, without risks life is nothing—a dream empty of dreams. What joy to see you take up anew the flight toward the light! May a beautiful dream of art carry you far, far away from here. *Mon coeur et mon âme sont remplis de vôtre grandeur.* For all the beauty I perceive in you, I thank you."

A deep-seated restlessness embedded in her nature, augmented by that constant torment gnawing at her vitals, impelled Isadora to leave the villa and her work. She had a sudden desire to go to Rome. St. Peter's with its great art works, the many fountains, the ancient ruins, the tombs along the Appian Way, all breathed eternal peace and calm. When Duse heard of this plan, she wrote:

Dear Isadora,

Since we must say farewell, I beg you not to say it tonight but rather tomorrow in the full light of day at noon. *Chère* Isadora, how sad to see you leave! But you must find your wings again all by yourself, then you will re-enter a state of grace which is your art, your strength, your nobility—for sorrow is everywhere in this world. . . . My thoughts are with you, recuperate, have a good rest, do not despair. Your benevolence and all the illusions of your heart will never be lost.

Adieu, et au revoir.
Eleonora Duse

Isadora later confessed that when she was in the depths of despair only the thought of her school, "my other child" as she called it, saved her reason. A supernatural voice seemed to whisper to her to continue to teach little children to dance in beauty and according to the divine law.

Paris Singer, concerned for her welfare, did everything in his power to help her regain an interest in her work. With this aim in mind, he presented her, around Christmas time, with a magnificent building of palatial proportions to house her new school. He had bought the former Paillard Palace Hotel, completely furnished including silver, linen, and china. A fifteen-minute drive from Paris, it was situated in the rural hamlet of Bellevue-sur-Seine, close to the forests of Meudon and Saint-Cloud. On a bluff directly above the river, where the Seine makes a big loop, the sixty-two-room house had a magnificent panorama of Paris in the distance and the Seine valley in the foreground.

Soon Isadora was busy remodeling the house to suit her purpose and preparing it for the influx of new pupils whom she expected.

In the meantime, we girls in Darmstadt had no inkling of these interesting developments. As usual, not a word concerning Isadora reached our ears. Early in the summer Augustin Duncan paid the school a visit, bringing with him his second wife, Margherita, and their little boy, Angus. As upon former occasions "Uncle Gus," as we called him, soon had an artistic project under way. In Grunewald he had taught us to recite and act small parts of Shakespeare's plays, such as *A Midsummer Night's Dream*. This time he wanted us to dance and mime the opera *Echo and Narcisse* by Gluck. He always took a great interest and an active part in furthering the artistic education of his sister's pupils—the only one of her brothers to do so.

While we were on tour with our new show, Augustin wrote to Isadora, who was then still living in Viareggio. In the hope of arousing her interest in our activities and thus taking her mind

off her sorrow for a while, he wrote from Hamburg on October
18, 1913:

My dearest Isadora,
    We have received some beautiful notices for "Echo and Nar-
cisse," that show an appreciation of what I have been trying to
realize. The lighting effects have been especially appreciated.
    We opened in Darmstadt with very good results. The Grand
Duke and Prince Henry of Prussia attended with their wives.
We repeated it in Mainz and had much better music.
    Now we are here for two evenings. The first performance is
bought out by the Lessing Society and the second is a public evening. It is being given in the new Opera House where they have
a very good orchestra and a director from the Stadt Theater in
Leipzig. This director is a famous man in Germany and is to
give a fifteen-minute conference to the press to prepare them.
    We travel from here to Munich on November 4th, and are in
Stuttgart Nov. 5th. Can't you come and see us at one of these
places? We are to appear in Zurich on the 27th.
    Margherita is coming on to see us at Stuttgart. The baby
[Angus] is splendid and runs about the place his nose scratched
up from tumbling. I do wish you would come either to Munich
or Stuttgart because we have a beautiful plan if you would like it
—without you it is unrealizable and must then remain a
dream. . . .
    I will write again more fully, am hurried this morning. We
have just arrived here and there is a great deal to attend to. I
will send you some clippings. It is a great success and a great
advance and a tiny step forward towards your great idea.
                                                Love from us all,
                                                        Gus

    Our tour ended in Berlin. The recently opened Hotel Eden
on the Kurfuerstendamm then represented the height in luxurious accommodations. We spent several weeks there over the
Christmas and New Year's holidays. Gus, who was well aware
of our love for Isadora and our antipathy toward his older

sister, gave us the best Christmas present in the world when he surprised us with the wonderful news that Isadora wanted us six older girls and her niece to join her immediately in Paris, where she had founded a new school.

We shouted for joy and could hardly restrain our happiness, when the door opened and Tante Miss walked in, accompanied by Max Merz. Our faces fell, and solemnity descended like a pall over our exuberance. She showed us Isadora's telegram, saying, "I have no objection to your going to my sister for a while to help her get started with the school in France. After all, the main thing is that she finds a renewed interest in life. And we must do everything we can to help her."

Mr. Merz, who had been impatiently stalking up and down the room, interrupted her. "This is absurd, Elizabeth, utterly senseless. Why must we send all the girls at the same time? Can't we simply send one or two, and keep the rest? You know very well that we have a command performance to give for the Crown Prince and his wife in Potsdam in a few weeks. And what about our plans for appearing at the Salzburg festival this summer? Have you thought of that?"

"Yes, Merzl, yes, they will be back for that," Elizabeth reassured him. She always called him "Merzl" when she wanted to have her own way. Red in the face with fury, he stormed out of the room shouting, "You don't know what you are doing! This is ruin for us!"

He went out, slamming the door behind him, and that was the last we girls saw of him for many years. He fully realized that, given a choice, we older girls without exception would prefer to remain with Isadora.

Elizabeth later came to Paris and tried to force us back for the command performance and Salzburg festival—without success, as far as I was concerned. I happened at the time to be ill with influenza. She found me in bed with a nurse in attendance. I had a high fever, but she imagined I was shamming and—disregarding the nurse's shocked protest—yanked me bodily out of bed. In my weakened condition, I fell down in a dead faint at her feet.

Isadora did not want us to go, and we, of course, resisted with all our might. The two or three girls that Elizabeth corralled for the command performance for the German Crown Prince insisted on coming back to Paris afterward. And that was the end of our association with Tante Miss. She functioned on her own from then on, with Max Merz beside her. For a few years she was in America, but most of her time was spent in Austria and Germany till her death in Stuttgart in 1948.

The night in January, 1914, when we arrived at the gates of Isadora's school on top of a hill overlooking Paris, our jubilance at being reunited with her cannot be imagined. In the train coming from Berlin to Paris, we practically sang all the way. And now, when we saw her again after her terrible tragedy, waiting for her "other children" at the top of a flight of stairs, we rushed up two steps at a time into her outstretched arms. I felt I had come home at last.

Life took on a fresh meaning for all of us, working here together in harmony in this "Temple of the Dance of the Future" she had named Dionysion, after the ancient Greek god of creation. Since Isadora did not teach beginners, the instruction of the new pupils (mostly French and Russian children) devolved upon us older girls. She expressed herself most pleased with the knowledge and confidence with which we passed on her teachings.

Because she was expecting the birth of her third child (it was to die a few hours after birth), she herself would teach the older group while reclining on a couch, using only her hands and arms. She had changed much in appearance. She had cut her hair, and with this simple act set a fashion soon to be copied by other dancers and women all over the world, chalking up another reform to her credit.

Immersed in her work and surrounded by happy, laughing children, she made a valiant effort to overcome the effects of the recent tragedy whose memory haunted her day and night. We six girls had nothing to offer her but our youthful enthusiasm for the dance, and our devotion. She said, "In the morning, when I entered the dancing room and they saw me, they would shout, 'Good morning Isadora!' It sounded so joyful. How could I be sad amongst them?" *

In April she sent Anna and me to Russia to choose some Russian children for the school. Her brother and sister-in-law accompanied us. And here I ran into an unexpected and curious experience. One had to have a passport to visit Tsarist Russia. The regulations demanded a baptismal certificate in order to obtain a visa. This necessitated my going back to Hamburg, as I had no documents with me and Mr. Merz refused to be co-operative. When Margherita, who chaperoned me, discovered by talking with mother that I had never been baptized, it did not faze her in the least. I myself had been completely ignorant of my heathen status all these years, and could not have been more surprised. Fearing this would prevent my going to Russia, I said to Margherita, "I am afraid we are out of luck and must return to Paris. There is nothing we can do about this now."

"Oh yes there is," Margherita retorted firmly. "We are going to have you baptized right away!"

In her breezy American style that would not admit to being thwarted in any undertaking, she picked up the phone and called the nearest Protestant church to arrange an interview with the pastor. The St. Petrikirche, consecrated in the twelfth century, is the oldest church in Hamburg. The pastor received us kindly in his study and, though sympathetic to our request, gravely refused to baptize me in a hurry merely to let me get a Russian visa. He insisted on a minimum three-week course of preparation and instruction in the Lutheran faith.

We persuaded him that this was impossible. Margherita explained in English that it was now or never. I suppose it was to save my soul that he then agreed to do it on the spot. While he

* Cf. *Life*, p. 302.

retired to don his vestments, I entered the old church, where someone began to light the candles by the altar. The very moment Pastor Poppe gave me the benediction, a ray of sunlight pierced the beautiful stained-glass window and fell directly on my head as I was kneeling by the altar rail. I suddenly felt very sanctified. I heard mother crying softly into her handkerchief, and then the pastor solemnly shook hands with us as we departed. Half-way up the aisle he called out, "Wait a minute! Haven't you forgotten something?" And he waved the precious baptismal certificate for which Margherita, who acted as my godmother, had paid ten gold marks. We rushed to get it, jumped into a taxi, and drove to the Russian consulate.

And here occurred the most ironic thing. When I handed in my passport, the clerk stamped on the Russian visa without demanding to see my certificate of baptism! Annoyed at his disinterest after all I had gone through to get it, I asked him why. He answered blandly, "Not necessary in your case. One can see at a glance you belong to the Aryan race."

Margherita and I met Anna and Augustin in Berlin and gaily continued on our mission to St. Petersburg. We stayed at the new Hotel Astoria, opposite the grand St. Isaac cathedral. Anna and I gave a small dance recital in the ballroom of that hotel. I remember how terribly thrilled we were to have the great Constantin Stanislawsky of the Moscow Art Theatre consent to introduce us to the audience and give a lecture on Isadora's art. At the end of our performance he personally presented each one of us with a lovely bouquet of flowers. Immensely proud and flattered, we took a snapshot of each other holding his flowers and posing with them on the window sill of our hotel room with the huge cathedral looming in the background. A nice souvenir of our only joint performance anywhere. We remained in Russia for two months. Later, some of the other girls and Hener Skene joined us so we could give a few performances before returning to Paris with a group of newly recruited pupils.

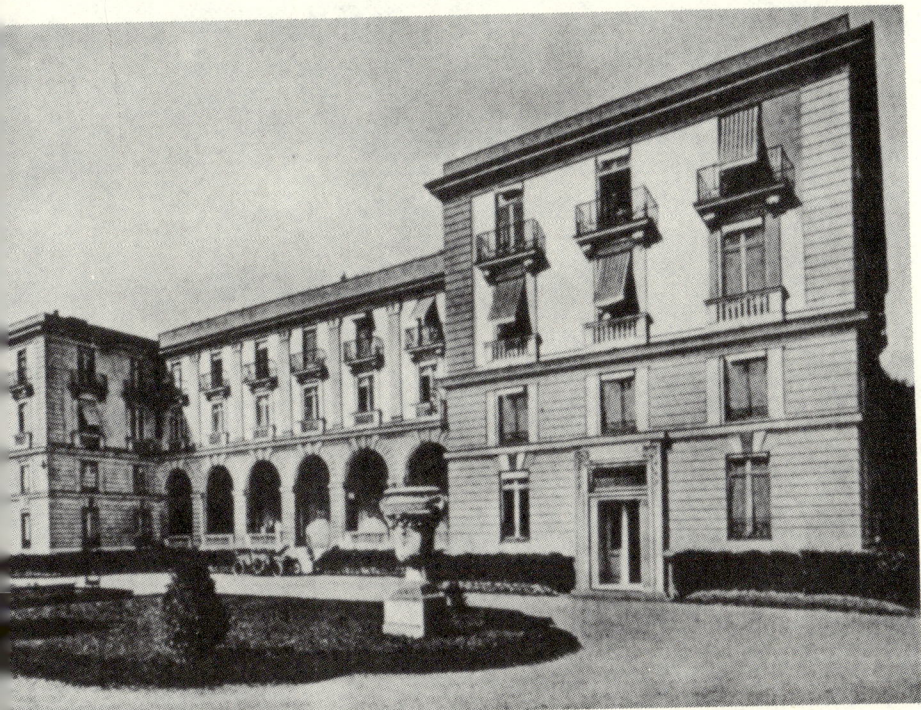

Dionysion, 1914.

Dionysion: the six Duncan girls with statue of dancing maenad.

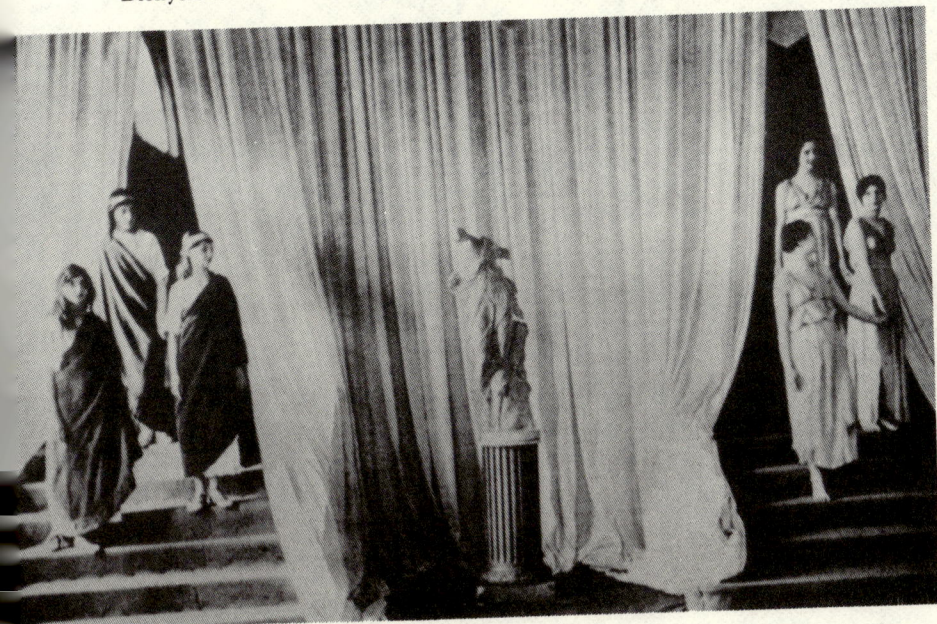

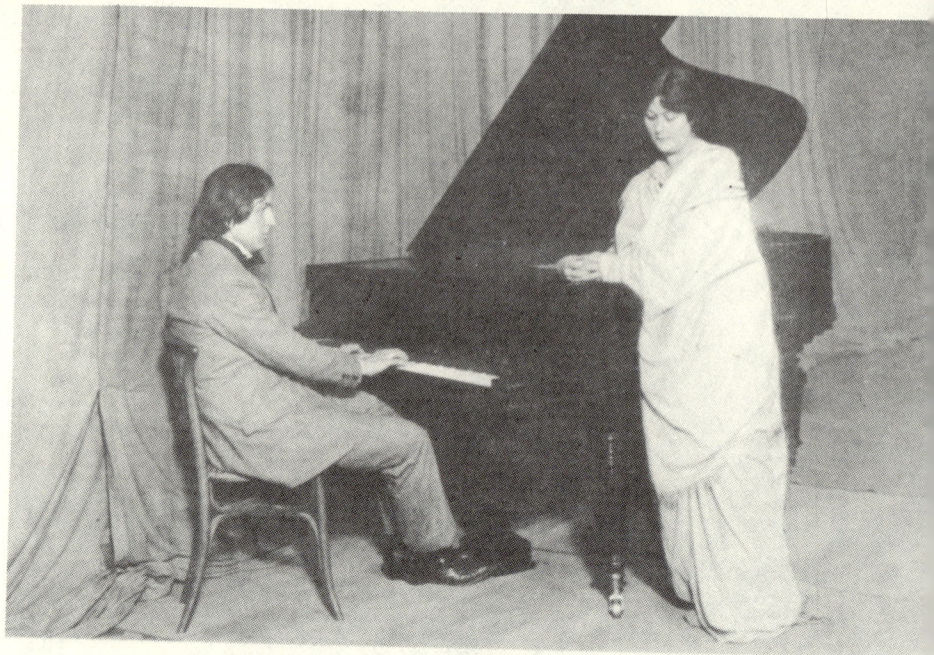

Walter Rummel and Isadora, 1919.

Duncan Dancers, 1920: Lisa, Irma, Margot.

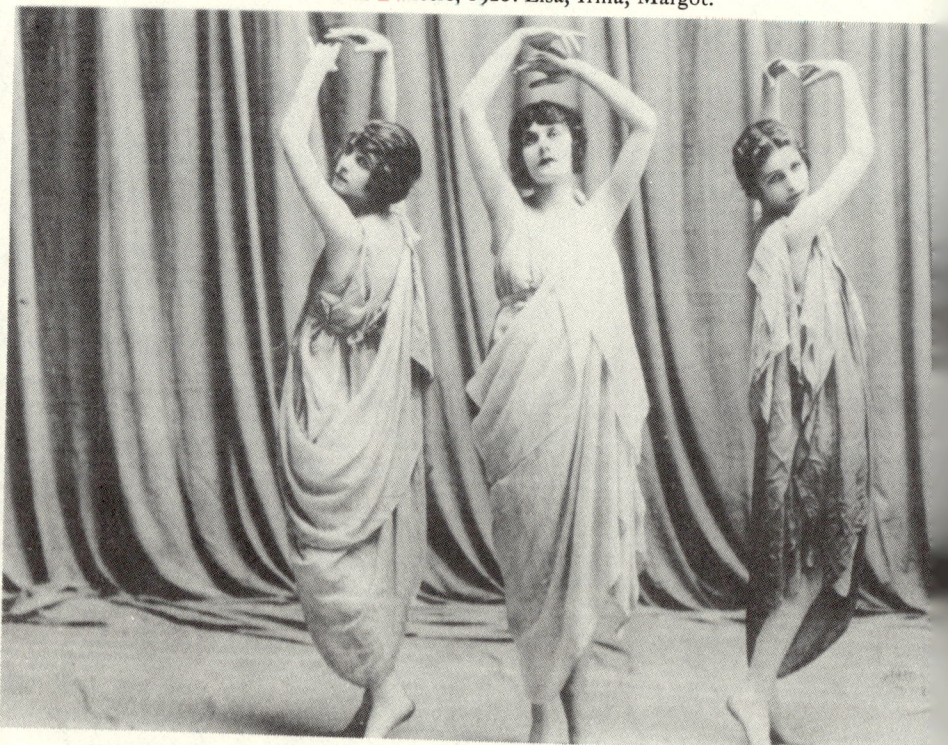

We all led a happy, wonderful life with Isadora in that beautiful school. The fact that she treated us like adults and allowed us each a room to ourselves started things off to our entire satisfaction. She told us of her plan to build that theatre of the dance and drama so long dreamed of, and how she intended to make us members of a company patterned after the Comédie Française. Our artistic future seemed assured. Isadora too firmly believed that Dionysion had taken permanent roots and that she would live there for the rest of her life, continuing to do creative work.

All these noble prospects came to an end when disaster struck once more—this time on a gigantic scale. In August the First World War set cannons to roaring over most of Europe, and the millions of soldiers wounded in battle needed help. Isadora gave her temple of the dance to the Red Cross for a hospital. She and her pupils fled to America, via London and Liverpool, where the streets were crowded with soldiers going off to war singing, "It's a long way to Tipperary."

The wild excitement engendered by those stirring times, added to the intriguing adventure of crossing the ocean to another continent, prevented my realizing what sad consequences the war would have for our school. In years to come, I have often looked back with deep regret that Dionysion existed for only seven short months. For it represented Isadora Duncan's ideal school, the perfect center and environment—now lost to posterity—for preserving the results of her work. And I regret also that she did not make more of an effort to keep it functioning despite the world-wide catastrophe. For wars have come and gone, and life is short, but art lives on forever.

~§ 10 §~

Growing Up

WE reached New York on September 13, 1914, after an uneventful voyage on the Cunard liner *Lapland*. But the moment we landed, all sorts of unforeseen and startling things happened in quick succession.

As soon as the immigration officials discovered that Isadora Duncan's school had arrived without the protection of a legal guardian, they barred our entry. To the great consternation of Mr. and Mrs. Augustin Duncan, who had safely brought us through war-torn Europe to America, we were not permitted to disembark, though their children were allowed to go ashore. With Alicia Franck, the school secretary, and Miss Baker, our English governess who volunteered to remain with us, we were locked up in that ignoble detention pen called Ellis Island. For this reason, my first impression of the United States was not a favorable one.

We remained incarcerated under armed guards, like a bunch of criminals, for two interminable weeks before the necessary formalities could be straightened out. I used to gaze in amazement at the heroic Statue of Liberty standing in the harbor nearby and wonder: Is this the land of the free?

New York at the time was in the grip of a formidable heat wave. This circumstance contributed no little to our extreme discomfort, for eighteen of us were crowded together in one small room with bath, sleeping on the bare floor like animals, without any covers or bedding. At that, we considered ourselves lucky when a kind immigration commissioner by the name of F. C. Howe placed his private quarters at our disposal, thus eliminating our having to sleep in the barrack-style dormitories with the rest of the unfortunate immigrants. We had also been accorded the privilege of eating in the public restaurant instead of having our meals at the community table, where fork and knife were chained to the tin plate in front of each person.

On the day of our release, I learned what a condemned person must feel when suddenly granted freedom. That first free breath of air tastes like ambrosia. After that unpleasant experience, nothing seemed more wonderful than Ellsworth Ford's house near the water in Rye, where we found a hearty welcome. Under the giant elms and maples, late summer flowers still bloomed in profusion. Mrs. Ford, whose husband had owned a large hotel on Forty-second Street, was a lady of some literary pretentions and loved to be in the company of writers and poets. Through her we met the poets Witter Bynner and Percy Mac-Kaye. And it was here that MacKaye wrote the following poem about the young guests, refugees from war-torn Europe:

THE CHILD-DANCERS

A bomb has fallen over Notre Dame:
Germans have burned another Belgian town:
Russians quelled in the East: England in qualm:

I closed my eyes, and laid the paper down.

Grey ledge and moor-grass and pale bloom of light
By pale blue seas!
What laughter of a child world-sprite,
Sweet as the horns of lone October bees,
Shrills the faint shore with mellow, old delight?
What elves are these
In smocks gray-blue as sea and ledge,
Dancing upon the silvered edge
Of darkness—each ecstatic one
Making a happy orison,
With shining limbs, to the low sunken sun?—
See: now they cease

Like nesting birds from flight:
Demure and debonair
They troop beside their hostess' chair
To make their bedtime courtesies:
    "*Spokoinoi notchi!—Gute Nacht!*
    Bon soir! Bon soir!—Good night!"
What far-gleaned lives are these
Linked in one holy family of art?—
Dreams: dreams once Christ and Plato dreamed:
How fair their happy shades depart!

Dear God! how simple it all seemed,
Till once again
Before my eyes the red type quivered: *Slain:*
Ten thousand of the enemy.
Then laughter! laughter from the ancient sea
Sang in the gloaming: *Athens! Galilee!*
And elfin voices called from the extinguished light:
    "*Spokoinoi notchi!—Gute Nacht!*
    Bon soir! Bon soir!—Good night!"

Isadora turned up unexpectedly in October. None of us had been sure she would come to America. By that time we were cozily and comfortably settled for the winter in an old brownstone house on Gramercy Park. We lived there under the benign supervision of Margherita and Gus, with a Southern mammy in the basement kitchen to serve up real American cooking. I had a room of my own on the top floor; it looked out on the small square called a park, to which we had a key though we never used it.

The one thing that stands out in my memory is Miss Baker's presenting me with a pink silk nightgown for my birthday. For a strictly brought up European girl, this was a sure sign—like the first kiss on the hand—that I had definitely grown up. I did not wear it for a long time, but kept it wrapped in white tissue paper, naïvely believing this to be the beginning of a hope chest.

Our days, as usual, started with early morning workouts

over on Twenty-third Street and Fourth Avenue, where Isadora had fixed up a studio in an old loft. Mary Fanton Roberts, a very good friend and editor of the art magazine *The Touchstone*, described it:

> A great space, silent and high, separated from the world by curtains of blue; soft lights streaming down rose scarves; back in the shadows low couches in brilliant colors—this is the setting for Isadora Duncan's school in the heart of New York.*

Into this setting one day marched the Mayor of New York, to a meeting arranged by a group of writers including Mabel Dodge, Walter Lippmann, John Collier, and others, who represented the Greenwich Village intelligentsia of that era. For some reason, Isadora was in a bad mood that day and refused to dance. She did, however, have the pupils parade in front of Mayor John Purroy Mitchel in their school uniforms. As an ardent advocate of dress reform, she tried to persuade the Mayor to make our costume official for all the children in New York. He gravely assured her he had no authority to enforce any attire on the populace, healthy or otherwise. Yet what no edict could enforce, the passing of time has successfully accomplished. Mayor Mitchel would be surprised if he lived today to see the many women and children on the sidewalks of his city clad in simple, sleeveless sheaths and with bare feet in sandals!

On a rainy November afternoon at the Metropolitan Opera House, Isadora's European school made its American debut. Since this was her first public dance performance after the death of her children, the program had a religious character. It opened with a requiem march and her première presentation of Schubert's "Ave Maria," the huge audience listening with profound reverence. Her hold on the mind of her spectators had not diminished with the years. Her older pupils did most of the dancing. As Minna Lederman commented later in the *Mail*, June 27, 1918:

* *Art*, p. 28.

I see them now, circling on the immense stage, six girls, the light falling yellow over their young heads and along their arms so gently linked. Something idyllic, something innocent, tender, something indefinably grave was the slow movement of these young people together.

Under Isadora's guidance we made much progress that season. Early in the spring of the following year, she undertook a very ambitious project. A New York financier and art patron, Otto H. Kahn, made it possible for her to use the former Century Theatre on Central Park West as an experimental Greek theatre. "The Greek was essentially a democratic theatre," Isadora once stated in a pamphlet she wrote on the subject.*

She removed the orchestra seats and covered the boxes with long draperies to make the old-fashioned theatre conform more closely to her ideal. Here she presented that spring season several shows composed of "Drama, Music, and Dance."

For me personally, the outstanding event remains my taking part in the speaking chorus of an English version of Euripides' *Iphigenia in Tauris*, written especially by Witter Bynner for Isadora's presentation. It was staged by Augustin Duncan, who persuaded me, much against my will, to take part in the chorus. The stage directions say: "The great bell rings. One by one the Temple Maidens assemble." As the first chorister I had the opening lines, and can still hear myself proclaiming:

> O ye who dwell upon these Clashing Rocks
> That guard the Euxine Sea,
> Keep silence now before Latona's Daughter,
> Artemis, Goddess of the pointed hills!

The whole thing was to be a wonderful surprise for Isadora —so Gus assured me when I voiced my qualms about accepting the speaking part. "I am sure she won't like it," I kept repeating, while he kept insisting, "Nonsense, she will love it; you are very good in the part."

* Cf. *Art*, p. 87.

And so I let myself be persuaded against my better judgment. At the initial rehearsal, the curtain went up on the big stage, where I suddenly stood revealed in solitary splendor high on a scaffolding representing the "Clashing Rocks." I had no sooner finished speaking when Isadora's voice rose in an angry pitch from the front row of the orchestra: "Take her away! Take her away! What is this, Gus? She can't do that; take her away!"

At her unexpectedly vehement outburst, I fled from the stage. Back in my dressing room I had an attack of hysterics. No sooner had I vanished than both Gus and Mr. Bynner rushed backstage. Both tried to console me and assuage my hurt feelings by telling me how effective my recitation had been. Bynner even threatened to withdraw his verse unless Isadora permitted me to act.

"I told you, I told you," I repeated over and over again to Gus, who had brought all this about. He urged me not to give up. He said very earnestly, "Isadora is jealous. She thinks I am trying to make an actress of you." I could not quite believe this. But it must have been true, because a year later, when Attmore Robinson—who owned the Philadelphia Opera House at that time—sponsored my singing lessons with an Italian maestro and offered me operatic parts à la Mary Garden, she reacted in exactly the same way. She accused him of trying to alienate me from her school and make an opera star of me—something I had never considered seriously. As a matter of fact, I gave up my singing studies altogether after that scene with Isadora.

But to return to the Century Theatre: the upshot of it all was that she gave in and I continued to perform the speaking part. As one of the four actresses (the others were Margherita Sargent, Helen Freeman, and Sarah Whitman), I had to have my name printed in the program. So far we all had performed anonymously whenever we danced with Isadora. She herself suggested that I use the name IRMA DUNCAN, and so it has been ever since.

Because we spent all our waking hours in the Century Theatre for rehearsals and matinees and evening performances, Isadora decided to give up the Gramercy House and have us
actually live there. The huge theatre had a complete set of
private rooms, including a library and a kitchen, on the mezzanine floor. A Greek chef was hired and everything seemed very
comfortable and most convenient. But there was one big flaw in
this ideal situation that no one had reckoned with: namely, the
Fire Department. One dark night after the show, when the
lights were doused and all of us were fast asleep, a whole
brigade of firemen forced their way in without warning and
rudely evicted us. The next day (April 24, 1915) the *New York
Tribune* related this story in detail. Here are a few excerpts:

> Twenty sleepy little girls, pupils of Isadora Duncan, the
> dancer, were routed from their beds in the Century Theatre
> last night and were forced to find sleeping quarters elsewhere.
> Art and the Fire Department had clashed.
>
> Shortly before midnight the youngsters were safely quartered
> in the Hotel Empire, Broadway and Sixty-third Street. Miss
> Duncan was at her apartment in the Hotel Majestic, Central
> Park West, ill and suffering from the nervous strain attending
> the ousting of her little dancers from their cots, and vowing she
> would leave New York forever.
>
> Yesterday afternoon, Commissioner Adamson declared that
> the Century Theatre could not be used as a dormitory under the
> law and that the girls quartered there would have to lay their
> curly heads somewhere else than on cots in the theatre building.
>
> The dancer was ill when the edict from Fire Headquarters
> was brought to her by Frederick H. Toye, her manager. She
> promptly gave way to her emotions. She refused to take the order
> to quit the improvised dormitories seriously, however and at eight
> o'clock last night, shortly before the curtain rose on *"Oedipus
> Rex,"* in which she and some of her older girls danced, the little
> ones were tucked into their beds in the pressroom on the prom-
> enade. Three hours later the nurses in charge awakened them
> with orders to dress quickly. Sleepy, and not knowing where they

were going, they were bundled into taxicabs and taken to the Hotel Empire to complete their night's rest.

Miss Duncan was beside herself with indignation. She could not comprehend why she was forced to remove her girls from the Century Theatre building which she said was as safe as any hotel or apartment house in the city, merely because there was a building law that forebade their sleeping there. Furthermore, she said she would terminate her appearance in New York this evening. She declared she was being persecuted by the city officials.

Lieutenant Gallagher of the theatre inspection squad of the Fire Department unearthed the violation of the law. Wednesday afternoon Lieutenant Gallagher took a stroll along the second floor promenade. He pushed open a door and found himself in a room that bore evidences of being a dormitory, although a sign above his head proclaimed it a library. . . . Right before Gallagher's eyes were seven neatly covered beds in an orderly row, with as many dressing-tables littered with the appurtenances of feminine adornment.

On the lower floor he found nineteen cots in the pressroom. The tearoom had been converted into a dining room and the kitchen bore signs of being used not many hours since. The larder and ice-box were well stocked. Wishing to be sure of his grounds before reporting to headquarters, Gallagher bode his time. He waited till after the night performance.

Making his way along the darkened corridor, he approached the room where the seven cots stood in a row. He stepped inside and, hearing soft breathing, switched on the electric light. Seven curly heads lay upon seven white pillows. Seven pairs of sandals stood beside seven little beds, while from the wall hung seven Greek togas. Here and there were seven times seven flimsy articles of attire. When seven pairs of sleepy eyes opened and gazed in astonishment and seven startled "Ah's!" escaped from the awakened dancers, Lieutenant Gallagher blushed and fled in confusion.

When our eight months' sojourn in the United States thus came to a sudden dramatic end, Isadora decided to turn her back on America and as one paper headlined it, "leave New York to

Philistine Darkness!" She made good her threat; we sailed late in May on the *Dante Alighieri* for Naples, Italy, hoping to find a safe haven in one of the neutral countries. As ill luck would have it, immediately after our arrival Italy entered the war. So Isadora had to look elsewhere to shelter her school.

Her next choice was Greece, where her brother Raymond lived close to nature, weaving cloth in the mountains. Wanting no part of that, we put our collective foot down on the proposition. But it took a real mutiny on her pupils' part before she would change her mind.

"Then where would you like to go?" she demanded, displeased with our insubordination, for Isadora always had her own way. "To Switzerland!" was our answer.

For a year and four months, she settled her refugee school in a *pensionnat des jeunes filles*, first in Lausanne, later in Geneva. In the latter establishment, called "Les Hirondelles" (all Swiss *pensionnats* have floral or bird or insect nomenclature), Madame Dourouze, the headmistress, had her hands full. When the monthly check stopped coming in regularly, her sixteen new pensionaires presented a real problem. Wartime communications, difficult at best, failed completely when the checks had to come all the way from South America, where Isadora was on tour. In the end, when her own resources failed to take care of all of us, Madame Dourouze and others suggested we give a benefit performance to make up the debt. I immediately agreed to that plan enthusiastically. But some of the other girls had grave doubts whether we could engage in a performance of that sort without authorization. Anna especially had misgivings and would not consent to the plan without consulting our friends, among them the composer Ernest Bloch and his wife, who then lived in Geneva.

But each and every one urged us to do it. In this way we pupils of the Isadora Duncan School undertook our first independent venture.

The successful outcome encouraged us to organize a tour

through Switzerland, which we did under the management of Augustin Duncan, who had meanwhile been dispatched by Isadora from Buenos Aires to rescue her school. She had given him strict instructions to discourage us from returning to America, as we all fervently desired to do. The ten younger pupils, when funds ran low, were forced to go back home to their respective parents. Thus only we six original Grunewald pupils (myself, Anna, Erica, Lisa, Margot, and Theresa) remained. And nothing, no edict from Isadora or anyone else, could turn us from our firm determination to return to New York.

We arrived at that crucial moment in world history when America was about to enter the war. New complications now arose because of our German nationality. Isadora, who was really delighted to see us again, said, "I have decided to adopt you girls legally as my daughters." And she added, "I should have done this long ago."

However, because of the war, the necessary papers from abroad could not be obtained. And so we only changed our names to Duncan * as she suggested, legalizing this act in the New York court. We also applied for American citizenship.

From this period dates the more intimate association I had with the woman who was now my foster mother. A growing, affectionate friendship would forge the already existing bond between us into an even closer one. This opportunity to get to know each other better arose after her break with Singer. His financial assistance had ceased abruptly, leaving her short of funds. Suddenly she found herself unable to keep up the style she was accustomed to. Nor could she maintain a school for grown-up girls. She gave up her elegant suite at the Ritz and reluctantly moved to a cheaper hotel. The six of us found temporary homes with relatives and friends.

"Irma, you come and live with me," she said. "We'll make out somehow."

So I roomed with her at the Woolcott on the west side of

* My original name was Irma Dorette Henriette Erich-Grimme.

town. We managed to share the same room for a while until things became too cramped and, flinging economy to the winds, she engaged a three-room suite. We now each enjoyed a room and bath with a nice sitting room between. She had a knack for transforming a banal hotel room with a few deft touches here and there, using a Spanish shawl or an embroidered cloth to hide some ugly piece of furniture; creating an attractive, personal atmosphere.

She always carried certain personal belongings with her on her travels. There was, for instance, the handsome Tiffany vanity set of vermeil silver and the tall flaçon of "Ambre Antique" by Coty—her favorite perfume. On the bedside table was a photograph of Paris Singer and their little boy Patrick in a red leather frame, beside a small cluster of books, her constant traveling companions—*The Bacchae*, *Electra*, *The Trojan Women*, and other plays by Euripides. Also there was a slim volume of Sappho's poems in a French translation and Gabriele D'Annunzio's *Contemplatione della Morte* with the inscription, "To the divine Isadora Duncan who dances along the lines of immortality." On the writing desk was her red leather case containing her personal note paper, a small bottle of black India ink, and an ivory pen with a very broad nib. And, of course, always the photograph albums of herself and her children, bound in striped leather.

Living and sharing things together, as any mother and young daughter would, I got to know her well. For the first time I got acquainted with the human side of the great artist who had always—from the beginning when I met her in that other hotel room in far-away Hamburg—been my sole inspiration.

Being temporarily deprived of the services of a personal maid, she was sitting on the bed sewing on a button when I happened to come in one day. Seeing her occupied with such a domestic chore gave me quite a start. It struck me for some reason as being very funny, and I started to laugh. "Why do you laugh?" she asked. "Do you think I am incapable of doing this sort of thing? I want you to know that I can also bake a very good peach pie. I bet that is more than you can do!"

She was right. We had been taught housekeeping at school, but not cooking. Our hands had to be beautiful for dancing. Since then, however, I have made up for that deficiency.

We also discovered we had much in common. "Have you noticed that we both react to things in the same way?" she would ask.

"I have noticed that we laugh at the same things, if this is what you mean."

"Yes, but there is more to it than that. It is curious how one often finds a closer relationship with people to whom one is not related by flesh and blood."

"I once read a book by Goethe," I said, remembering my literary class at Madame Dourouze's *pensionnat*, "in which he expounds the same idea. It is called 'elective affinities.' "

She did not generally take life too seriously—only her art. She had a nice sense of humor and liked to tell amusing anecdotes that had happened to her. My own sense of humor is fairly acute and I could not live for long with anybody who totally lacked it. As for that anecdote which connects her name with George Bernard Shaw, he himself admitted that the "dancer" in question was not Isadora. The latter had no occasion to meet G. B. S. nor did she correspond with him. Her letters and writings give ample proof of her own native intelligence and wit.

That summer Isadora rented a small beach cottage on Long Island. We girls, reunited once more, had an apartment next door. I remember coaxing her into a movie house one evening when I discovered she had never seen a moving picture. "What, me! Set foot in there?" she exclaimed, horrified, but went in anyway. "How did you enjoy it?" I asked when it was over. She laughed and said, "It was more fun than I imagined—but what an awful picture!"

Soon thereafter a movie company offered her a contract for a dance film. They were willing to pay a high price for it, and though she needed the money badly she adamantly refused. No one could persuade her to sell her art to the "flickers." In those jumpy pictures she was afraid her art would appear like a St. Vitus' dance. "I would rather not be remembered by posterity like that," she said.

She had a great craving for speed and for being constantly on the go. She liked to ride in her open touring car, a Packard with chauffeur, *en grande vitesse* (in those days, forty-five miles an hour was fast), over the narrow, dusty road all the way out to Montauk Point and back. The fresh air soon aroused her healthy appetite and she would say, "Let's stop at the Inn and get a nice rare steak and a bottle of red wine—unless you would rather have some steamed clams and Guinness stout."

Her enormous vitality and energetic stamina often left me completely worn out. I weighed only a hundred pounds then and did not feel very strong.

A continuous flow of visitors came to her beach cottage that summer of 1917. There we met such avant-garde artists as Marcel Duchamp, Francis Picabia, Edgard Varèse, and the Russian diplomats Count Florinsky and Baron Ungern-Sternberg. A frequent visitor was Elsa Maxwell, who played tangos for us that she had composed herself. The famous Belgian violinist Eugène Ysaye came, and Andrés de Segurola of the Metropolitan Opera, and of course always our old friend Arnold Genthe with Stephan Bourgeois, in whose Fifth Avenue Gallery I saw the first abstract sculpture. At about the same time we made friends with Wienold Reiss, the painter of Blackfoot Indians, in whose Greenwich Village studio we met such artists as Fritz Kreisler. And then of course Olga and Hans von Kaltenborn when the latter was still with the Brooklyn *Eagle*. Then there were Stuart Benson, editor of *Collier's*, and his friend Bill Hamilton. Later also our acquaintances included Max Eastman and Eugen Boissevain, who eventually married Edna St. Vincent Millay. It was a cross-section of the "people about town" during the war years. Most of them were more or less contemporaries of our foster mother. The marriageable men of our age—alas—were all in uniform "over there," fighting in the muddy trenches of the Argonne.

I suppose the most important factor in the process of growing up is the age-old story of falling in love. The sheltered life we girls had led so far, despite our many public appearances (and this was during the innocent years when the word "sex" could never be mentioned openly), prevented us from coming in contact with young men of our own age. We did not attend social affairs or organized dances as young people do nowadays. I imagine our professional existence acted as a hindrance. Everywhere advertised as a highbrow concert attraction, we had little opportunity to run into even that common garden variety called a stage-door Johnny.

But never underestimate the power of love. Love always finds a way. In my case, stringent wartime circumstances unfortunately imposed a long separation. In the end, it turned out to have been an ill-starred romance, which caused me a great deal of unhappiness.

In order to find a few moments of forgetfulness and distraction at that time, I used to frequent a small nickelodeon at the intersection of Broadway and Columbus Avenue on the west side, where I spent hours almost daily watching Lillian Gish, Norma Talmadge, Theda Bara or Pauline Frederick emote. And my favorite, the one I considered the most beautiful of all (though not the moving picture) Priscilla Dean in *The Darling of Paris*. Watching these stars of the silent pictures, I became quite screen-struck and harbored a secret ambition to become a moving picture actress. However, that youthful ambition is buried with the past together with the heartbreak of my young and romantic days. That nickelodeon is no more. In its stead, like Phoenix rising from the ashes, on that same spot there now stands the magnificent monument dedicated to the performing arts—Lincoln Center.

Despite our close relationship Isadora knew nothing about

this unhappy state of affairs that put a blight on my youth. Though she and I talked freely on many subjects, I did not care to discuss so private a matter concerning one's heart emotions with anyone. I put on a brave front. Outwardly I maintained a cheerful attitude in the company of others and so successfully learned to hide my tears.

This, I also learned, was one of the sad penalties for having at last grown up.

❦ 11 ❧

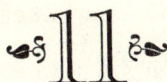

Isadora Duncan Dancers

By the above title the Isadora sextette eventually emerged as
an independent group. Because of Isadora's constant opposition
to our ambitious aims, it proved not at all an easy matter to
accomplish. Our successful Swiss tour, where we appeared on
our own and gave ample proof of being able to support ourselves, had encouraged us to continue in that path and had also
bolstered our youthful self-esteem. We had reached a point of
no return.

Much as we loved Isadora and venerated her as an artist
and teacher, knowing she would spare nothing to keep us well
and happy, we nevertheless ardently wished to be independent.
Not merely financially but also artistically independent. With
growing maturity, we came to realize that our franchise constituted a vital development in our character as creative artists
and self-respecting human beings. A God-given right, so to
speak. This overwhelming motivating force in our new relationship with Isadora, unfortunately, placed us in opposition to our
mentor. It unavoidably became a constant cause of friction and
contention between us which, with the passing of time, threatened to come inevitably to a head-on collision of wills. For she
continued to treat us like children, subject to her every whim. I
found it irritating that she persisted in looking upon her grown-
up group of young girls as her "little pupils" from the Grunewald School, and not as individual artists developing to whatever degree each one could hope to reach. Whenever we aired
our opinions on this subject of greater freedom and independence, she invariably voiced her objection. She insisted we stay

away from the city and urged us to continue our studies. "New York is no place for young girls," she said.

The same old story of children rebelling against parental authority repeated itself; the big city exerted a powerful fascination and drew us like a magnet. In the fall, while Isadora toured the West Coast, our wish was granted. Before leaving, she rented a large studio on the top floor of the newly constructed Hotel des Artistes on the upper west side, just off Central Park. Artists such as Alla Nazimova, James Montgomery Flagg, and the eccentric Russian timpano player Sasha Votichenko, also had studio apartments there. We got to know them well.

Here I resumed teaching children's classes, with little Marta Rousseau as my first American pupil. The idea of devoting my entire time to teaching had no particular appeal to me then. Most of the other girls were in complete accord. We confided our discontent to dear old Uncle Gus, who as ever had our best interest at heart. He warmly sympathized with our longing for greater freedom of expression in the art for which we had been trained since childhood. Our education as "dancers of the future" needed to find fulfillment, even as Isadora promised years ago. Now the time had come.

Without special authorization by his sister, Gus organized some performances for us at the Booth Theatre, in the heart of New York's theatrical district, under Charles Coburn's management. When the news reached Isadora in California, she instantly voiced her severe disapproval of Gus's action. This caused a serious disagreement between them for a while. I believe it left a wound that never quite healed on the part of Augustin Duncan. She sent a terse wire saying: "I forbid it. The girls are not yet ready for performances of their own in New York."

She chose to ignore completely the inescapable fact that her pupils, ever since the early Grunewald days, were used to giving public performances on their own. Had she forgotten the special matinees at the Duke of York's Theatre in London in 1908?

And, much more recently, the memorial performance she herself organized at the Trocadéro in Paris before the outbreak of the war, when she occupied the stage box and proudly watched her pupils dance? Or the performances she permitted us to give in Russia in the spring of that same year? Hardly possible. Whatever her motives, the Booth Theatre engagement came to an abrupt end, placing Gus in an awkward position for having negotiated the whole thing with Coburn. And there was our displeasure. If she did not consider us ready now at the age of twenty, she probably never would, we told ourselves. Her explanation always remained the same. She had "not trained her pupils for the stage."

Fate often has a way of accomplishing what cannot otherwise be changed. One need only cultivate enough patience. Disillusioned with life in her native land, ever homesick for France—though the war still raged there—Isadora decided at the end of her California tour to return to Paris.

"I am going back to France, because I find conditions here more than I can bear," she announced one day in February of 1918. "My struggles to establish a permanent school here have been to no avail. I feel utterly disheartened and much too discouraged to continue. Perhaps in France, where I have certain properties left, I may be able to raise some money and return in the fall."

Here it was again—that eternal question of finding the money to finance the school. Why would she not let us support ourselves? I began actually to resent my utter dependence on her for sustenance and support. Her objection to our making our own way and contributing to the school, rather than being a burden, was incomprehensible to me. Feeling just as discouraged on our own part, we queried, "What shall we do while you are abroad?"

Her answer really floored us and left me dumbfounded. She gave us a searching look and said nothing for a minute or two. Then came the bombshell, as far as we girls were con-

cerned. She announced in a serious tone, "I want you all to return to Elizabeth's school here in Tarrytown."

We were up in arms at once at the very thought of having
to come under Elizabeth's thumb again. We all refused, point
blank. "Oh, no! Isadora, not that!" we shouted angrily. "That
is impossible!"

"I for one won't do it!" I pronounced flatly, stamping my
foot. "You can bet on that!"

"Don't be impertinent!" she flashed back. "This is my
earnest wish, because I know you will be safe there until I
return."

We angrily argued back and forth, really frightened at the
thought of having to submit once more to the unreasonable discipline of Tante Miss, especially now when most of us had
come of age. The proposition seemed utterly preposterous. Re-
senting our foster mother's treachery—as we called it—we furiously stomped out of her room. Our adamant refusal to obey
aroused her anger too, for her word had hitherto been law.
Our insubordination made her so furious that she left a few
weeks later for France without seeing us or saying goodbye. It
was most unusual for her generous, kindhearted nature.

Gus once again stepped into the breach. Finding ourselves
suddenly completely penniless and on our own, we listened
to his sage advice when he suggested that we find shelter at
Elizabeth's school for the present, just long enough for him
to get us another engagement.

"I know how you girls feel about Elizabeth. I have spoken
to her and she is quite agreeable to the idea that you merely
board with her as paying guests, not pupils."

That clinched the deal, and we moved to Tarrytown without further protest. Hearing of our move, Isadora wrote to her
sister:

Dearest Elizabeth:

The first letter I received from any of you was April 20th—
so you see I was more than two months without news. If the

girls had only told me the last evening that they would go to Tarrytown we could have enjoyed four weeks of pleasant work. But human beings, contrary and cussed—and such a pity. It would have been such a comfort to know.

Our citizenship papers had not yet become final and, theoretically at least, we could still be considered "enemy aliens." Very conscious of this twilight-zone status as far as patriotic sentiments were concerned, with the red-lettered headlines screeching hatred for the enemy every day while General Foch and his valiant army made a desperate stand on the Marne, our utter surprise can be imagined at the news Gus brought to us.

"Guess where I have booked you," he asked with a twinkle in his eye. "On a tour through the soldiers' camps!" And he added, "With the full approval of the War Department Commission on Training Camp Activities, of course."

In this way we were happy to be able to contribute our mite to a patriotic cause and to do what we could through our art to make the American doughboy happy. Camp Dix, Camp Upton, and all the other camps had their first cultural entertainment. I am afraid not many soldiers had a hankering for this spiritual sort of uplift; for the halls were nearly always half-empty. But we girls, on our way to becoming full-fledged citizens, got a great kick out of it and a wonderful sense of belonging.

We had engaged the well-known pianist George Copeland to accompany us. Isadora Duncan was not at all aquainted with George Copeland, nor had she ever heard him play. The only thing she had heard about him was his reputation as the foremost interpeter of modern music, especially Debussy, in this country. Under the erroneous impression that we too interpreted Dubussy's music and being ever so watchful of our artistic presentation of her dance, she wrote to her pupils the following epistle:

Please don't let anyone persuade you to try to dance to Debussy. It is only the music of the *Senses* and has no message to the

Spirit. And then the gesture of Debussy is all *inward*— and has no outward or upward. I want you to dance only that music which goes from the soul in mounting circles. Why not study the Suite in D of Bach? Do you remember my dancing it? Please also continue always your studies of the Beethoven Seventh and the Schubert Seventh; and why not dance with Copeland the seven minuets of Beethoven that we studied in Fourth Avenue? And the Symphony in G of Mozart. There is a whole world of Mozart that you might study.

Plunge your soul in divine unconscious *Giving* deep within it, until it gives to your soul its *Secret*. That is how I have always tried to express music. My soul should become one with it, and the dance born from that embrace. Music has been in all my life the great Inspiration and will be perhaps someday the Consolation, for I have gone through such terrible years. No one has understood since I lost Deirdre and Patrick how pain has caused me at times to live in almost a delirium. In fact my poor brain has more often been crazed than anyone can know. Sometimes quite recently I feel as if I were awakening from a long fever. When you think of these years, think of the Funeral March of Schubert, the *Ave Maria*, the *Redemption*, and forget the times when my poor distracted soul trying to escape from suffering may well have given you all the appearance of madness.

I have reached such high peaks flooded with light, but my soul has no strength to live there—and no one has realized the horrible torture from which I have tried to escape. Some day if you understand sorrow you will understand too all I have lived through, and then you will only think of the light towards which I have pointed and you will know the *real* Isadora is there. In the meantime work and create Beauty and Harmony. The poor world has need of it, and with your six spirits going with one will, you can create a Beauty and Inspiration for a new Life.

I am so happy that you are working and that you love it. Nourish your spirit from Plato and Dante, from Goethe and Schiller, Shakespeare and Nietzsche (don't forget that the *Birth of Tragedy* and the *Spirit of Music* are my Bible). With these to guide you, and the greatest music, you may go far.

Dear children, I take you in my arms. And here is a kiss for Anna, and here one for Therese, and one for Irma, and here is a kiss for Gretel (Margot) and one for little Erika—and a kiss for you, dearest Lisel. Let us pray that this separation will only bring us nearer and closer in a higher communion—and soon we will all dance together *Reigen*.

All my love,
Isadora*

Duncan Dancers on Their Own at Last read the headline of an article written by the distinguished music critic Pitts Sanborn of the *Globe*. He went on to say:

> It might seem incredible that one of the rarest and most enchanting events of all the musical year should be reserved for the twenty-seventh day of June, but in time of war, at any rate, the Isadora Duncan Dancers gave last evening an entertainment truly exquisite in its charm and artistic quality. For the nonce let comment stop with the general impression of a ravishing performance—altogether a memorable evening.

And Sigmund Spaeth wrote for the *Mail*:

> It may truthfully be claimed that no dancing in the world today has more of truth and sincerity in its appeal than has the dancing of these six adopted daughters of Isadora Duncan. When people thronged about the stage of Carnegie Hall waving hats and handkerchiefs with loud shouts from the gallery and no inclination or any desire to go home, it was a spontaneous demonstration of approval. There can be no doubt of the fitness of the Duncan Dancers to carry on the unique art created by Isadora Duncan. It makes little difference whether they appear singly or in groups, always they impart the same involuntary thrill that comes only when art is based on something very real.
>
> Whether it is Anna's interpretive art, or the rhythmic certainty of Theresa, or Lisa's airy leaps, or the dramatic eloquence of Irma . . . there is always the effect of a youthful spontaneity,

* *Isadora*, by Allan Ross Macdougall, pp. 173–174.

a direct challenge to everything that is artificial and insincere. There are no cut and dried methods in this art and there is little evidence of the stupendous technique that underlies it. A technique of which one becomes aware only in seeing the clumsy efforts of untrained and uninitiated imitators. This individualizing of the dancers is making them for the first time in their careers, distinct artistic personalities.

I would like to stress here that his last remark proves what Isadora years ago predicted and hoped would come to pass. Observing her apprentice pupils in Grunewald developing her new idea of the dance, she said, "While forming part of a whole, they will preserve a creative individuality."

We lived at the time in a large studio on the top floor of the Carnegie Hall annex which we sublet from Alys Bently. To have emerged finally from our chrysalis (from "a moving row of shadow shapes in imitation of Isadora," as one severe critic remarked of our previous joint appearances with her), and to have, at long last, gained individual recognition, was a great source of satisfaction to each one of us. Now that we were free to dance to the music of our own choice (apart from the modern composers), the music of Chopin especially afforded us a wider scope for individual interpretations, some of them based on our teacher's choreography, some on our own. For she had previously—on the advice of Hener Skene—encouraged her pupils to compose their own dances.

I still recall the initial lesson in dance composition she gave me privately and how miserably I erred in interpreting the Brahms song she had chosen. It began "If I were a bird," so I flew about the room as if I were a bird. When I stopped, I saw "that look" on Isadora's face. I was terrified. No, she explained, the song did not say "I am a bird," it said "If I *were* a bird." It meant, "I wish I could fly to you, but I am earthbound." From her couch, she demonstrated with beautiful gestures how the dance should have been done. She had really thought out the language of movement. There and then she taught me a valuable lesson, which I subsequently used as an example whenever I tried my hand at choreography.

We six Duncan girls knew we had definitely "arrived" as a distinct artistic ensemble when—the day after our successful New York debut—a lady reporter asked for an interview. As an outsider's point of view, it may be of some interest here to show how each girl impressed her:

Modest and charming are these young women, ranging in age from a little under to a little over twenty, with a pleasant affection for one another and single in their ambition to dance anywhere, everywhere, so long as they can appear uncompromisingly as interpreters of music. . . .

They speak many languages. . . . Anna, the black-eyed, the black-haired, is the leader in their lives as in their dancing. She is practical, she always plans. She has a way of saying "We children," and her voice carries great authority. And she is very beautiful, beautifully made, with a most exquisite modeling of chin and neck and shoulders. Though she is not tall there is something heroic in her structure.

All of them are rather small, surprisingly fragile to see after their dancing, which leaves the impression of long bodies. Lisa of the famous leapings, and Margot, both unusually slender, are still more delicate in repose than in motion. . . . Erica is the youngest, a quiet dark-eyed child, who looks upon the world with great solemnity and on rare occasion smiles.

Theresa is to my mind the loveliest of all—a simple maiden with long, blond braids wound round her head. She is complete in her response to music, and when she dances, her face, alight with joy, gives me great pleasure. Waltzing, she is more than anyone like Isadora, lost ecstatic, whirling through an immense quiet. . . .

Irma is another very slight girl, perhaps the most distinctive member of the group, in whose mocking grey-eyed face there is mingled wisdom with a mischievous gaiety. She has an amusing wit. She is gifted; the others speak of a singing voice which she, however, has neglected. To see her dance is to have a feeling that some day she may make of herself an actress. . . .

When Isadora passes, nothing of her will remain but these young girls. After her own dancing they are her greatest contribution to art. They are the mould into which she has struggled to pour her genius. . . . Through their magnificent bodies, Isadora has projected a new ideal of woman's beauty. . . .

Today, Isadora, who assembled and brought them here, is far from them. . . . And today they are making their first large venture unguided by her. From under the protecting wing of genius they emerge to test themselves, to feel their own weight and the space about them.

Though they are the offerings of Isadora's spirit, each one begins now to measure her lot and her fame alone.

One engagement led to another and eventually to a transcontinental tour. We also did our bit for various war charities. The major event of this kind was an open-air recital with the Barrère Orchestra for Italian war relief that was staged at Kenilworth, the George Pratt estate in Glen Cove on Long Island Sound. Mr. Pratt, an amateur color photographer, took many pictures of us the week end we stayed with him and his wife. He posed us in graceful attitudes holding aloft garlands of roses or standing among the tall Madonna lilies and among the blue iris reflected in the limpid pool of the sunken garden where we danced.

Even while dancing for Allied war relief, I could never quite forget the "other side." In my mind's eye I saw mother living in Germany, now an enemy country and my homeland no more. With a heavy heart, I wondered what her fate might be, for I had not heard from her since America entered the fray. I worried a great deal over her. And then one glorious morning I awoke to the ringing of bells and blowing of whistles. The shrieks of sirens brought me rushing to the window. There, in the street, was the strangest sight. Grown-up people holding hands like children and dancing for joy down the avenue! Then I knew. The war was over, the armistice had been signed. Overcome with long-pent-up emotion and utter relief that the horrible, bloody nightmare was terminated, I sank down on my bed and cried, thanking God for PEACE. That same day, the eleventh of November, I wrote two letters; one to my German mother, the other to my dear foster mother. Weeks later I received answers from both. Mother had survived the holocaust but was very ill. I sent her money and food packages, doing what I could from that distance to help. Isadora wrote from the Riviera Palace Hotel in Nice:

Dearest Irma,

If you knew how happy it makes me to receive letters from you, you would all write oftener. Now you must admit I am a good prophet—since the beginning I predicted the Republic of Germany. What good news! And think how wonderful, for you all can now hope to dance the Marche Lorraine at Munich!

I started bravely to make a tour of the French provinces but after three evenings was stopped by the Grippe closing all the theatres so have come back to Nice where, as usual, am living on Hopes.

I think now, if you wish it, I can arrange for you all to join me very soon. Passports etc., will be simplified.

I have given up writing to Elizabeth and Augustin as they never answered even *once*—it is true many letters are lost. Tell me your plans, how far is your tour booked and what prospects, and send me your programmes. Everything you are doing interests me. I have the promise of a beautiful large hall to work in here. Perhaps you would all like to come in the spring? But tell me frankly your ideas and wishes.

It is a beautiful morning the sun is sparkling on the sea and *warm*. I take long walks by the sea and my heart goes over to you. Do write me news of all our friends. . . .

If you were here we would study the 9th Symphony [of Beethoven] to celebrate the Peace. Here is a kiss of Peace and Hope for each of you.

With all my love—
Isadora

Our reunion had to be postponed for more than a year. We girls had contracts for a second tour. During the season of 1919–1920 our tour brought us all the way across the country to California, Isadora's birthplace. She had been born in San Francisco, and that lovely city exerted a special appeal for her pupils. We tried to dance our very best at our first matinee at the Columbia Theatre to make her fellow Californians proud of us. We must have succeeded, for Redfern Mason of the *San Francisco Examiner* wrote:

> One goes to see these six girls in a mood that has a note of reverence in it. During the trials of the war they have not yielded to the voice of those who would commercialize their art. They have closed their ears to the gilded seduction of vaudeville. Their ideal has remained inviolate and uncheapened. . . .
>
> Gluck, Chopin and Schubert; that is the lyre of three chords from which they drew their inspiration. . . . The Chopin group brought out the personality of each individual dancer. Anna danced a mazurka and a valse. Irma gave us the "Minute Valse." In another life I think she danced at the Feast of Reason during the French Revolution. She has the tenseness and clean-cut emotional suggestiveness of Yvette Guilbert.
>
> Lisa of the golden locks is kin to Undine of romantic legend. In the Schubert dances we saw the other girls. Nothing is more beautiful than are those Schubert waltzes with their old-time memories and their sentiment of "Heimweh." The girls put their hearts into the dancing and the house simmered with contentment.
>
> In the audience was Mrs. Duncan, the mother and first teacher of Isadora, happy to see her daughter's art pulsating and young in another generation. It is wonderful to have revitalized an art and that is what Isadora and her disciples have done. . . . Today the Isadora Duncan girls dance in Oakland, next Sunday they will again be seen at the Columbia. Not to see them is a misfortune; carelessly to miss them would be a crime.

We had not seen Isadora's mother since we were children in Grunewald. She used to sit on the garden steps in the pale northern sun and tell us about her home—California; of the abundance of flowers and fruit growing there, and the glorious hot sun shining every day, and of her longing to go back. "Some day you will go there and love it too," she said. Her prediction had now come true. She seemed happy to see us. A very ancient lady then, she nevertheless accepted with pleasure when we invited her and her Norwegian companion (who in the old Grunewald days had been our governess for a while) to spend the two weeks of Christmas with us at the St. Francis Hotel.

We received a hearty welcome everywhere in the larger towns of California. The only prudish place was Santa Barbara, where the mayor refused us permission to dance with bare legs. When I think of the bikini suits currently *en vogue* there, I feel quite proud of having been a martyr for the adoption of a more enlightened attitude by the present generation. Not only that, but considering that we encountered nowhere a real dance audience such as exists nowadays, we Duncan girls can be proud also of having contributed our share toward bringing about a greater appreciation of that art in this country.

I am not able to recall the many details of our grand tour through the States. I kept a little diary at the time, and a few pages from it may give a better idea of what was involved in such one-night stands as it mostly turned out to be. Our return trip started with the end of the holiday season.

Saturday, Jan. 3, 1920.
Goodbye California! We are taking 6 o'clock train to Colorado Springs.

Tuesday, Jan. 6.
Arrived 1:30 Colorado Springs. Antlers Hotel. A health resort kind of a place. Surprise! Wienold Reiss showed up, he is on his way to paint Blackfoot Indians in Montana. In the evening saw a vaudeville show at the Burns Theatre.

Wednesday, Jan. 7.
A nice day. Took a motor drive out to the Garden of the Gods, huge, red water-washed rocks in various shapes of corrosion. 8:30

performance at the Burns Theatre. A very small but select audience.

Thursday, Jan. 8.
A magnificent day, snow on the mountains and sunshine. Took a train to Denver and arrived at 5 o'clock. Brown Palace Hotel. A horrible place. 8:30 performance at the Auditorium with an enormous stage and a correspondingly large audience. Had supper afterwards at the hotel with Judge Lindsey and his wife.

The Judge, of course, was Ben B. Lindsey of the Juvenile Court, whose ideas about "companionate marriage" caused something of a national sensation when he published them in book form several years later. Our Denver performance seemed to impress him, as it did at least some others of the audience. But we were working against a real handicap. The *Denver Times* reported the circumstances the next day:

> Those who did not attend the performance of the Isadora Duncan dancers and George Copeland, pianist, last night at the Auditorium missed a rare combination of the terpsichorean art with that of the musician and deprived themselves of a share in one of the most restful, refreshing evenings that has been offered Denver concertgoers this season. The Lions Club of Denver sponsored the event. . . .
>
> The huge stage was so effectively draped and curtained that it gave the impression of unlimited space, and the slender figures stole from its recesses like nymphs slipping thru wondrous woods.
>
> So carefully are the dances and the music blended that the portrayal of emotion is absolute and distinctive. One of the most effective was the "March Funebre," by Chopin, in which five of the graceful figures draped in purple robes glide forth in slow, steady rhythm truly typifying a funeral cortege, while one of the figures in a filmy shroud portrays the dead for whom they mourn and the resurrection. . . .
>
> Unfortunately the Auditorium grew so cold during the performance that it was impossible to sit thru the entire program with any degree of comfort and many left before the end for that reason. One shivered in sympathy for the bare-footed dancers in their filmy attire.

Friday, Jan. 9.
Judge Lindsey invited us to visit his court this morning. Only Theresa, Margot, and I went. He is presiding over the "Stokes Case." Mrs. Stokes is suing for the custody of her children and she will get custody too if Judge Lindsey wins out. After lunch listened to more Juvenile cases of boys and girls in trouble with the law. Very, very interesting. It gives one a different slant on life. Had dinner with the Judge and his lovely wife.

Saturday, Jan. 10.
The Lindseys invited us to see Trixie Friganza in "Oh Mama!" We met her backstage. She is amusing off as on stage.

Sunday, Jan. 11.
The Judge and his wife called on us this morning and drove us up through the mountains covered with snow for a wonderful view down on Denver. We all lunched together at our hotel. Leaving at 8 o'clock for Kansas City.

Tuesday, Jan. 13.
Kansas City is a big, sooty town. Had a 3 o'clock matinee at the Schubert Theatre. A lovely audience, very appreciative but we had to rush our performance on account of the Sothern-Marlowe show that followed immediately.

Wednesday, Jan. 14.
In St. Joseph. All hotels overcrowded because of convention. Had to stop at a second rate Station Hotel. 8:30 performance on a rotten stage. No more St. Joe for me! Tomorrow we dance in Topeka.

Friday, Jan. 16.
Arrived late in Newton and on account of a train wreck had to motor over to Hutchinson. 8:30 performance at Convention Hall with a fine, big stage but a very noisy audience. Dogs barking, children screaming, first George made a speech asking them to be quiet and then Anna did the same.

Saturday, Jan. 17.
Leaving for Wichita on the Interurban. Catastrophe! Found there was a strike on and our stagehands are not allowed to work. The Theatre manager himself and several other gentle-

men volunteered to help set the stage (lay the carpet, hang the curtains, set the lights, move the piano) and work during the performance at Forum Hall. For some reason the lights worked only on one side the other pitch darkness but we didn't care the audience was large and most enthusiastic.

Sunday, Jan. 18.
We spent all day in a day coach on the Santa Fe which is invariably late and uncomfortable. Arrived after midnight in Oklahoma City. Hotels had no vacancies—drat those conventions—and so we were forced to spend the night in what looked suspiciously like a disreputable house, dirty as Hell.

Monday, Jan. 19.
A perfectly glorious day, warm and sunny spring-like weather. We decided to enjoy it and rented an open car for an hour's drive to get some fresh air in our lungs after those long train rides and soak up the sunshine. Evening performance at Overhulser (what a name!) Opera House and leaving immediately afterwards for Tulsa, another big "oil town."

One had to be very young and healthy for that kind of a life. The dancing was always a pleasure but oh, those train rides! And the incessant packing and unpacking, since we had no maid and had to do everything ourselves. We always envied George Copeland, whose traveling companion acted as his valet. He went through none of the frenzy of having to change costumes while performing. He always appeared cool and collected. His favorite pastime during the interminable train rides consisted in a game of cards; he was also a collector of fine antique jewelry. In the end, he came out far ahead of us girls financially. We had to pay not only our own traveling expenses but his and those of a stage crew of three men. We carted our own décor with us everywhere.

From Tulsa we proceeded to St. Louis, and from there to Ohio, via Hamilton, making large jumps through the Middle West. When we arrived in Detroit on January 27, we discovered to our great annoyance that we had a whole long week to wait

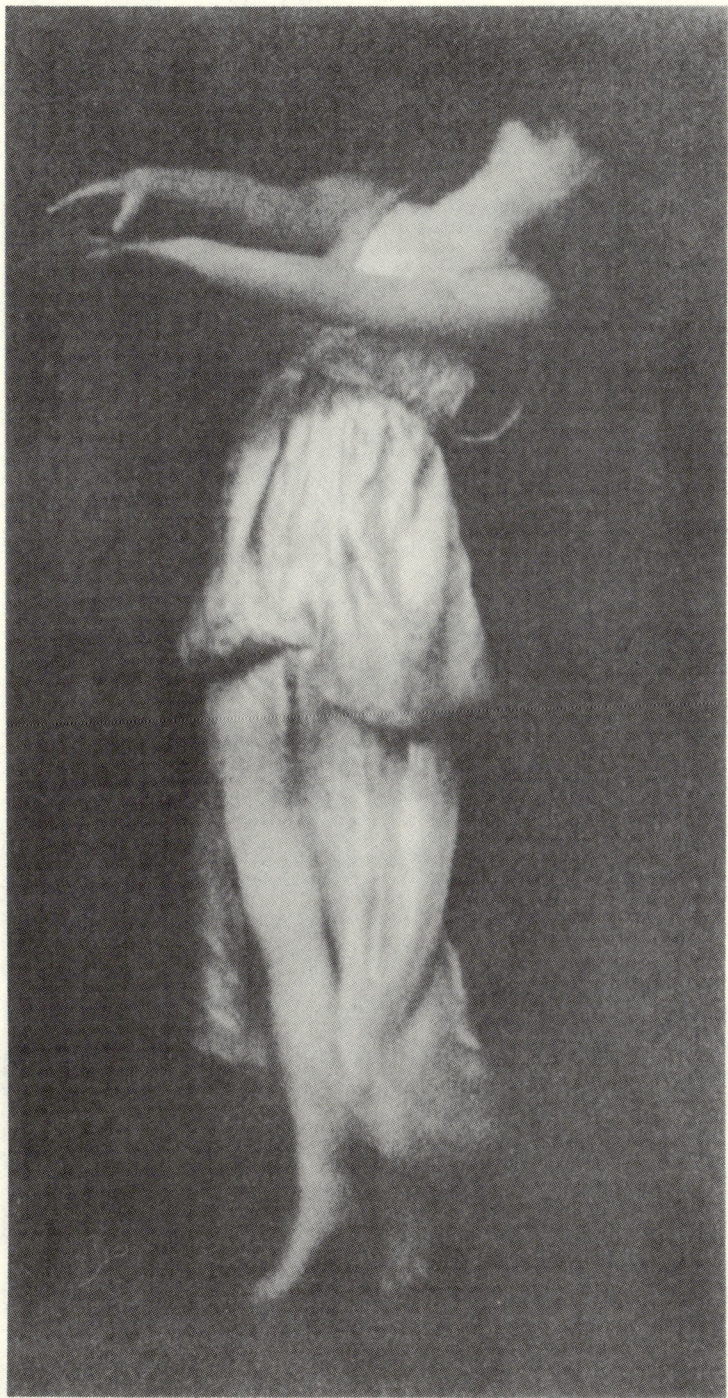

Irma Duncan: dance photo by Arnold Genthe, 1917.

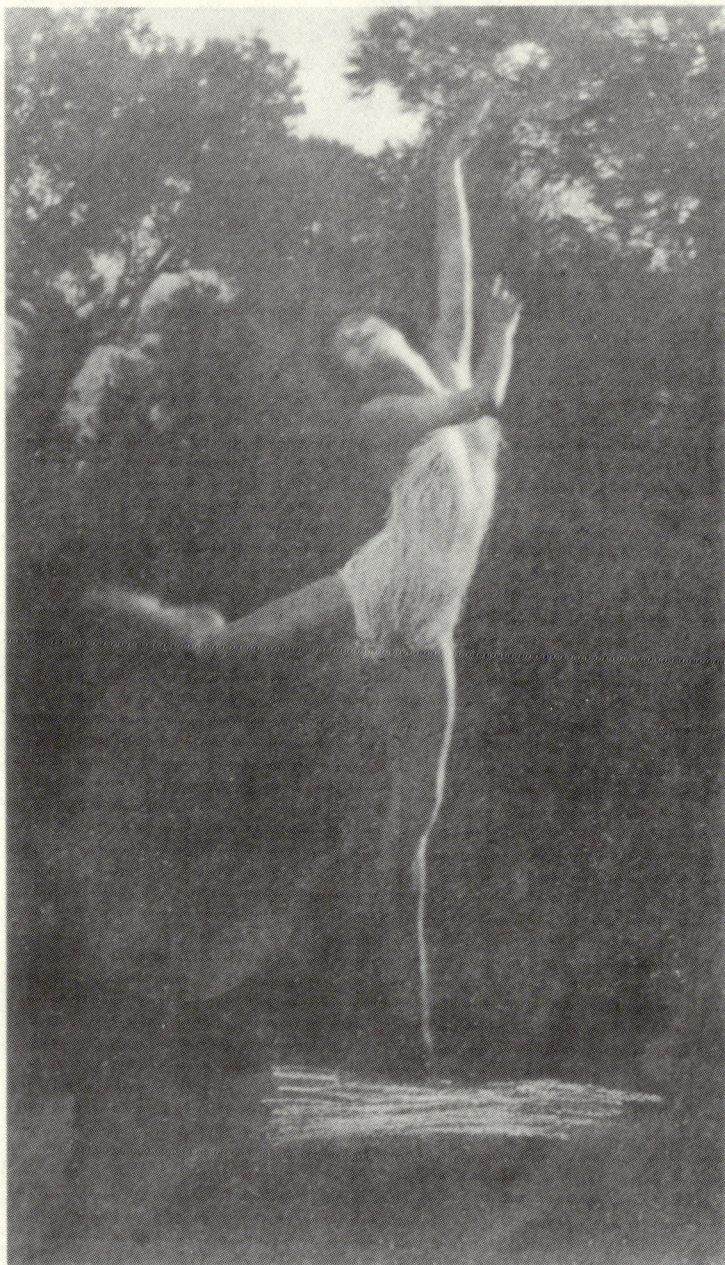

Irma Duncan dancing outdoors, Greece, 1920.

before our performance there. A full week's delay meant more expense, and it also increased our impatience to return home as soon as possible.

Wienold Reiss had been commissioned by Otto Baumgarten, the owner of the new Crillon Restaurant on East Fifty-third Street in New York, to paint our individual portraits. On his way north, he told us that they had been installed in the blue and gray "Duncan Room" at the fashionable restaurant. We were dying to see this, for fame seemed to have caught up with us.

Wednesday, Jan. 29.
Snow and very cold here in Detroit and found an influenza epidemic raging. Oh, how I long for sunny California! We shall have to stay at the Tuller Hotel for a week, with nothing to do but go to the movies. They are showing Theda Bara in "The Blue Flame" and "Don't Change Your Husband" with Gloria Swanson and my favorite—Tom Meighan.

Tuesday, Feb. 3.
Evening performance at the Powers Theatre in Grand Rapids. A sold-out house! Erica became suddenly very sick; we called doctor and he says she has to have her appendix out at once! Erica went to the hospital alone, for the rest of us had to leave for Toledo. Poor Erica!

Wednesday, Feb. 4.
Toledo. We received a wire from Erica's doctor. The operation was successful and she is O.K. Gave a performance at Coliseum Hall. It is freezingly cold here and for that reason had not a big audience.

Thursday, Feb. 5.
In Cleveland at the Hotel Statler. Danced to a sold-out house at the new Masonic Temple with a nice ample stage but, alas, poor lighting. Many of the music critics here are Copeland's friends.

Saturday, Feb. 7.
The critics wrote only about George; didn't mention us girls at all. Heard from Erica. She is quite out of danger and sitting up

in a chair already. I see in the papers that they are having terrible blizzards in New York. Am not too anxious now to return would much rather go back to California. Depart for Utica on Sunday.

Monday, Feb. 9.
Encountered a heavy snowstorm in Utica. Tonight we are giving our 62nd performance on this trip. Full house and a nice audience. Left for home.

Tuesday, Feb. 10.
We arrived an hour late at Grand Central Station. Back at last! Nearly all our friends there to greet us. Gus and Margherita, Stephan, Bill, Arnold, Stuart etc. We all had dinner together in the famous "Duncan Room" at the Crillon. Otto Baumgarten gave us a fine dinner with wine and liqueurs. Grossing seventy-five thousand dollars on this tour we only deposited twelve thousand to our credit at the Guaranty Trust.

We rented a small furnished apartment on West Fifty-eighth Street near the Plaza. Our former English teacher from Geneva, Miss Annie von Stockhausen, acted as chaperone. Here we often entertained our various friends for tea, cocktail parties being unknown in those days. We were celebrities in our own right and attracted much attention wherever we went as a group. The fashionable, glossy magazines frequently reproduced our photographs, most of them by Arnold Genthe. Like other attractive young women in the limelight, we too had a number of admirers; some with serious intentions, others not. Of the latter species Isadora, who always acted much as any bourgeois mother toward her adopted daughters, would warn us by saying, "They are men who only care to profit by your youth and give you *nothing* in return. It sickens me when I think of it and raises my indignation."

However, none of us had any immediate plans for marriage. Too immersed in our burgeoning careers, anxious to build a little financial security for ourselves, we were quite content to turn all our efforts in that direction. Everybody made much of us on our return from a successful tour. For a while we led a gay social life, as can be seen from my diary notes:

Feb. 12.
We had tea at Stuart Benson's place. Johnny Aubert [Erica's beau from Geneva] is in town. He has already given several piano recitals. We shall hear him on Saturday.

Feb. 14.
Went over to Brooklyn to hear Johnny Aubert with the Symphony Orchestra, Stransky conducting. A concerto by Grieg. He seems to have put on some weight but otherwise looks the same. He is a good musician and very charming young man, I like him. He is going to dine with us on Thursday, the day Erica returns from Grand Rapids.

Sunday, Feb. 15.
The other girls have all gone to Tenafly for a visit with the Rousseaus and their two little children Marta and Theodore Jr. I have the blues and remained at home. Freddo Sides who works for Alavoine's called and invited me to luncheon. We talked about Isadora, he admires her tremendously. Likes my dancing too.

Feb. 17.
Expected Johnny for tea but he never showed up. W.R. came instead. Freddo sent me two seats for the Opera to see the Sakharoffs dance. They used an exact copy of our stage setting. Their dance had no continuity of movement—nothing but poses.

Feb. 25.
We all had dinner at Albert Rothbart's. He engaged an Egyptian necromancer to amuse us with tricks evoking spirits, etc. Quite funny.

Feb. 26.
I received a lot of flowers for my birthday. Miss Annie served tea. Arnold presented me with a new dance photo of myself.

Feb. 28.
Gave a children's matinee at 10:30 A.M. over in New Jersey at the Lyceum Theatre with Beryl Rubenstein at the piano. Miss

N., the manager, a beast of a woman, spoiled the whole show by insisting on interrupting our dances in order to explain things to the children. When Anna objected she insulted her in front of the audience. Oh, it was dreadful. The stage and lights were pretty awful too and Beryl didn't play too well either—anyhow, what can one expect at ten in the morning!

Sunday, Feb. 29.

Rosenbach, Genthe, the Sigmund Spaeths, came to tea with us here at our diggings. Our primitive way of making tea on a spirit lamp is quite interesting to watch. In the evening we girls had dinner at Billy and Mary Roberts' apartment on East 18th Street. (How their wooden stairs do creak!)

March 1.

Johnny Aubert played for us tonight at our studio in Carnegie Hall. Bach, Mozart, Schumann and Chopin, very beautifully. He has much improved since we heard him in Geneva. . . . Tomorrow afternoon we have a dress rehearsal at Aeolian Hall with our conductor Edward Falck. We are going over the orchestra music.

Sunday, March 7.

Rosenbach, Ordinsky, Johnny, Max Eastman and Eugene Boissevain for tea. Afterwards we girls had dinner at Max Eastman's apartment in Greenwich Village that he shares with Boissevain. He recited poems all evening by the fireside.

March 10.

Worked at the studio. Gene and Max came around later, and Lisa and I went for a drive with them out to the Bronx Zoo.

March 13.

At 8:30 performance at Carnegie Hall with orchestra. A wonderful performance to a capacity house. The audience actually cheered at the end. Supper party at Voisin's with friends afterwards.

The following day all the New York papers carried rave notices. Just for the record, it may not be amiss to quote a few lines. Heywood Broun, writing in the *Tribune,* said:

The Isadora Duncan Dancers made their first appearance of this season. . . . They have just got back from the Pacific coast and in the year of absence have made great steps towards artistic maturity. . . . The program was largely of ensembles from Gluck's Iphigenia, the Schmitt waltzes and a war horse of Johann Strauss's called "Southern Roses." For encores there were Chopin's Polonaise and the Marche Lorraine.

In the ensemble dancing the personal idiosyncrasies of the dancers were properly subdued, but that Lisa must needs show off her jumping. . . . The dancers in the Gluck Amazon dance and the two encores gave the finest thrill that the present stage in this country can afford. . . .

A capacity audience first applauded, then cheered, then sat motionless at the end of the program till it got more dances. These children, who two years ago were pleading at our doorstep for attention, have gone in with tremendous blessings.

Another reviewer, writing under the pseudonym *The Listener*, observed:

Without the aid of Isadora, the Isadora Duncan Dancers have, in a swift, hard working year, become the chief champions of that art which she revived. Today they are undoubtedly its most inspiring interpreters too. Youth, Grace, Beauty, a thorough schooling in aesthetics; a year ago they had all these as their assets. Today they have that one thing more necessary—a power of imagination which enables them to create, actually to create a sheer and independent beauty from out of the moments of their faithfullest interpretations.

Carnegie Hall held an audience of amazingly large size on Saturday night to see these young dancers . . . an audience which thundered and thirsted for more through a blue darkness and which found in the dances, both separate and ensemble, to Chopin's music a succession of glowing explanations. No explanation of Chopin alone—for that would be a sorry task to ask of youth—but for life itself and all it hides of poetry and beauty.

Sunday, March 21.

Gene has sent me a lovely Java Batik. He and Max invited Lisa and me to lunch at Longue Vue by the river. A sunny day, the first day of spring. B and I heard Jascha Heifetz at Aeolian Hall. We all had dinner together at St. Luke's Place and then went to another concert at the Hippodrome with the Ampico piano . . .

March 27.

Margherita and Angus went with us to Boston, at the Copley Plaza. We gave a 3 o'clock matinee at Symphony Hall. Full house, great success. Beryl Rubinstein made good music at the piano for us. Many prominent people in audience including Senator Lodge. Leaving on the midnight train.

March 28.

We arrived early in New York on a beautiful day. Had luncheon at the Crillon with Otto, Miss Annie came too. Later we heard Galli-Curci at the Hippodrome.

Sunday, April 4.

Left early this morning for Croton with Anna, Lisa and Margot. A nasty, rainy day. Had lunch with Max Eastman at his bungalow and went for a drive afterwards, called on Isabelle and her baby. She is the same as she always was at school. After dinner went up the hill to Dudley Field Malone's house. Had drinks and danced. Motored back late at night. It was fun.

April 6.

Performance at the Metropolitan Opera House with orchestra, danced Symphony by Schubert. A big success. What a thrill it was to dance again at the Met, what memories of our appearances together with Isadora! Had supper party at Reiss' studio in the village.

April 10.

We received a cable from Isadora. She wants us to come over and work with her in France from June to October on new programs and also give performances.

Happy in the thought of seeing Isadora again and craving the fresh inspiration working with her would bring us, we girls nonetheless found ourselves in a quandary. Should we accept her offer or decline it? We had several important factors to consider. Knowing our foster mother as well as we did, we had no assurance that she would let us return to the States at the appointed time. Sol Hurok, our new manager, had signed us up for another season, a commitment we intended to keep at all costs. Our newly won emancipation and financial independence had to be maintained, come what might. There was also the question of citizenship papers. Would the State Department allow us to leave? I especially held back from committing myself to this trip abroad. I voiced my doubts to Gus, who wrote his sister: "All the girls are willing to accept your offer. Only Irma is 'holding out.' "

I insisted on a written contract from Isadora, stating the conditions and guaranteeing our release at the end of the season, so we could return in time for our winter engagements. Being a bit psychic, I could not suppress a distinct feeling that, once in Isadora's grip, we would not be able to extricate ourselves. To my utter surprise, she readily agreed to signing a contract with us. But once I held it in my hands, I instantly realized the complete futility of this gesture. It was just a piece of paper.

In my diary for May 15, I noted, "Our last performance of the season at Carnegie Hall"—not suspecting in the least what my inner voice kept trying to tell me: namely, that this was indeed the end of the Isadora Duncan Dancers as a group of six. The first link in the chain would be broken by Erica. She and Margot never having been particularly outstanding in the dance, Erica decided to make an end of her own dance career. Her ambition now was to study painting with Wienold Reiss. This she did after a summer vacation in Switzerland. As for myself, little did I dream that with destiny pulling unseen strings, I would not set foot on American soil for many years. Here are the last entries of my diary before I left:

April 20.
To Baltimore. It is always lovely in Baltimore, but we had a poor house. And this was a Benefit performance for our manager Mr. Hurok at the Lyric Theatre.

April 21.

Took an early train to Washington. Gus went with us. Matinee at Poli-Schubert Theatre—an old place but a good house. The audience not quite so enthusiastic as last year. Here we met Mr. F. Howe again former Immigration Commissioner when we landed on Ellis Island. He wants to help us with obtaining passports for France. We have still two years to go before we become citizens. So it is necessary to get special permission in order to leave the country.

April 22.

It is so lovely in Washington, everything green and in blossom. Went for a long drive into the surrounding country, after a bit of sight-seeing. Leaving on the midnight train for Altoona. Saturday we dance in Lancaster, Pennsylvania. And then home.

Sunday, May 2.

Got up early to go to Yonkers by train where Gene and Max met us with their car. We motored over to Connecticut to visit Art Young than back to Croton for lunch, out of doors picnic style. Dudley Field Malone came. He promised to help with the passports.

May 27.

Anna returned from her trip to Washington where she had an interview with Secretary of State Polk. He gave her a letter with permission to leave the country only temporarily for the purpose of engagements abroad. So all is well. This is Isadora's birthday.

May 29.

Motored out to the Untermeyer estate in Yonkers to have our pictures taken for *Vogue* in the Greek Garden by Arnold Genthe. We have another cable from Isadora saying she sent the contracts for us to sign.

June 22.

Goodbye America. Sailing at 1 o'clock on the S.S. *Leopoldina* for France.

Demeter and Persephone

EVER since she went to Greece in 1904, when she thought of founding a school, Isadora had dreamed of bringing her pupils there some day. Soon after we joined her in Paris, she said, "Let us all go to Athens and look upon the Parthenon. I may yet found a school there."

With the sale of her property at Bellevue-sur-Seine to the French government (something she had been trying to negotiate unsuccessfully for a long time), her dream was to be realized. Her plans called for our departure at the end of July. I remember Paul Poirêt giving a fancy farewell party for us with some of his beautiful models at the Oasis Club—a very chic place. As bad luck would have it, that same night poor Anna was stricken with an inflamed appendix. This necessitated a change of plans.

Isadora had to stay, but she sent Lisa and me, chaperoned by Christine Dalliès, ahead to Venice. She told us to wait there. The rest, including her friend and pianist Walter Rummel, intended to follow when Anna could make the journey. Once again, exact details of our trip to Italy and Greece escape me, and I must needs consult my faithful diary.

July 31, 1920.
Departing for Venice tonight via Milano. Arrived on Sunday Aug. 1, in a downpour. To make matters worse I caught a painful cinder in my eye. Eager to catch my first sight of the Queen of the Adriatic, I leaned too far out of the train window completely disregarding the warning below, "*E pericoloso sporghesi!*"

A motorboat whisked us out to the Lido and the Hotel Ex-

celsior. Got only a glimpse and even less because of the cinder
which inflamed my eye. But what a mysterious, fascinating place
is Venice!

Aug. 2.
Sasha and Dolly Votichenko are also staying at the Lido. Could
hardly wait to get back to Venice. St. Mark's is perfectly ador-
able, the Palais des Doges lovely. I am crazy about Venice and
its atmosphere of an operatic stage setting. Had tea at Florian's
on the piazza. Did some shopping and had dinner at Bonevechiatti's. Wonderful moonlight ride in gondola along the Grand
Canal.

Aug. 3.
Went bathing in the blue Adriatic at Lido Beach directly in front
of hotel. After lunch returned to town. Tea at Florian's. Some
more shopping and a lengthy promenade around town. Dined
again on the little open terrace of Bonevechiatti, an excellent
restaurant. The risotto is superb, exactly the way I like it.

Aug. 5.
To Venice and stopped at Florian's for an ice cream. Then down
the canal to the station to meet Margot and Theresa. The others
won't be long in joining us, they said. Anna is rapidly mending.

Aug. 7.
Visited the church of San Marco and the Palais des Doges. At
Florian's as usual. We expected Isadora today but no sign of her
yet.

Sunday, Aug. 8
They came today. We all went bathing together except Anna
who still looks frail and very pale. Isadora invited me for a gondola ride. We dined at the Danieli and watched the Tombola
on the piazza afterwards. She appeared to be in a state of shock.
Very taciturn and morose. It seems she and the Archangel
[Walter Rummel] had a serious quarrel.

Aug. 10.
Who would surprise us today but George Copeland and his
friend Arthur. Both have been in Venice for weeks. We intro-

duced him to Isadora since they had not met before. We invited
them to luncheon. There is dancing on the terrace tonight.
George made a date with us for tomorrow's lunch at Vapois in
Venice including Sasha, Dolly and Isadora.

Friday, Aug. 13.
Unlucky Friday! And how!! Seems that Anna and the Archangel have fallen in love. Isadora is awfully jealous. She made
us all move to the Danieli, forsaking the Excelsior and the Lido.
I told Christine: *"Cette histoire avec Anna et l'Archangel est
vraiement embêtante. Il parait qu'elle est amoureuse de lui, mais
lui aime encore beaucoup Isadora. Grande tragédie!"*

Aug. 14.
After a good luncheon at our favorite place—Bonevechiatti—we
went, accompanied by Sasha to show us the way, to the famous
Fortuni Shop. We each bought a different color dress. Mine is
rose-colored. I love it.

The pleated Fortuni gown came into existence in 1910,
when Signor Fortuni designed the first one for Isadora, in the
hope she would display it in her performances and help to
make him famous. She did not, however, consider his gowns
suitable for dancing professionally, and never wore one on the
stage. She did invariably wear them at home or to parties and
frequently was photographed in one of Fortuni's creations made
of fine India silk, often gold-stenciled and with Venetian beads
along the sides.

It amused us to see how the gowns were twisted together
and tied with a belt—an exact imitation of the way we treated
our dance tunics. To achieve the same pleated effect observed
on Greek statuary, we started out by sprinkling the tunics with
water. Two girls then got hold of the ends, folding one tiny
pleat upon the other, and then gave the whole thing a twist,
held together by a ribbon. This had to be repeated after each
performance, so the tunics would be in proper shape for the
next one. With so many tunics involved, it was a laborious and
patience-demanding process. Isadora herself taught us this trick.

She must also have shown it to Fortuni, who invented a secret process to keep the gowns artificially though not permanently pleated.

We girls always longed to own one of these long, clinging tunics that give women the beauty of archaic Greek statues. Only now could we afford to buy them. We soon discovered their one big flaw. It was absolutely fatal to sit down in these gowns—the pleats all disappeared! If I may be allowed a bad pun: an un-fortuniate situation, indeed, which permanent pleating corrects in modern dresses.

Society ladies with an artistic bent eventually took up the fad of wearing Fortuni dresses, another instance of the influence exerted by Isadora Duncan on the world of fashion.

Monday, Aug. 16.
After luncheon we rented a gondola for the Lido where we met Isadora. At sunset we returned and had dinner on Isadora's balcony at the Hotel Britannia. Steichen arrived tonight. We are getting ready to leave for Greece tomorrow.

Aug. 17.
We got up at six A.M. only to find that all the motorboats are on strike. Were obliged to rent gondolas with all our baggage and row way out into the middle of the harbour in order to board the Austrian vessel, S.S. *Canonia*. Luckily it was a lovely warm day. The Adriatic's deep blue color is quite startling to see after the dull, muddy waters of the canal.

Aug. 18.
Reached Bari late in the day. A hot little town. Had dinner and went to the hot little theatre where we saw a Neapolitan group of actors perform a completely incomprehensible play with all the exaggerations of a Polichinelle show. Didn't like it. Tomorrow we expect to reach Brindisi.

Aug. 19.
Brindisi looks exactly the way I remembered it from my last visit on our way to Egypt. Same old place with same old stairs leading up to an uninteresting town.

Aug. 20.

Stopped at Corfu for a few hours, visited the former German Kaiser's villa—the Achillion. Wonderful view from up there. The sea so blue and the islands in the distance like rosy clouds.

Sunday, Aug. 22.

Passed the Isthmus of Corinth very early in the morning. At high noon in ferocious heat set foot on Attic soil. Landed at Piraeus and immediately motored out to Falerone near the sea. Not much of a place. I didn't care for it nor did the other girls. We returned to Athens and engaged rooms at the Grande Bretagne. The ones that face the square and open into a long balcony-terrace. Isadora occupied the end suite on the right. At the Zappeion Garden we bought the fragrant white jasmine blossoms for our hair from the boy flower vendors who followed us—shouting with shrill, high voices: "Smeen! Smeen!" until we gave in. Had a gay dinner there. Greek food—caille aux riz, black olives, stuffed eggplant washed down with Resin wine and to the accompaniment of Greek zither music. Afterwards looked at the Temple of Zeus in the moonlight. Beautiful!

Aug. 23.

I forgot to record yesterday that the first thing Isadora did after we unpacked at the hotel was to show us Copanos, the Greek house she started to build in 1904 when she first visited Athens. It was never finished and only one room has a roof over it. There is no water, and goats were stabled here, by the looks of things. She wants to have it cleaned and to furnish it with a grand piano for a studio. What optimism. The heat is atrocious, I nearly succumbed to it. Only the marvelous view of the Acropolis opposite made it all worth while.

Aug. 24.

Modern Athens is not particularly attractive, I noticed going shopping. Saw some lovely Amazon statues at the National Museum. Isadora and the rest went up to the Acropolis to look at the Parthenon. I refused to go. She was displeased. I intend to wait till there is a full moon and, if possible, go up there alone. At a moment like that I don't relish crowds.

Aug. 27.

Full moon! As luck would have it, the nice young man I met on the boat coming to Greece called on me after dinner. He asked me to see the Parthenon by moonlight. By a strange coincidence, no other visitors were up there.

Overcome himself by the glorious sight, he let me wander off in silence as I wanted to be alone. An unearthly vision of beauty —no words can describe it. In the moonlight the marble shimmered snowy white, the way it must originally have appeared. Its daytime color is orange.

Sunday, Aug. 29.

Early this morning, Isadora, showing herself very restless, suddenly ordered an open touring car. She invited Edward [Steichen], Lisa, Margot and myself to accompany her on a trip to Aulis and Chalcis. We rushed northward raising a cloud of dust behind us. Coming down the mountain near the island of Euboea we stopped to gaze at one of the most surprisingly beautiful views in the world—the seashore of Chalcis. There, in Euripides' legend, Iphigenia and her handmaidens played on the shore. How often, in our imagination, had we simulated their Attic games there in our dances to the music of Gluck! What a thrill actually to see it there below us in the sunlight.

Were in time for luncheon at the hotel. In the evening walked along the shore where Iphigenia and her maidens trod of yore. Had a nice dinner at San Stephan by the sea.

Aug. 30.

Continued down the coast to view the Temple and Theatre of Dionysos. Just a few stones left, and overgrown with vegetation. Steichen, having forgotten in the hurry of sudden departure to bring his camera along, asked me to lend him my little Brownie. He snapped a few pictures of us three girls and Isadora in the ancient theatre.

After lunch we motored back to Athens via Thebes. There is great excitement in Athens over the arrival of Venizelos. We watched him pass from the hotel balcony.

The month of August had passed pleasantly. But in September all sorts of unpleasant things occurred. To begin with,

Theresa had a nearly fatal sunstroke. I nursed her day and night applying cold compresses over her feverish body till a doctor could be summoned, it being a holiday. He said my treatment saved her life. Then Anna had to go to the hospital with an infection and Margot, too, was unwell. Lisa caught a bad cold, and later I myself came down with a strep throat. The Greek doctor told me to gargle with lemon juice. Isadora suffered mostly from bad humor on that never-to-be-forgotten trip to Greece.

So it happened that she only started to work with us on September 25, in the Zappeion Museum, where the government provided her with a large hall. Three years had elapsed since last we worked together. She started on the Seventh Symphony of Beethoven, parts of which we knew and had performed with her in New York. Following that, she taught us the Scherzo of Tchaikowsky's Sixth. Two weeks before we began to work with her, she told us quite frankly that she opposed our return to the States. This was my turn to say to the other girls, "I told you so!" It did not exactly come as a surprise to me.

Several days later, when we failed to show up in New York on the prescribed date, we received a cable from our American manager. He threatened us with breach of contract and heavy costs. Lisa and I offered to come immediately, but he wanted all six or none. A huge argument resulted with Isadora. I suggested quite logically, so it seemed to me, in order to evade a lawsuit, that we fulfill our contract and then return to her. But she would have none of this.

"I did not bring you up and teach you my art, only to have you exploited by theatrical managers," she admonished us.

She wanted us to perform only under her guidance and to help her found a school for a thousand children in Greece. Most of the other girls had meekly given in to her wishes. I made the big mistake of growing more obstinate and infuriated by the minute. And when I do, I am bound to say almost anything. This unreasonable attitude of hers aroused all my ire. In the heat of the argument, which developed into an angry dialogue, the other girls not saying a word, I really lost my temper. She said I had an ugly Broadway spirit and if I felt that way I had better return to America. With that, I stormed out of her suite and rushed straightaway to the steamship office, still smarting from the verbal blows. Back at the Hotel d'Angleterre, where we girls lived, I sat down and tried to be calm. My anger is soon spent; I seldom harbor grievances for long. I regretted the vehemence of my unguarded utterances. On calmer judgment, I sat down and wrote her a letter, trying to explain my motives and all those things one really can't explain, that remain the secrets of a human heart.

Hotel d'Angleterre, Athens, Sept. 30, 1920.
Dear Isadora:

I inquired at the steamship office and there is a very good boat sailing for New York on the 10th of October. I think I had better book a passage on it—this will be the most convenient way to get rid of me. I quite understand that a "cheap Broadway spirit" has nothing to do with your art. Because, if that is all you see in me, I should certainly not remain another day with you.

Words are futile. I really cannot explain my true nature to you. It is, at times, even too complicated for me. Your art which is the highest expression of all that is pure and divine in man, makes those who practice it—if they are pure at heart—purer. And if they are great—greater. But a spirit that is fundamentally not simple and naive cannot so easily be molded. I cannot change my inner self, nor can you.

One thing I am unable to comprehend: How is it that you, with your intelligence and intuition, have not been able correctly to judge my character before? I think it is rather too late now. What a waste and what a crime! For another person might have profited in my stead and been of real help to you. Someone to be proud of, and of real value to you, who could be a fine example to those hundreds who are going to follow.

I don't feel I can thank you for what you have done for me, since it has apparently all been in vain. On the contrary, I would rather curse the day you took my hand and led me to your school. Your hand has always pointed upward. This made us sense there is something beyond—something more important than life. And willingly I wanted to be led. Now, you turn around with a frown on your face and point a finger of scorn at me and say that you see into my soul and what you see is . . . Isadora, do you really think you have the eyes of God?

Maybe only very earthly, petty things are obscuring your vision. Perhaps, if you had tried to peer into my soul with a little more understanding, you would truly have been able to see. I am a queer girl, one must take me as I am. If you could have done so, who knows, I might have been of genuine service to you until my death. But I don't believe in sacrifice. You did not sacrifice your life either for the sake of your school. The idea of the school has always been your salvation. In your worst moments of anguish and misery it has been your only joy and inspiration. *But it has not been everything in your life!* How then can you expect that I should devote mine *entirely* to the future of the school?

Two days later I received a message delivered by hand:

Dearest Irma—

I have just received your letter. I can't answer it now but will tomorrow. I think there is a great deal of *misunderstanding*. At any rate, you must confess that the things you say sometimes would make a saint angry. Whatever you decide and whether you really want to go back to New York or not, please don't doubt of my very great love for you who are to me exactly like my own little girl. And if I become so *furious* it is only that I want your future to be splendid. I am probably stupid to take the small things you say in earnest.

I will answer your letter tomorrow. With a kiss and all my love—

Isadora

I waited anxiously for her letter, glad that she held no rancor and much comforted by her nice note. When the messenger appeared next day at my hotel, he handed me an envelope that contained not only her letter of explanation but also a picture. The picture was self-explanatory. It portrayed the Greek goddess Demeter, Mother Earth, handing on a torch to her young daughter Persephone, the new life, bringing light to the world.

Dear Irma—

I answer your letter. In the first place, do not believe the words which were wrung from me in anger by your extraordinary exasperating attitude. Blot out the "Broadway" phrase, it has nothing to do with you or me. And as for "Getting rid of you," it is *because* you are so precious to me and to my art that I have made such an effort to tell you the *real* future of the work, which is not for *you* or *me* but for the *generations to come.*

As for *sacrifice*—take one example. When in December, 1914, Paris Singer said to me, "If you have the courage to start your school now, I will give you the house in Bellevue and 100,000 francs a year to do it with," I hesitated, for the idea of seeing *little children* at that time meant absolute torture to me. But I answered, *"yes,"* for the thought this opportunity might never come again and it would be a crime to deprive those children.

No one will ever know what it cost me to teach those children at Bellevue. Often, in the midst of a lesson, I went upstairs and cried with agony, "No, I can't look at them!" But the next day I tried again.

I think in fact it was this fearful struggle that killed the little Baby that was my only hope. And you know since then I have not been able to look at a child without bursting into tears. And yet, I am willing to take them again and teach them. Is not that sacrifice?

And such a useless sacrifice, as all Bellevue is gone and the little children that were there have come to nothing.

I only have a few more years to do it. Won't you help me? Before I die, at least one hundred beings must *understand* the work and give it to others.

You irritated me the other day by the stupid things you said until I would have said *anything.* But my expression and tears often when you dance must have proved to you that I found it *beautiful.* I want it to be more so and *glorious,* especially the Beethoven.

I don't ask any of you to sacrifice all your life for the school. I only want you to give me a part of each year to helping me. The rest of the year you may tour as you like. And above all, I want you to learn the Iphigenie, the Orphee, the Beethoven and all to a state of perfection, or as near it as possible, before dancing it in a theatre.

Come this morning to work. Forgive anything I have said that wounded you—I did not mean it. You are for me always my little Irma whom I love most dearly. And I am for you—your *friend.*

Isadora

Dear, dear Isadora:

I read your beautiful letter and I think if we don't speak to each other we understand each other better. I also want to ask you a hundred times pardon for everything I have said—it must all have been very insulting to you. For there is nothing in this wide world too beautiful that I could say or do to compensate you for all that you have given me spiritually and materially. I do want to aid you in *every way* possible so that your wonderful idea shall be realized. And on the day we actually see a hundred children dance, I too will shed tears of joy. You are right; we should all agree to work part of the time together as you suggest. I am willing to wait and not perform till we have perfected our work. We look up to you to guide us and let us know when the time has come.

I want you to know that I love you more than my own mother. I cannot show you my affection but it is all in my heart.

—Love,
Irma

October 1, 1920.

Dearest Irma—

Your letter has made me *happy.* Now, hand in hand, we will go forward and conquer the world in *harmony* and *love.*

—Isadora

13

The School Is Dead, Long Live the School

THE bite of a pet monkey that killed the King of Greece decided our departure. The performances we planned to give in Athens had to be canceled. We left toward the end of October for Paris.

There is a street in Passy, which George du Maurier describes in his *Peter Ibbetson* as the "Street of the Pump," winding its way to Paris through the Arc de Triomphe at one end and to the river Seine at the other. He called it a delightful street where the "butcher, the baker, the candlestick-maker" still had their *boutiques* within the residential quarter. Here Isadora bought a house because of the large room in the rear, called "Salle Beethoven," where *intime* concerts could be given. She converted it into a studio with the same blue curtains and carpet. We girls had rooms in a small hotel nearby.

What little money we had saved from our tours in the States dwindled alarmingly. In order to economize, we rented a small furnished apartment on the Rue Eugène Manuel, in Passy, a short distance away from Isadora's house. Here we were left to struggle along financially as best we could; for one moment our foster mother lavished everything on her adopted children, the next she withdrew her support. That is why we were so eager to give performances. As always, we had to wait for Isadora's consent. We chafed under this inactivity, having no outlet for our pent-up energies. But, being young, we managed to enjoy life from day to day, whatever it might bring. We hired a cook from the provinces, a *bonne à toute faire*, who went on her daily errand dressed in a black shawl with a market basket on her arm.

Like all French women, she had the culinary touch with a Gallic flavor, and I can still see us girls sitting at the round table in our tiny *salle à manger*, relishing every savory morsel. The lamp with a green shade suspended from the ceiling directly over the dining table created a warm, homey atmosphere. As soon as the table was cleared, with no neighborhood movies available to attend, we sought amusement in a game of whist.

Working at the studio on Rue de la Pompe, we frequently lunched with Isadora and Rummel. On those occasions she would take the precaution of drawing the dark velvet curtains over the windows to shut out the brilliant spring sunshine, which left us in the dark except for a red Japanese lantern burning on the side table. She said it created a more restful light. But it also erased all those fine encroaching lines and wrinkles on the face of any woman in her forties, a little vanity on the part of the famous dancer that fooled no one. Sunday was her day at home when friends dropped in for tea. I often went with her to shop in an American bakery on the Rue de Bac for her favorite—coconut cake. Afternoon tea was a daily habit with her.

That winter and spring of 1921 turned out to be quite a social season. We attended the theatre frequently, concerts galore. The Ukrainian Chorus was the big attraction in Paris that season, and the elegant Bal Noire et Blanc at the Champs Elysée Theatre. We often had friends take us to night clubs such as the Peroquet, where the American Negro entertainer Josephine Baker held forth.

I must interrupt my story here to point out and correct some popular misconceptions. In all my life with Isadora I never attended a so-called "orgy," staged either by her or by anyone else, as the newspapers loved to misrepresent. A champagne party and supper where guests dance, cut funny capers, and generally enjoy themselves in public cannot exactly be termed an "orgy"! That happened every day in the social world I used to know and is a festive occasion most people have enjoyed at least once in their lives.

Outside of an occasional cocktail before meals, none of us girls, nor Isadora, ever indulged in drinking or especially craving hard liquor. Our European tastes were conditioned to wines. Only in her late forties, after her marriage to a Russian and under his malign influence, did she acquire a habit for stronger stuff. But no one who ever knew her intimately in her day-by-day existence could ever honestly accuse her of becoming an alcoholic in her last years. That, to my certain knowledge, represents a gross calumny.

Now to go on: Afterward we continued on to Joe Zelli's opening with Maurice and Hughes, the popular ballroom dancers of that period. Maurice had lately dropped his former long-time partner Florence Walton, which created a sensation. Isadora, in a short Chanel gown covered with gold beads, liked to dance to tango music rather than the fox trot. She knew none of the conventional steps; she always improvised her own, much to the confusion of her male partners.

I recall her telling me that once in San Francisco in 1918, when she appeared there in a Chopin recital with the pianist Harold Bauer, the audience as usual clamored for an encore at the end. Tired of hearing more Chopin she decided on a sudden, whimsical impulse to dance a tango. The tango was then the latest craze in popular dance. Harold Bauer protested, not knowing any popular tunes as a concert pianist of the first order. He considered it below his dignity but Isadora urged him along saying, "Oh just improvise on the rhythm and I'll do the same," adding slyly, "The public won't be able to tell the difference!" She was right, they loved it and wanted her to repeat the "Duncan Tango" but she never did that again.

In Paris that year the tango was still very popular, thanks to the expert ballroom dancers who specialized in this Argentine dance like Maurice and the American movie star Rudolph Valentino. A place called El Garron on Montmartre caught her fancy. It was a small room, with banquettes upholstered in red velvet along three walls; the fourth was taken over by two rows of sixteen Argentine accordion players in red coats. And how electrifyingly they could play those exotic Latin tunes. I learned to dance the Argentine tango very well, with a professional partner as tutor. Even today, my feet can't resist beating the measure whenever I hear one played. We usually danced through the night and at dawn sped over to Les Halles for the traditional reveler's *soupe à l'oignon* and crusty French bread warm from the oven. Ah, *sacrée jeunesse!* What exuberant fun we had! Curiously enough for one so young, those diversions did not make me forget the more serious ambition then nagging at my psyche—to make a name for myself as an artist.

The year before, in the fall of 1920, it all had seemed so promising when Isadora and Rummel and we girls worked in artistic harmony and enthusiasm on a new project, the study of *Parsifal*. She taught us the Flower Maiden Scene, while she portrayed Kundry in her bewitched garden enticing Parsifal. And a beautiful etherealized choreography for the Holy Grail music.

The world première took place on November 27, 1920, at the now-vanished Trocadéro. That evening, at the theatre, she summoned us to her dressing room a few minutes before curtain time. It was an event for her pupils, because this joint appearance was the first in two years. Her dressing room had the familiar look I had seen so many times since my childhood, for she always liked to say a word or two of encouragement and give us inspiration. She sat in front of her dressing table which was covered with a lace cloth and littered with an assortment of makeup. Leaning against the frame of the mirror and pinned above it were reproductions of Greek sculpture and friezes. On a table beside her, still partly wrapped in green tissue from the florist's box, lay the fresh flowers she used as wreaths or decorations for her various dances. The open wardrobe trunk spilled over with a profusion of tunics and scarfs needed for the performance. The chaise longue in a corner held her white and red Indian shawls, so she could stretch out and rest during the intermission. A three-hour program of uninterrupted dancing is a most strenuous affair. The throat gets parched, and to quench one's thirst with water is fatal. Aqua pura has a funny way of jumping around inside with every lively step, a horrid sensation. For that reason, to ease the maddening thirst, she preferred a glass of champagne during the intermission. She never touched a drop of anything stronger.

A pleasant perfume of flowers and cologne enveloped us six girls as we entered, dressed in flesh-colored Flower Maiden attire with blooms in our hair and a garland from shoulder to waist. Each one was different. My floral adornment consisted of large anemones in a combination of vivid red, purple, and white. She smiled and looked us over critically. "You all look ravishing," she whispered. Then she fixed her glance on me with a small *moue* of dissatisfaction and said, "I do wish, Irma, that you would not wear your hair so low over the forehead. It hides your nice wide brow." She got up and brushed my forelocks back as far as they could go, tilting my anemone wreath to the back of my head. Inwardly I seethed with annoyance, just waiting to push it all forward again as soon as I left her dressing room. She insisted in having her own way even in such trifles. Then she did something she hitherto had refrained from doing. She offered us a large goblet of champagne and urged each of us to take one sip. "It won't hurt you and may put you in the right mood for the seduction scene," she whispered. (It was her habit to keep complete silence for hours on the day of a performance.) She herself looked like the Goddess of Seduction, in a long cream-colored satin gown, a flowing red velvet cape, and a crown of red and white roses in her auburn hair.

She reminded us that we had a truly magnificent orchestra of a hundred musicians to play Wagner's glorious music for our dancing, so we must give our very best performance that night. She changed after the intermission and donned the gray, drab shift of a *penitente* to pray for divine grace and forgiveness. She danced to the Good Friday music—and danced it as no Wagnerian Kundry of the great master's imagination ever interpreted this role. The program ended with the Venusberg and Bacchanale from *Tannhäuser* in which she danced the part of Venus, with rose petals floating down over her throughout that sensitively imagined scene. Here all the love and sensuality inherent in the score were merely indicated by her, brought to life in the imagination rather than the flesh. It was one of her most perfect choreographic masterpieces.

Thrilling as was this experience at the Trocadéro—it eventually proved to have been the culmination of our artistic collaboration—it left me strangely dissatisfied. Isadora tolerated no solo dancing by her disciples in our joint appearances. However humble my own efforts compared to her genius, I chafed at remaining part of the chorus all my life. The artist in me longed for self-expression.

Isadora arranged several performances during the winter season—the opening one, with an all-Wagner program, took place on November 27 as already mentioned. It was our first public appearance since we girls had come abroad five months before. The famous contract we signed with Isadora, being of no further value, we tore up and threw away. Dissension was in the air. One of the causes, which we resented and which disrupted the harmony that should have prevailed, was the discovery that she had tried to enter into negotiations with Hurok, our New York manager, without consulting us. Her secretary, Norman Harle, inquired of Augustin Duncan what the prospects might be. Gus, still annoyed about the contract which he had once arranged for his sister and which she did not keep, answered:

Nov. 25, 1920

My dear Mr. Harle:

Your letter received, but I have had no opportunity of replying to it until now. I had occasion to see Mr. Hurok the other day and he asked me to write you the following and to give you his address in case you cared to write to him. He expresses a willingness to arrange some appearances in this country, with or without the girls, after the first of January. Even as late as March running into April and May provided the negotiation was completed by Christmas time.

Orchestra is only possible for New York (Metropolitan); piano on the road. Isadora could get a large fee, possibly $2,000 a performance, if she appeared with piano. But even $1,000 is unlikely if orchestra is insisted upon, outside of New York. In the latter case Hurok would not guarantee but only share on percentage. However, I advise you to write to him direct and leave me out of the negotiation. Do not ask less than $2,000 guarantee with piano. You can get it. Turn that into francs at the present rate of exchange and realize what that would mean. H. also offers a tour of the Orient. My advice is that you deal with him direct and not any representative, as they do *not* represent him.

My own opinion is that Isadora should not come to this country. The conditions are worse than ever before and I do not believe she would fulfill her contract. No one else in the business is more hopeful than I am on that point and therefore she could not make advantageous terms. For instance, payment in advance and steamer fares paid—entirely out of the question. She would be forced to stand all the risk of failure to carry out the bookings, as confidence in the likelihood of fulfilling a contract once made, is down to Zero.

Very truly yours,
Augustin Duncan

Nothing came of this plan. What little money we had saved from our American tour, even changed into francs at the then favorable rate of exchange, soon came to an end. The only way we knew to earn a living was by giving public performances, though every time we did, we ran counter to our teacher's wishes. Naturally we resented this situation, which caused much unhappiness. Money matters are notorious for causing trouble and ruining the best of friendships. To make up for our financial deficiency, we entered into negotiations with a French concert manager, who was willing to arrange a tour of the provinces for us. Because of her personal estrangement from Isadora, Anna had left the group. Thus only four girls remained—Lisa, Theresa, Margot, and myself.

Being careful to obtain Isadora's consent, I wrote to her. She was at that time in London, giving joint recitals with Walter Rummel. She agreed, providing she received 33 per cent of our fees after expenses had been paid. Her wire to me stated: "Programme Lyon: first part selection Iphigenie; second part Schubert Waltzes, Marche Militaire. Pianist playing solos Bach, Mozart, or Beethoven. No Chopin or any modern music."

As artists in our own right, we did not like her dictating to us. We considered it unreasonable and unjust on her part to interfere with our own mature judgment on such matters. We could not go on forever performing the same dances. She tolerated no solo dancing when we girls appeared with her. To me, the freedom of expression provided by a solo dance was necessary to my own artistic satisfaction. I suggested we call the whole thing off. Feeling frustrated and chafing under this constant control, we foolishly let off steam by talking the situation over with close friends, such as Mary Desti (formerly Mary Sturges) and Dolly Votichenko. We had no one else to help or advise us. As usual under such circumstances, where dissension is in the offing, the inevitable gossips—who simply itched to carry a tale and to embroider it in the telling—came to the fore. On hearing these exaggerated reports about us, our foster mother dispatched a letter from London:

> My dear Children—
> This is a message for all of you. Please reflect that all the things you say to my discredit reflect eventually on yourselves. And the people to whom you give your love and confidence have never done for you and will never do for you one per cent of what I have done, and am still willing to do for you. But it is discouraging when I hear from all sides that in return you only try to break all my relations in Paris and cut all my friendships.
> I assure you that this can do you no good and my patience is

almost at an end. If you could only learn a bit of discretion. Please work and live simply—read and study—and either be true to me or leave me on your own names and your own responsibility. Please write me. With love,

Isadora

In our apartment on the Rue Eugène Manuel in Passy, we immediately held a council of war. Isadora had offered to pay our rent but had failed to do so. The landlord threatened to evict us. Not knowing what to do, our own funds being depleted, Lisa managed to borrow enough to tide us over. Borrowing money was not to our liking. We aspired only to achieve independence, to earn our own living as we had done in the States. This could, under no provocation, be construed as showing ingratitude to our dear foster mother. I wrote her again of our financial dilemma and the trouble with the landlord, mentioning the loan we had to get. She immediately sent word through her secretary for us to move into her house at 103 Rue de la Pompe. But she sent no funds to pay off the loan.

Meanwhile Dolly Votichenko made a special trip to Brussels, where Isadora had a dance engagement. Within a short space of time, we received another sharp letter from our foster mother, written from the Hotel Metropole and dated April 30, 1921:

My dear Children:
I had a great joy and some hope in receiving Lisel's letter which I confess has been rather dampened since meeting Dolly Votichenko here who says that the way you all speak of me made her think that I was possibly some sort of monster. And in fact she repeated to me word for word what Mary had already told me. This is really too much and my patience is at an end. That you should speak of me this way is simply disgusting.
First, she says, you accuse me of having "left you to starve" in Geneva. Whereas you know perfectly well that I sent you by telegraph all the money I had in the bank in Buenos Aires and left myself not enough to pay my hotel bill. When on account

of the war conditions this money did not reach you, I sent Augustin from Buenos Aires to Geneva to rescue you, leaving me alone and without aid in a strange country.

Second, it seems you accuse me of having "deserted you," in New York. You will please remember that I sold all I had, even my shawls, and only left New York when *you were successfully launched* at Carnegie Hall, with a lucrative contract before you. I arrived in London ill and penniless and telegraphed to Augustin that I had no money to reach Paris but received no answer from any of you.

Third, it seems you accuse me of not procuring you engagements. On this score I am writing Mr. Harle to write you an account of money spent and time and cables amounting to 800 francs, to America trying to fix contracts for you. Also he will give you the true account of the contract which you seem to ignore.

Fourth, it seems you accuse me of not teaching you, when I have given you the very secret and most holy of my art. And to crown this you tell Dolly that I am *jealous* of you as an artist. Really, my poor children, I think you have all taken leave of your senses. And to *comble* that you say I owe Lisel money. This is *shameful!*

That I should hear all this from a stranger—really my affection for you and my patience is about at an end. As for the way Anna has spoken of me, I think she must be demented. My only crime toward her was a too great indulgence and affection for her. But my patience is at an end. If you can not understand that talking of me in this way you are doing me a great deal of harm and in doing me harm, are doing yourself harm . . .

In the meantime I beg you learn not to tell every little stupid idea in your heads to strangers. If you wish your tickets to America or elsewhere, Mr. Harle will arrange them, as your present attitude toward me seems to me to make further relations very difficult. I am, as Harle says, "fed up."

Isadora

Merely to set the record straight, I want to point out that Isadora left four months before we were "successfully launched at Carnegie Hall" in New York, and with "a lucrative contract" ahead of us.

However, these recriminations were not getting us anywhere. Isadora returned from her successful tour of England and Belgium in May. On the twenty-sixth, the day before her forty-third birthday, the French papers fairly brimmed over with the news that she had decided to go to Soviet Russia. Reporters swarmed all over her house, jostling each other in order to obtain a first-hand interview. Apparently, while she was in London, the head of the Russian Trade Commission, Leonide Krassine, hearing of her desire to go to Russia under the Communist regime, promised to help her obtain an official invitation. Her idea of founding a great school of the dance there appealed to the Bolsheviks, primarily as a wonderful piece of propaganda.

Her desire to go to Soviet Russia was no news to us girls. Her reason for this move was made quite explicit in an interview she had granted a woman reporter in Paris even before we left America. The article, which appeared in an English paper, stated:

> She received us graciously, with all the ease and naturalness which characterizes her dancing. In a dark, loose-fitting dress, her mink toque on the table beside her and fur coat thrown back, Isadora looked most charming. Her bobbed coiffure is most becoming and harmonizes with the expression of Irish sympathy and humour alternating with the warm California sunshine laughing in her eyes and mouth. There is in her face also—behind its vivaciousness—that indefinable mystic or spiritual quality which is so peculiar to great teachers. Asked, if she expected to start a new school of dancing this was her reply:
>
> "Nothing would please me more, but this time it must have a government guarantee. There must be some protection against the pupils of the school leaving and commercializing their knowledge before it has reached the stage of perfection. And this can only come about through the cooperation of a government. You may recall how under the Czar's regime that very thing was accomplished for the Imperial Russian Ballet. It is the only assurance of success."
>
> "What about the French government? The French have al-

ways been liberal patrons of art and they have admired your dancing," was the interpolated remark.

"Pouf! It's a question of money. The state of French finances . . ." and she dismissed them with a broad comprehensive gesture.

"And this story of your going to Russia to receive help from the Bolsheviki, what about that?"

"I did say that it didn't matter to me what the government was and that if Russia offered me a school I would go there and accept it. But of the Bolsheviks and their politics I know nothing. So contradictory are the stories concerning the Bolshevist attitude toward art, that one doesn't have any conception what it really is. I most certainly wouldn't hesitate to accept an offer from Russia. . . . Four fortunes have disappeared in this effort of mine to re-create dancing as the Greeks knew it—a natural expression of the spirit or the soul. Out of the twenty-five children whom I trained, only six were loyal. . . . These six girls could teach hundreds of pupils. But people say, they are beautiful and I suppose they will marry."

She smiled sweetly though a bit sadly at this conclusion. Miss Duncan, during the course of afternoon tea related the history of her school which has never before been published. It is a fascinating tale.

"Who wants to go to Russia with me?" Isadora asked us when she came back from London. I unhesitatingly said I would. The other two girls (Lisa and Theresa, for we were only three now dancing with her) seemed less interested. She smiled at me and said, "I knew I could count on you."

"I'll go wherever you want to go," I assured her. "I'll even follow you to Mars, if that is the place you have chosen to found your new school. Providing you are serious and really mean to go through with it."

She triumphantly produced a telegram she had just received from the People's Commissar of Education, Anatole Vasilief Lunacharsky, officially inviting her to Moscow. Overjoyed, she immediately thought of giving a party for her friends to tell them the good news. Among them were several Russian immi-

grants who had fled from the Revolution. When they heard that
Isadora had really made up her mind to go to the land of the
Bolsheviks, they seemed terribly shocked. One of the women
went down on her knees before Isadora and implored her by all
the holy saints not to go.

"You don't know what you are letting yourself in for! Food
is so scarce that the Communists are slaughtering four-year-old
children and eating them! Look, I have a letter here, smuggled
out of Russia, telling us about this. Please, please, don't go, Isadora!" she implored her.

"Well, if this is true," Isadora responded, looking pale and
grim, "then I *must* go."

After the guests departed, and she and I remained alone in
the studio where the planned festivity had turned into a session
of horror tales, she looked ruefully at me, trying to gauge my
reaction. By way of laughing the whole thing off, she said as a
joke, "Don't worry, Irma; they'll eat me first anyway. There is
a whole lot more of me than you. In the meanwhile, you'll
manage to escape!"

I confess the stories made my flesh creep. However, having
heard the worst about the Communists, I still could not quite
believe that they officially sanctioned cannibalism.

On the last day of May, Isadora gave another reception, a
far pleasanter one, for artists and writers. The pianist de Renne-
ville played, Jacques Copeau read his poems, and we danced.
Cécile Sartoris, a woman journalist who was present, later wrote:

> This evening Isadora dances for us; a dozen friends. It is her
> *adieu*. She is off to Brussels, then on to London. And after . . .
> Here she is then, surging out of the shadow, she who thought
> to resuscitate in our midst the play of noble attitudes, the rhythm
> of grace in the movements of life! Under the vaporous envelope
> of her veils she embodies, successively inquietude, melancholy,
> doubt, resignation, hope. Her face is like the surface of a lake
> where the ripples pass, like a mirror reflecting the rapid race of
> clouds.

Isadora to Irma, October 1, 1920: "Your letter has made me <u>Happy</u>—"

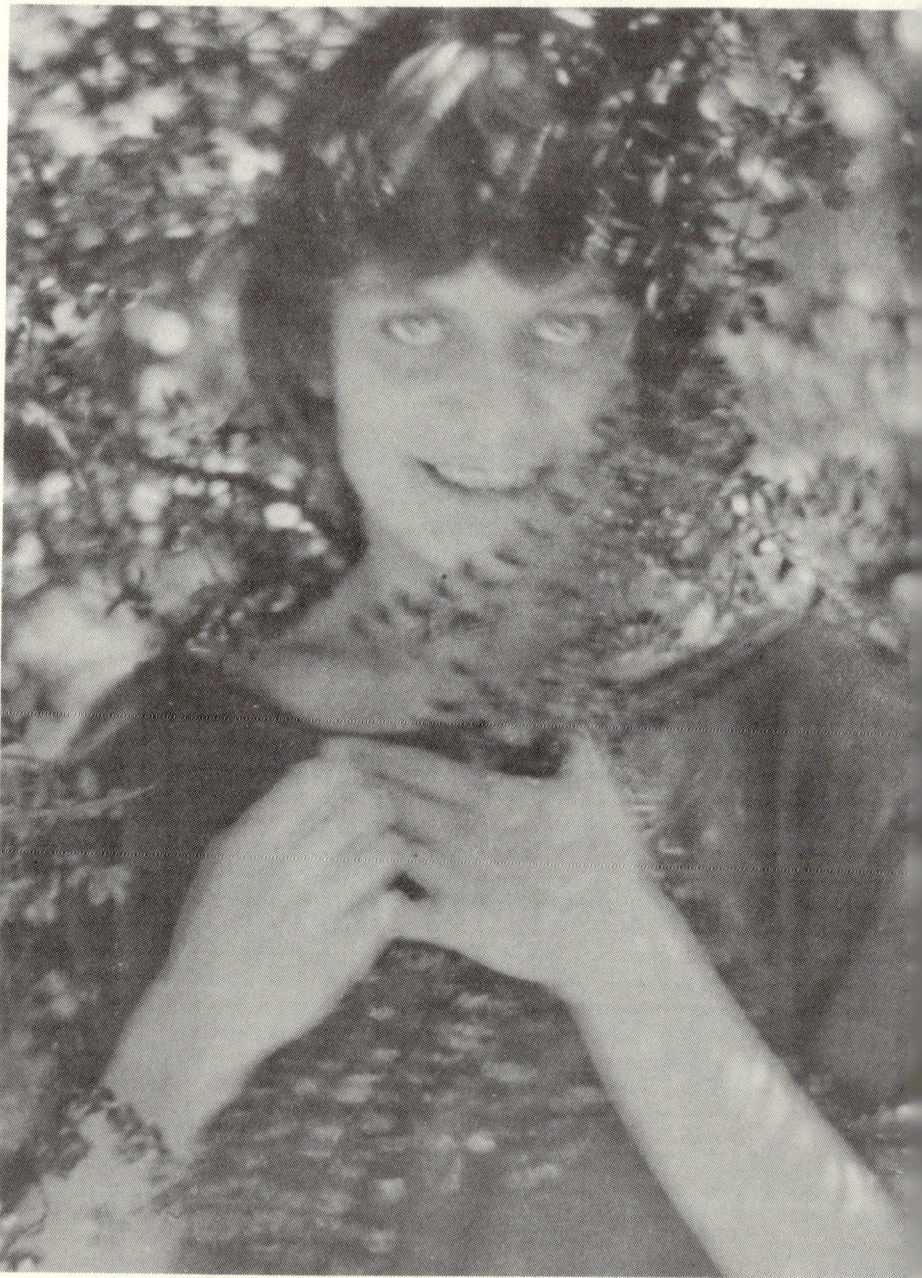

Irma Duncan: portrait photo by Edward Steichen, Versailles, 1920.
Inscribed: "Gay dancing eyes of the eager dancing faun girl. With a
vivat—Edward Steichen."

It is so beautiful that we do not applaud. Only our oppressed breaths reveal in the silence what our dumb enthusiasm bears of anguish.

Then she calls her pupils. There are only three, on this evening before departure, but it seems as though the Graces of Falconnet have left the pedestal where they have stood for more than a century. And these graces here have more than line; they have the charm of life. They come and go, dancing a rondo, while over them and about them floats the scarf with which Proudhon encircled the delicate face of Psyche.

It is incomparably charming, youthful and gay. Isadora leans over to me: "And if they were five hundred, if they were a thousand, don't you think that they would be lovelier still; don't you think that they would give the people something to rest them from their blackest care? For there will not only be us; my pupils will teach all the little ones. They will know how to dance as they know how to read: there will be joy for all!"

"And if you are hungry?" asks a sceptic.

Isadora shrugs her magnificent shoulders, and with an accent made grave by conviction: "We will dance so as not to think of it!"

O cricket! Delicious cricket that puts to shame the ants!

Isadora sublet her house on the Rue de la Pompe, and two days later we got our visas. I noted in my diary: "June 3, 1921. Leaving on the 4 o'clock train for Brussels. Poor little Gretel has to stay behind all by herself. I don't believe we girls shall ever live together again. Lisa, Theresa and myself are all that are left of the Duncan Dancers."

Isadora considered Margot (or Gretel as we called her) too frail to make the trip. The number of Isadora's disciples was rapidly dwindling. We gave several performances in the Belgian capital before proceeding to England. The London *Observer* wrote of our recital at Queen's Hall:

> Last night Isadora Duncan with her three pupils, Irma, Theresa and Lisa, appeared . . . in a Grand Festival of Music and Dance. But Dance is surely hardly the right word; what we

saw was Keats' Grecian Vase come to life—with some moving
tragedie added to its living grace. Tchaikovsky's Symphony
Pathetique teems with emotion—not pure musical emotion—but
emotion that can be expressed in bodily action and facial play. It
was very interesting to observe the interpretation of this by the
great artist and her three pupils.

The first movement she took alone and made it a wonderful
example of the beauty of slow motions . . . it became intensely
tragic rather than merely "pathetic" as indeed it should.

On the five-four movement that followed the younger artists
alone took the first section, the elder appearing and the younger
disappearing as the second and contrasting section began. (The
effect was perhaps that of Care driving away the Graces). . . .
In the Scherzo all were on the stage together. The last movement (the Lamentoso) Isadora Duncan alone . . .

The experience last night was a very interesting one, and as
the music was played exactly as in a fine concert performance,
one did not feel the objection that one does when one hears some
of these Chopin and Schumann ballets that have become so popular, where music is rhythmically and orchestrally sacrificed in
order that set forms of bodily movement and an arbitrary story
may be made of it. . . .

It was really in every way a great evening and one is amazed
that the hall should be half empty. Will it be full next Saturday?
This will be the last opportunity of seeing Isadora Duncan before she goes to her work in Russia—to return when?

Thirteen years had passed since we girls had last danced in
London in the Duke of York's Theatre. What childhood memories it brought back! The golden watch that turned out to be
pure brass; the famous luncheon party at the Duchess of Manchester's house, and the purloined peaches; dancing for the King
and Queen; and oh! my lost sovereign! We reminisced about
these things in our dressing room after the performance when,
lo and behold! who should suddenly open the door and walk in?
As if conjured up from the past by our talking about it, like
some specter of our childhood days, the tormentor we all loathed
and feared—our former English governess!

She stood there and silently looked at us, even as a serpent hypnotizes its prey. We stared back in stony silence, then we turned around and left. After all these years, she still personified the serpent in our childhood paradise.

That last performance in London spelled finis to Isadora's original school. Theresa and Lisa confided to me their fears and their resolve not to accompany Isadora to Soviet Russia. "What has gotten into her!" Theresa wailed. "Why, of all places, revolutionary Russia?"

"It must be perfectly awful there," Lisa chimed in. "The people are starving, disease is rampant, and they walk about in rags. At least, that is what the papers say. What sort of place is that for her to found a dance school in? I cannot understand her!"

"How shall I ever have the courage to tell her?" Theresa worried. "I know she is going to have a real fit when she hears we have decided not to go with her. It is going to be awful."

"Yes, please, Irma, be present when we tell her tomorrow morning," Lisa said. "You may be able to help us explain our reasons better than we can. I don't want her to think I am refusing my help, but I am willing to do anything she asks—except go to Russia. I am simply plain scared of the Bolshies—and that is the whole truth."

I sympathized with the girls and their reluctance to embark on so dangerous a mission. Few people in those days expressed a willingness to enter, much less live in a country where law and order as we knew it in the West had been completely abolished. The dictatorship of Lenin and Trotsky had created an unholy blood-bath in their unhappy country ever since the October Revolution four years earlier. Certainly it was no fit place for a group of young, sensitive girls, who were concerned for their immediate future. I agreed to support them in their dreaded interview with our foster mother.

It turned out exactly as we had feared: grand hysterics on her part and a flood of tears on theirs. "Ingrates," she called them. When they finally left her angry presence, pale and shaken, I turned to leave also, intending to see the girls off at the station. She called after me, "And you, Irma, are you also leaving me?"

I hastily assured her I had given her my solemn word and that I meant to keep it. She embraced me, visibly moved, and with tears in her eyes, softly whispered, "Thanks. You are all I now have left in this world."

That afternoon I saw the girls off, saying a sad farewell, since none of us knew when we would meet again. Theresa was planning to marry Stephan Bourgeois, and Lisa was planning an American tour with Anna and Margot. I returned to find Isadora in the midst of a gay party. Dressed in a French gown of lace over blue satin, she sat surrounded by English friends all imbibing champagne. The moment I entered somebody shouted facetiously, "Here comes the *school!*"

Everybody laughed and joined in nicknaming me "the School." Only Isadora remained serious. Into my mind flashed the silly game we children in Grunewald used to play with our identification numbers and I always proudly ended up with the best prize—number 16, the house number of our beloved Duncan School. And now I myself had to laugh, for here I was actually personifying it. At that instant, Isadora slowly rose from her couch and solemnly called for attention. In the silence that ensued she raised her glass and said, "I propose a toast to Irma." Everybody stood up and Isadora continued, "Here is to the school. God bless her!"

PART III. 1921–1933

❦14❧

Exile

BEFORE leaving London, I visited the British Museum. I wanted to have a look at the Elgin Marbles, especially the caryatid that was taken from the Erechtheion in Athens. What a sad sight it was to see that noble statue confined in a somber hall in an alien land of rain and mists and separated from her five companion figures, who still stood together in the open air, under an Attic sun, forever gazing out to the blue Aegean sea.

I could not help but commiserate with her unhappy lot. I too would soon be exiled to another alien, northern country, whose language had a strange sound that I could not understand.

Being more of a skeptic, I could not share Isadora's enthusiasm for Communist Russia. Her idea of what it represented was naïve in the extreme. As someone once remarked, "Good sense travels on the well-worn paths; genius never!"

In her idealized conception of Russia, Isadora envisioned a new Utopia where mankind lived in love, beauty, and harmony. What a rude awakening was in store for her!

"Life in Europe is passé," she would say. "It is too hopelessly bourgeois ever to understand what I really am after. Of course, I realize that present conditions in the Soviet Union are difficult for a regime in the throes of stabilizing itself. But it can't be as bad as the papers make out, or the Bolsheviks would not have sent this friendly invitation."

She had accepted the "friendly invitation," and now we were in for it; there was no turning back. Theresa had said to me on the day of parting, "Dear Irma, I wish you good luck, and I do hope you will find a little happiness. I really do not like to think of you being all forsaken and exposed to Isadora's caprices. But I know you'll get through all right and your temper won't permit anybody to abuse you. So farewell—and may the gods be with you!"

The day prior to our departure, Mrs. K. (a member of the Soviet Commission in London), taking pity on us and our impending adventure, took me aside and said, "Poor Isadora! She has no conception of what she has to face. It will be very hard for her. I don't want to discourage her, but I am warning you. You will all have a very difficult time."

July 12, 1921.
Went aboard the S.S. *Baltanic,* but are not sailing today. Very small boat but clean. Mary and Harle saw us off.

July 13.
Sailed at 9 o'clock in the morning for Reval. The weather is lovely, the sea is a bit rough. There are some nice passengers on board, and Miss Ruth Mitchell from New York is sailing with us.

July 16.
Having heaps of fun on board with some jolly new friends including the General. Playing Isadora's portable gramophone and dancing with the "Tiger Man." We arrived in Danzig at 10 P.M. It was very dark but mother waited for me on the dock. She appears to be the same. We motored into town with the General, Miss Mitchell, and others to have supper at the Danziger Hof. Danced to Viennese music. We spent the night at the hotel. Isadora and I shared a room.

Sunday, July 17.
This far north it remains dark for only a few hours. I got up early, drove back to the boat where I met mother at the dock. She returned with me to the Danziger Hof and we had breakfast together. Just then Isadora and Miss Mitchell left the dining room. When Miss M. asked Isadora, "Who is that woman Irma is with?" I heard her say, "That is Irma's mother." And turning to me said, "You know I love your dear old mother. I wouldn't cross the street with mine, but with yours—I could travel around

the world." [Isadora had been estranged from her mother for many years.] I told mother about this. Later we all drove back to the *Baltanic*. Brought mother home to the place she is staying at. Poor mother, I was so glad to have seen her again. We sailed in the afternoon. Though it was quite light at midnight, I slept soundly, being very tired.

I had written mother about my prospective trip to Russia and told her the boat would stop at Danzig. Despite the late hour, there were many people on the dock when we made fast, mostly stevedores and men whose business it was to unload the freight. I did not exactly expect mother to be there. I leaned against the railing on the upper deck and watched the scene, which was illuminated by a few dim lamps. Suddenly there was a slight commotion in back of the crowd, as of someone trying desperately to push her way through. It was a frail old lady dressed in black, holding onto her hat with one hand and holding up a huge bouquet of flowers with the other. At first I was not quite sure, but as she managed to push herself through the crowd toward the front I recognized mother. The gangplank had not yet been lowered, so she had no way of coming aboard. I was about to ask the captain for permission when the friendly stevedores, hearing she had come all the way from Hamburg to see her daughter off to Russia, made short shrift of the situation. Lifting her bodily up in the air, they passed her on to the sailors on deck, while she still clutched both her hat and bouquet. I led her away from the stares of the curious into my cabin.

Not having set eyes on each other for seven years (not since that day of my christening before the war), we naturally had much to talk about. The strange thing was that neither of us could find any words. We just sat and held hands and looked at each other for a long time. What really was there to say? Living on another continent, divided not only by the whole width of an ocean but also by a completely different mode of existence, and speaking a different language now, I had grown away from her to such an extent that we met as strangers. The war years and suffering had taken their toll of my mother. She had aged considerably since last I saw her. She too must have had difficulty recognizing her little girl—a child no longer. Her first words were to chide me for looking so thin and pale.

The next day, after the boat sailed and passed a narrow spit of land jutting out into the harbor, I was surprised to see a small figure dressed in black with a long white shawl across her shoulders, standing below the lighthouse. Through a pair of binoculars I recognized mother. As the boat slowly turned out to sea, she removed her white shawl and waved and waved. . . . I waved back, but she could not see me. No sooner did we meet than we parted again; it had been like that ever since I left home. Mother waved that scarf as long as the boat was visible. And I seemed to hear her say, sadly but hopefully, as when we said goodbye to each other, "*Auf Wiedersehen! Auf Wiedersehen!*"

July 19.

After dinner, at 8 o'clock, we anchored at Reval. A very picturesque town on a hill with many church steeples. Mrs. Litvinoff of the Soviet Embassy came to meet us. Isadora was disappointed to see only her and not a red automobile full of black-haired and black-eyed Bolshies. All our luggage was sealed for shipment to Moscow. They took us to headquarters where Mrs. Litvinoff, who speaks English and is the ambassador's wife, had put us up on cots in her husband's study. Isadora refused to stay there. "Let's return to the boat and get Ruth Mitchell and the General and have dinner in town," she said. Had vodka, crabs, and danced all night at Mon Repos, a nice restaurant by the sea. Spent the rest of the night on the boat in Ruthie's cabin.

July 20.

Next morning Isadora and I took a droshky to the hotel where we had a hot bath together, there being only enough hot water for one, and a hot breakfast. The General invited us to lunch. Lovely food—chicken salad, good cold beer, and fresh raspberries with sour cream. Walked through the town. The General very thoughtfully, in fear we would starve on our trip, had a food basket prepared as a goodbye present. I hated to see the little *Baltanic* sail off without us. Isadora hugged me and, smiling bravely, said, "Well, we are in for it now!" Leaving on the midnight train for Petrograd. Mrs. Litvinoff saw us off. Funny feeling to ride in a Russian train again. The same candlelight and firing the engine with wood I remember from my two previous visits.

July 21.
Stopped all day at Narva. We are now in Red Russia. They inspected our luggage but did not confiscate anything. Artists are exempt. Isadora went to the market, bought some flowers and raspberries, and we lunched from the General's basket in our compartment, which we share with a young man, a diplomatic courier. Went to the village and returned followed by a group of children who were curious to see some strangers. Isadora turned on her gramophone and made them dance on the platform. Then we gave them all the candy and fruit we had. Train finally got going again after midnight.

July 22.
We arrived at 10 in the morning at Petrograd, as it is now called, and were driven to headquarters, the former Hotel Astoria. We walked along the Nevsky Prospect. How changed everything is! The town appears dead and infinitely sad. Empty shop windows, but the people do not look starved, though they are all dressed in dirty rags. Glad to leave for Moscow.

Sunday, July 24.
At a snail's pace crawled into Moscow at 4 A.M. Nobody at the station to meet us. Took a cab and drove to the foreign office and who should we meet there? Our first Bolshevik, none other than Count Florinsky from Long Beach! What a joke! Elegantly dressed in dinner clothes, he had just come from a party. He invited us in to his rooms. Isadora and I couldn't stop laughing, it was really too funny.

Isadora noted in her memoirs:

> I went to Russia accompanied only by my pupil Irma and my faithful maid Jeanne. We had been told such terrible things that as the train passed the red flag at the frontier, we would not have been surprised if the pictured Bolshevik with red flannel shirt, black beard, and a knife between his teeth, had appeared to violate us all three and then cut our throats as an evening's amusement. We all confessed to some shiver of excitement. . . .
>
> Our first night at Moscow we left Jeanne in the one room available at the hotel, in the one bed, weeping hysterically because she had seen "des grands rats," and we spent the night (with the young man from the train), wandering about the mystically beautiful city of the many churches and golden domes. He talked, more and more inspired, of the future of communism, until dawn we were also ready to die for Lenin and the cause. Then some clouds blew up and it began to rain. Our guide seemed supremely indifferent to the wet and I also noticed now that we hadn't eaten anything for fourteen hours. I found, after meeting others, that a real Communist is indifferent to heat or cold or hunger or any material sufferings. As the early Christian martyrs, they live so entirely in ideas that they simply don't notice these things. But Irma and I were worn out; and so we tramped back to the train.

July 25.

We have been waiting all morning to hear from Tovarish Lunacharsky, who invited us here, but didn't get word till noon. They conducted us to Madame Geltzer's apartment. The well-known ballerina is away on a tour.

There we met Ilya Schneider, a journalist and an intimate friend of Ekaterina Geltzer. He wrote in his reminiscences:

> The telephone on my table rang, and Lunacharsky's secretary said that the NARKOM wanted to speak to me. Lunacharsky had reported the arrival of the famous dancer, Isadora Duncan, who wanted to give her labor and experience in the artistic education of children to Soviet Russia.
>
> "We expected Duncan in three days from now," Lunacharsky

said to me, "but she came unexpectedly yesterday and had to stay at a room in the Savoy Hotel, which, at the present time, is not at all well built, one can even say it's a wreck. While we are looking for other lodgings, couldn't we put her up for a while in Ekaterina Vasilyevna Geltzer's apartment who is away and has, so I hear, entrusted her apartment to you?"

I didn't doubt Geltzer would agree to this but nonetheless I asked permission to call back in a few minutes while I consulted with Geltzer's sister, the wife of Ivan Mikhailovich Moskvin. She of course agreed and I informed Lunacharsky about this.

"Please go to Geltzer's apartment," Lunacharsky replied, "settle her there and look after her for a while."

When I entered Geltzer's apartment . . . we were introduced. I asked our guest if she was satisfied with her quarters and how she felt. . . . Isadora, dissatisfied, frowned, but I couldn't understand why—maybe my German pronunciation was at fault—I thought. However, I found out later that her displeasure arose on account of my addressing her as "Miss Duncan." Despising all remnants of the world she had left, she wanted to be addressed as Comrade or Tovarish Duncan. . . .

In the first conversation that sprung up between us at the tea table Duncan told me that she saw the "Look of the new world" only in the expression of the faces and eyes of the Red Army men whom she saw marching in the streets. . . .

A young woman noiselessly entered the room.

"This is Irma—the only one of my pupils who has decided to come with me to Moscow," Isadora said. "You know, they frightened us with endless horrors which we would have to live through and see here."

A big, full-bosomed person flew headlong into the room, babbling quickly in French and making "big eyes" while clapping her hands together. This was Jeanne, her French maid without whom Duncan did not travel. It turned out that Duncan's baggage had arrived. I stepped out onto the balcony of Geltzer's apartment and saw below baskets and suitcases and trunks rising up like a tower on the cart. . . .

At the time of our talk, Jeanne was bustling about the table serving tea and unloading jars of jam and marmalade, chocolate bars, sponge cakes and small packages wrapped in oil paper which she noisily tore open. . . . I peered into the huge basket and saw that it was filled with bread.

"Why did you bring so much bread with you from behind the border?" I asked Duncan. She had no time to answer when Irma blurted out with a laugh, "We still have two more such baskets!"

Isadora indignantly explained that these small loaves of bread were dietary . . . she burst out laughing and said in her special German language in which she sprinkled French and sometimes English words, "They all insisted that we take a lot of bread with us since there isn't any in Russia."

At this point the bell rang. Lunacharsky made an appearance. I was not going to hinder their discussion (for they spoke French together) and left.

Lunacharsky commissioned Ilya Schneider to look after us for a while. This he did for the rest of the time we lived in Russia; first as interpreter, then as business manager of the Moscow school. He was a slim young man of medium height, with dark eyes and dark hair slicked back. We all became inseparable friends. Lunacharsky, Commissioner of Education, a cultured author and playwright, published an article shortly after his interview with Isadora, which he titled "Our Guest." The article is too long to be quoted in its entirety, but a few extracts may be of interest:

What end had she in coming to Russia? The main end was an educational one. She came to Russia with the approval of Narkompross and Narkomindel, who made her an offer to organize in this country a big school of a new type. . . . Duncan believed with all her soul that, in spite of the famine and the lack of necessities, in spite of the terrible seriousness of the moment and the consequent preoccupation of the government officials with other vital questions, a beginning of her idea could be made. . . . Her vision reaches far. She is thinking of a large government school with a thousand children. She is willing for the moment, however, to begin with a smaller number. They shall receive elementary education through our teachers. Their physical and aesthetic education shall be under Duncan's sole direction. . . .

At present Duncan is going through a phase of rather militant communism that sometimes makes us smile involuntarily. . . . In one instance she was asked by some of our Communist comrades to a small, one might say, family fete. She found it possible to call their attention to their bad Communist taste, because of the bourgeois surroundings and because of their behavior, which was so far from the flaming ideal she had painted in her imagination. It would have developed into a small scandal, if our comrades had not understood how much original charm was contained in the naïve criticism which was in substance true.

The People's Commissariat of Education greets Russia's guest and believes that, on the occasion of her first public appearance, the proletariat will confirm the greeting. Duncan has been called the Queen of Movement, but of all her movements, this last one—her coming to Red Russia in spite of being scared off—is the most beautiful and demands the greatest applause.

When Isadora and I arrived in Moscow during the third year of the Red Revolution, we were the first foreign women, except for Anne Sheridan, to come to that country since the uprising in 1918. The rest of the civilized world trembled to come near it. America, and most Western nations, had not yet recognized the new regime under Lenin and Trotsky. Lenin, the father of the Bolshevik Revolution, once advocated that all the streets should be paved with gold, for as a means of exchange that metal would be made obsolete. We found the streets littered with every conceivable object *but* gold. Money in any kind of currency was out of circulation, throwing the whole economy into chaos. Everything could be had free—if it was available. In this short period of practical communism, people received sustenance and other commodities necessary to their existence according to their individual needs. Wherever one looked, one saw endless lines of people queuing up for food. We, too, were put on rations, or *paiok* as they called it for artists. Once a fortnight Jeanne went with her big market basket to the distributing center in the Kremlin to collect the rations consisting of white flour, pressed caviar, tea, sugar, and potatoes. For the rest of that first year we lived chiefly on potatoes, a diet we shared with all those lucky enough to obtain them, for elsewhere—outside of Moscow—a terrible famine raged. The famine would have caused a national disaster but for the food distributed from America through the Hoover Commission.

Most of the month of August we spent in the country in a small *isba*, or peasant's cottage, fashioned of rough-hewn logs. Living simply off the land, drinking goat's milk and eating goat's cheese, we waited patiently for the government to find a suitable house for the school.

At last, on August 23, two carriages drove us and our luggage back to town. They stopped in front of No. 20 Pretchistenka, formerly a fashionable street running from the Cathedral of the Savior, visible from afar, to the Zoubovsky Boulevard. We entered a house of palatial proportions done in the rococo style. It had belonged to Ushkoff, a wealthy tea-plantation owner, whose wife, Alexandra Balashova, had been a leading member of the Bolshoi Ballet. She had only recently fled the country.

One entered by a rather small door—small, that is, in relation to the immensity of the building—from Pretchistenka and came upon a terra-cotta-tinted Pompeiian room that had four marble columns and marble benches, whose backs were decorated with bas-reliefs of nymphs and satyrs. In a niche stood a marble statue of the goddess Venus. From this vestibule, one ascended by a broad white marble stairway to the grand hall. This hall had tapestries affixed to its four walls and a ceiling painted with murals depicting scenes from Greek mythology.

The upstairs rooms were decorated in a surprising variety of styles. There was the Empire room, the Louis XV boudoir, the oak-paneled Gothic dining room, the Turkish smoking room that led into a winter garden, and so on—but there was only one bathroom. Isadora installed herself in the master bedroom, which was decorated with every conceivable Napoleonic emblem from bees to swans in red and gold. I occupied the Louis XV boudoir next door, and we shared the bathroom between.

Of course all these elaborately decorated rooms were completely denuded of furniture. The last official occupant, Bela Kun, had filched everything including the bric-a-brac; he had even stripped the silk damask off the walls. The only fixtures remaining in my room, apart from the large marble fireplace (which was a comfort to me during the arctic winters), consisted of a tall mirror in an elaborate gold frame over a rosewood and ormolu commode, and the delicately constructed Saxe china chandeliers. My bed stood on a raised dais, enclosed by a gilded wooden balustrade, in one corner of the former boudoir. Two large double windows opposite opened onto the spacious courtyard, enclosed by additional wings of the house.

This private sanctum was home to me all the years I lived in Moscow.

On the third of December we officially opened the school with twenty-five children especially chosen for their dancing talents. Often in the beginning the dance room could not be heated, and classes had to be canceled. Frequently we went hungry. But the enthusiastic little pupils clamored for their lessons, and we taught them to dance "so as not to think of it," as Isadora had prophesied to Madame Sartoris.

The government had originally intended to settle us in the warm south, the Crimea, where the Tsar's old summer palace could easily accommodate a thousand children. For that reason, we had come to Russia without sufficient warm clothing. As the days began to get more sharply cold, we began to wonder about the winter when temperatures sink below zero. An official suggested we go to the fur storage warehouse and there choose garments for ourselves. He obtained a written order, and in great excitement Isadora and I set out for the warehouse. "We must be like the other working people," Isadora said. She had admired the sheepskin coats—or *shubas*—the peasants wore into town on market days, and suggested we get similar ones. However, that was not my idea of a proper fur coat.

At the warehouse we saw rows on rows of magnificent furs of every description—enough to make one's head reel. I quickly whispered to my foster mother, "Don't take anything but Russian sable!"

Isadora looked shocked. She picked the most modest specimens she could find. For herself she chose a long mink coat lined with ermine and for me a mink coat with a sable collar. With these over our arms, we marched out of the warehouse. But guards stopped us at the door, explaining that we had to leave the coats until they could be properly evaluated.

A week passed without any sign of the fur coats arriving at Pretchistenka. When we called up the warehouse, we were informed of the fantastic price we had to pay. Simply out of the question, we could not afford them. I turned to Isadora. "You see! You should have let me have my wish. I would at least have owned a sable coat once in my life, even if only for a week!"

She laughed and told me to have patience, that I would eventually receive a fur coat. For Christmas she presented me with a nice coat of silver-gray squirrel to keep me from freezing to death in that arctic climate.

The fourth anniversary of the Russian Revolution was to be celebrated on the seventh of November, 1921. Lunacharsky asked Isadora if she would dance at the gala performance at the Bolshoi Theatre. All the tickets were to be distributed free to the various workers' organizations and the Red Army. She accepted the honor with pleasure and decided to dance Tchaikovsky's Sixth Symphony and his "Marche Slav." Interwoven in the composition of the "Marche Slav" are several bars of the Tsarist Hymn. Several officials objected to her dancing to that music, fearing it might call forth a counter-revolutionary demonstration among some of the people. Their fear was completely unfounded. They had not seen Isadora's interpretation of the theme and did not know that she used the Tsarist Hymn motif to express the utter oppression of the masses beaten down by the knout. Her dancing and miming of the "Marche Slav" had a tremendous impact on the audience. It was a magnificent performance, not in the least "pretty"—which may be the reason people schooled in ballet found it shocking—but its stark power was obvious to everyone else. A critic wrote in *Isvestia* the next day:

> Isadora Duncan depicted in moving gestures a bent, oppressed, burdened, fettered slave, who falls exhausted to his knees. Now see what happens to this slave at the first notes of the accursed Tsarist Hymn. He lifts his weighed-down head, and his face shows an awful grimace of hate. With all his force he straightens himself and breaks his chains. Then he brings from behind his back his crooked and stiffened arms—forward to a new and joyful life. The allegory was understood by everyone. . . .
>
> The thrill of the evening came when after the emotion of the "Marche Slav" calmed, the orchestra began to play the "Internationale," and Isadora moved to the center of the stage, draped in red . . . when the dancer had mimed the first stanza, the singing audience, standing up, saw Irma come from the side of the stage leading by the hand a little child, who was followed by another and another—a hundred little children in red tunics, each with the right hand held high, clasping fraternally the left hand of the one before, moving against the blue curtains, forming a vivid, living frieze, and then circling the vast stage and surrounding, with childish arms outstretched toward the light, the noble, undaunted, and radiant figure of their great teacher.

The allegory was understood by everyone, the reviewer said, all, that is, except the confraternity of the Russian Ballet whose sole concept of the kinetic art represents the PRETTY dance. Of course Isadora's March Slav was not meant to be pretty, on the contrary. But that did not seem to penetrate their limited understanding of what the true art of the dance should represent in all its multiple facets. Isadora Duncan's individualistic approach to the dance was apparently entirely incomprehensible to their narrow, drilled-in conformity of thinking. Since then, some leaders of the Russian Ballet have publicly voiced their total incomprehension in really quite vulgar and stupid criticism of her unique art, obviously motivated by envy because of their own lack of creative originality.

Isadora's grand scheme of founding a free school supported by a generous government slowly began to disintegrate. Financial assistance was not forthcoming. The spacious building was about the only thing the government provided free of cost to further the work for which Isadora Duncan came to Soviet Russia. Lenin, the ruler of Red Russia, being above all a realist, found it necessary to abolish War Communism in order to put his country on its financial feet again. In December of 1921, he inaugurated the New Economic Policy, called NEP. A money system was re-established, standardizing the ruble on a gold basis, and workers again became wage-earners.

Lunacharsky himself came to Pretchistenka to inform us of these important matters and to tell us that the serious financial crisis made it impossible for the government to support the school. Isadora's idealism was blown sky high. She was right back where she started—saddled with the enormous upkeep of the newly installed school housing more than fifty people. As of old, she saw herself once more forced to give paying performances in order to support her idealistic enterprise. "*Plus ça change, plus c'est la même chose.*"

At this moment in the history of her school, Isadora met the young Russian poet Sergei Essenine, to whom she was married in May of the following year. From that time, she became more and more restless in Moscow. She felt that she must leave Russia. This was necessary for the simple reason that she needed desperately to replenish her private coffers. She asked me to go with her. "You know yourself that there is no future here for us and our idea," she confided to me while in a discouraged mood. "Come with me to America, half of everything I have

is yours." But she quickly added, jokingly, "Half of everything
—but my husband!"

I advised her not to take her husband to either Western
Europe or America, foreseeing nothing but disaster, for he was
a neurotic man, not the type to be suddenly uprooted from his
familiar environment. She would not listen to me, and I certainly wanted no part of that mad ménage. I much preferred to
stay in Russia. Besides, what about the children? The thought
of sending them back to their miserable homes after they had
become used to the school (and loved it) was more than I
could bear. Remembering my own childhood and what dancing
with Isadora meant to me, I had not the heart to forsake them
now. And so I stayed, come what might, for better or for worse;
resolved to do my utmost to make this thing I helped to start
a success.

Before leaving, Isadora handed me a check for a hundred
dollars. "That is all I can spare," she said, "but I shall send
more from America."

The trouble was that these one hundred dollars did not last
very long. So when they were gone, here I was, in my early,
hopeful twenties; left stranded in a strange, forbidding land
without a kopek to my name. What would the future bring?

❧15❧

Little Dividend

To celebrate the official opening of the Moscow school, some friends had invited Isadora and myself to a night club. Situated in the basement of an apartment house, it was the only *sub rosa* night club in town. Being foreigners, we always created a mild sensation wherever we went. The populace would approach as close as they could and silently stare at us, as if seeing creatures from another planet. As a celebrity, Isadora was given the red-carpet treatment at the night club. When the master of ceremonies saw her seated at a ringside table with her entourage, he focused the spotlight on her. Then he made a little introductory speech to the assembled guests. In an allusion to Balashova's secret flight from Red Russia and Isadora's candid arrival, he said, "Now that the New Economic Policy is in force, our government has recently made a very smart deal by exchanging worthless Russian rubles for valuable American *valiuta*. Comrades, I have the great honor of introducing Isadora Duncan!"

When the applause died down, he continued, "It appears they obtained not only valuable American *valiuta*—but even a little dividend!"

The little dividend was me. Would this dividend, reinvested, bring forth a goodly sum some day? That was the question. Confronted with the biggest challenge of my career so far, I asked myself whether I really had it in me to make good. Isadora had left me in charge of the artistic direction of the Moscow institution. But I must explain that without Ilya Schneider's clever business administration and the devoted help of the other co-workers associated with me in this difficult venture, I could not have achieved what I did.

Let no one imagine that it was an easy matter to earn a living in those lean early years of Revolutionary Russia. Apart from my free room and keep, I received no salary. Any money I could possibly hope to earn would have to come from paid performances. Up to this point I had appeared only as a member of a group. Would the general public care to see me dance alone? At one of her own recitals, Isadora had once introduced me at the end to the public, who gave me a few cheers. That was all. Except for leading the pupils onto the stage in the "Internationale" as a sort of grande finale, I was not permitted to dance. I therefore decided it would be of importance for my future work in Russia that I should show the people what I could do, both as dancer and as teacher. To achieve this, I forced myself to cultivate patience and to concentrate on working hard for a whole year with the most talented of my pupils. In Russia I had done all the teaching because Isadora never instructed beginners. Every so often she would show them a gesture, but nothing else. I had no doubt whatever that I would attain good results. Here is where my practical experience in developing my own method of teaching in Darmstadt proved to be of great help. And, more important, my foster mother fully endorsed it, for Isadora herself once said, "I have watched you work. You never speak about it. You just quietly go in there to teach every day for an hour or so, and the next time I see the children—they can dance!" Her saying this gave me hope and bolstered my courage in pursuing my goal.

To increase my effectiveness as a teacher, I had to study Russian. Luckily I pick up foreign languages easily. By the end of my third year in the Soviet Union, I spoke and read this difficult language fluently. My knowledge of German and the Greek alphabet were helpful in getting me started. Being able to converse freely furthered my acquaintance with the Russian people, whom I came to understand and know more intimately than do most foreigners.

A month after my foster mother left, I received a letter from her, from Wiesbaden, Germany:

Dear Irma—
I have been expecting every day to leave for London, and passports each day delayed. Therefore I telegraphed you three times but waited to write from London. We are so tired with all the waiting that we have come here to rest and recuperate. London performances are all arranged . . . only the waiting on account of formalities.

Berlin is very quiet and dull—was delighted to leave it. The house in Grunewald was lost through the war, etc. The lawyer handed me the absurd sum of 90,000 inflation marks for it. All my moneys, properties, etc., in Paris were attached so we have nothing but difficulties. Therefore I could not send you money from Berlin. Hope everything can be cleared up soon. I am enclosing check of ten pounds as experiment; if you succeed in cashing it I can send you others. To send money through bank is impossible.

From then on, I received no further funds from her. Nor did I hear from her again till she returned to Russia a year later. That summer and the following winter, I lived on the simple fare the school provided, with an occasional dinner out with friends; while my foster mother toured the States. All my efforts were concentrated on my forthcoming debut as a solo performer in Moscow.

In the spring of 1923, on the twenty-ninth of April, I made my debut with a group of my little pupils at a Sunday matinee. It took place in the Comedia, the former Korsh Theatre, situated on the Petrovka in the center of Moscow. What a lovely, sunny day! Driving to the theatre in the morning in an open carriage for this important event in my career, I thought of Isadora, and how she must have felt once. Was she as proud then as I felt now—on that date in July in 1905 when she

showed off her pupils for the first time to the public? I remember what a thrill I experienced seeing the elegant cream-colored
posters with my name spelled in Russian in huge gold letters,
splashed on the walls all over town. Pierre Luboshutz, a well-
known Russian pianist, played for us. What can I say about the
artistic merit of my debut? Let the reviewer speak:

> Anyone who sees this performance for the first time can imme-
> diately appreciate its enormous value in an artistic and educa-
> tional sense. It has immense public significance. What strikes one
> above all is the extraordinary physical control of the dancers.
> Irma Duncan, herself, is a very distinguished artist. She trans-
> mits the interpretation of this dance of the future with great
> ease and is besides full of temperament. She has a wonderful way
> of using her draperies to excellent effect. She danced Schubert's
> "Marche Militaire" beautifully, and with great skill manipulated
> a big silken scarf that floated in the wind. Irma is the light, love,
> and animating flame of her encircling young students.
> The strong, healthy, uncomplicated art of the young dancers,
> and the splendid mastery of Irma Duncan herself, harmonize
> with the problems of our modern age. We are very glad that
> the Duncan Dancers came here and we recommend to everyone
> who has the means to invest a poltinik [fifty kopeks] to go and
> see them dance.

Two weeks later we danced in Leningrad. It amused me to
see how the history of the school repeated itself when I led my
little group to the station on our first tour. Each girl carried
her own little suitcase filled with dance tunics. Remembering
my childhood as a fledgling dancer and the discipline admin-
istered to me, I saw to it that a more enlightened attitude prevailed while I was in charge. Every problem was explained to
the children intelligently, and they gave me their whole-hearted
cooperation without anyone's needing to take drastic disciplinary
measures. My main concern for these citizens of an autocratic
dictatorship was for them to grow up and develop in a congenial,
friendly atmosphere, free of too much restraint. The first Rus-

sian word I used when teaching them to dance was *svoboda*—freedom. Freedom in movement and in expression and—most important—freedom of thought. They understood, and gave me their love and devotion in return for my genuine interest in their welfare. They always called me "Irmushka."

Though postal communications between Russia and the outside world were extremely uncertain, I nevertheless sent pictures, articles, programs, and posters to my former colleagues to inform them of my work. I knew they would be interested to find out how the Moscow school was progressing. The three of them—Anna, Lisa, and Margot—planned a tour through the United States in the fall.

Lisa told me later that she had attended Isadora's all-Wagner program on July 3—quite marvelous, though it contained two numbers she had never rehearsed. The "Bacchanale," Lisa said, had been wilder than ever—"as though Hell itself had entered on scene." Isadora had also spoken to the audience—in the dark, for the police had turned out the lights—saying she was going back to Moscow because *"la bourgeoisie m'a tuée."*

Lisa added that Essenine had received some Russian papers, in one of which was a long and enthusiastic article about me and my work. Reading it, he screamed at Isadora with all the malice of which he was capable, "Oh, Irma *bolshoi* success! Bravo Irma!" But Isadora made no reply.

At about that time I received a letter from Anna. She had recently come out of an unhappy experience, which made her look at the world with bitterness and melancholy. She wrote:

> Paris, 6 Avenue Montaigne
> June 11, 1923
>
> My dearest Irma:
>   Although I did not write to you, dear, I often think of you and we frequently speak of you. Especially since we received your nice letter and you told of your plucky work and doings. I certainly am more than astonished and admire you for what you have accomplished with the school and what you call so cutely "My

children." My heartiest congratulations and good wishes, dear, for your own future as well as that of the school.

I need not tell you of many things Lisa wrote you already. It is a great tragedy that is now passing with Isadora and I think the final curtain will come soon. Alas, the best intentions of the already so few friends cannot bring help, unfortunately. She was wonderful at her two performances and if only she would just do that—live for her work and dance as only she of all people in the world knows how.

We are struggling to go on with what she gave us, in spite of her. And I hope we shall be able to do as much and more than we did last time in America, when we return in the autumn. Dear, it would be lovely to go and spend the summer with you as you suggest, but of course you know the reasons . . . you will perhaps understand me, Irma dear, but I am another person in my inner self. And I am only trying to do what I can to continue with our own work as long as it is still good and strong enough.

Go on, dear Irma, you have found a great hold in your new work, and I admire you for it. All the luck in the world—and take much love from your always affectionate, old friend,

Anna

That summer in Moscow, Comrade Podvowsky, the Minister of Sports and Physical Culture, taking due note of my successful appearances with my pupils, told me, "What a wonderful thing it would be if you could make this fine work available to many more children of our working population—to all those thousands of boys and girls who cannot leave the hot and dusty city in the summertime. It would be a real boon to them to have some outdoor activity for their benefit and pleasure."

He promised to place the big sports arena, an open-air stadium just outside Moscow, at our disposal. Willing to try this experiment in mass teaching, we put an advertisement in the papers, offering free lessons. The response was tremendous! It seemed as if all the children in town wanted to dance. Podvowsky supplied a brass band. With the musicians leading us and with my own pupils setting the pace, we carried a banner with the slogan of our school emblazed in crimson letters on white—"A free spirit in a healthy body"—as we proceeded from the Pretchistenka to the stadium. A steadily mounting crowd of children dressed in short red tunics and bare feet, waiting to join us at each street corner, swelled the ranks of our parade.

With the assistance of my young pupils, I taught five hundred children the entire summer long. It was an inspiring sight to see them all dancing together—"like a field of red poppies swaying in the wind," as Isadora said when she saw them. They made immense progress in so short a time. The Communist officials took notice, and Lunacharsky wrote an article in *Isvestzia,* saying:

> The Duncan School, conducting important work with hundreds of Moscow workers' children, presents one of the priceless and interesting artistic-educational institutions of the U.S.S.R. The students of the Duncan School, renouncing their own summer vacation under the guidance and direction of Irma Duncan, conducted throughout the summer open classes in the sports arena of the Red Stadium. This occupation gave brilliant results. The children, who looked weak and timid, soon became healthy, tanned and literally reborn.
>
> The Duncan School itself was created under immense difficulties. But today I read with pleasure the delighted opinions of the central press about the work they are doing. Recognizing for the Duncan School extraordinary significance and an enormous future in the matter of harmonic development of a new generation in Soviet Russia, the workers count it extremely desirable and necessary to send large groups of their own children to the school.

Other and equally appreciative articles appeared in the press, many with pictures showing the children in action. All this publicity could not escape the top leaders in the Kremlin, though Lenin himself—popularly called "Ilyich"—was living in the country, recuperating from a severe illness. The entire Duncan School was taken completely by surprise one day when a car drove up with a couple of military men in uniform and a little girl, holding a large bouquet of flowers in her hands. The little girl, in Pioneer uniform, held out the bouquet and made a little speech: "These flowers are from Ilyich for Duncan with his compliments." "From Vladimir Ilyich?" we inquired incredulously, "You mean Tovarish Lenin?" "Yes, he picked them this morning in his garden and told me to present them."

Since Isadora was not there, I accepted them with thanks. "Is there a card with them?" I inquired. "No," retorted the little Pioneer, whose father was military aide to Russia's ruler. "Only his good wishes for the wonderful work the Duncan school is doing."

I placed Lenin's flowers, such as grow in any man's garden, in cool water in a crystal vase on the mantel in my room. During the long ride from his *dacha* in the country they had wilted a bit in the open car under a noonday sun. I hoped they would revive. But like the great man who had sent them, they did not last long. Six months later he too faded away, to lie embalmed forever in Red Square under the Kremlin wall, worshiped by the masses as a god.

The highest award in Soviet Russia is the Order of Lenin. After his death, everyone in our school felt proud that our work had been given this lovely award on the order of Lenin himself.

Somehow this seemed to crown my own efforts with success. It does not appear unduly boastful, I hope, if I confess to having felt a thrill of real accomplishment. For the benefit of all those children who profited from it, the "Little Dividend" had at last turned into a worth-while investment indeed.

❧16❧

A Last Visit

"LENIN is dead!"

I can still hear these words spoken when my train stopped at the frontier the day he died. My instant reaction was that maybe now, with the great leader of the Communist Revolution gone, the unfortunate Russian people could anticipate a more liberal regime. Alas, history has shown that the next ruler turned out to be even more of a despot than Lenin had been.

I recalled the early days of our coming to Soviet Russia. When, stirred by a wild enthusiasm for the new idea that was born here, Isadora who then saw everything through red colored glasses, as it were—cried out, "Isn't communism wonderful!" And I, politically every bit as ignorant as she though not as gullible, cried out in disgust with the unrealism of this new ideology, so incompatible with my own common sense, "Communism is the bunk!"

"How can you say that," she protested, "when all the theatres and concerts are free for the common people to attend? That is something I have always dreamed of!"

"That is exactly what I mean," I retorted, "when I maintain communism makes no sense. Everything is free—but the people!"

I was definitely not receptive to my new environment. I steadfastly refused to share my foster mother's vision of a contented proletariat, happily building a new life for themselves. Or, as she expressed it in an article she wrote at the time for *L'Humanité:* "All men will be brothers carried away by the great wave of liberation that has just been born here. . . . The prophecies of Beethoven, Nietzsche and Walt Whitman, are being realized."

As I look back now, I recall the utter sense of boredom with which I contemplated living among the Bolsheviks. In my eager youth, I expected a finer life than this to be my lot. Impatience to be gone and to return to the civilized existence I had led before was a feeling I had to suppress. I thus started out to fulfill my mission in Russia in a state of utter mental depression of which I never spoke to Isadora.

In my effort to keep the establishment functioning during Isadora's absence of more than a year, I had exerted myself too much and I was not accustomed to such a meagre, unbalanced diet. The strenuous physical work and deprivations had undermined my health. Never very robust, with a delicate nervous system, I lost so much weight that I was a mere shadow. Nightmares kept me awake at night, and the many worries and frustrations upset my metabolism, so that I suffered from a severe stomach ailment. The doctor prescribed a special diet and ordered me under the care of a nurse. It so happened that the mother of one of the pupils, Elisaveta Gregorievna Mysovsky, was a registered nurse. During the First World War she had been stationed at the military hospital in Tula, under the direction of Grand Duchess Maria Pavlovna. She cared for me day and night.

At this time, my foster mother returned from America. Seeing how my health had suffered while she was away, she suggested I come with her to the south for a cure. To start out, we headed for the Caucasus where in Kislavodsk—a watering place as famous as Vichy in France—I took the baths in sparkling Narzan waters. To replenish her coffers, Isadora decided to give performances while I acted as her helper backstage. It was there that I had the famous fight with the two armed Tcheka men when they tried to stop her from dancing the "Marche Slav" because of the Tsarist Hymn. While Isadora stepped in front of the curtain and notified the audience that members of the police had come backstage to arrest her, I forcibly pushed the armed and uniformed Tcheka men (forerunners of the dreaded GPU) off the sacred blue dance carpet, not knowing how close I came to being shot for doing so. Only because the president of the local political bureau happened to be in the audience, we got off scot free, and Isadora received permission to proceed with her program as planned.

After that episode, she felt it might be better and safer for us to move further afield. That summer of 1923, we went on to Baku, the famous oil city on the shores of the Caspian Sea. From there we continued our journey to Tiflis. I loved this beautiful old Georgian capital—the wonderful hot sulphur baths and daily massage, the excellent wines, and the excursions in the mountainous countryside way up to Mount Elbrus. There was a nice little restaurant, overhanging the wildly rushing river Kura, that we liked to visit in the evenings. There, over a bottle of Zinandaly, with shashlik, we enjoyed listening to the orchestra playing native music on native instruments and watching the Georgian dances.

The Caucasian tour ended at Batum of the Black Sea, which lay blistering under the scorching heat of the last days of August. The government placed a beautiful little villa high up on a cliff at our disposal. In this same villa Trotsky had lived during his stay at the Black Sea port. And before the Revolution it had been the property of a wealthy Frenchman, who had planted the garden with a magnificent profusion of European and tropical flowers. Unfortunately the rainy season began to spoil our sojourn, and we proceeded to Yalta in the Crimea.

We resumed life at the Pretchistenka school early in October. Separated from her mad poet husband, Isadora got down to serious work with the pupils. Though the memorable trip to the south of Russia—where living seemed easier and pleasanter for both visitors and population alike—had restored my strength sufficiently for me to continue my classes, it had not helped me get rid of my mental depression. After two and a half years of Russian exile, what I needed most was to get away from it all. Like a caged bird, I desperately needed to escape, spread my wings, and inhale for a while the heady air of freedom. With some of the money I had saved from my performances, I decided to take a long vacation by myself.

I left in January, via Warsaw, for Berlin. In my hurry to make contact with the outside world after my exile, I rushed into the station buffet at the Polish frontier, not merely to eat but to buy up all the newspapers and magazines that were unobtainable inside Soviet Russia and that I had missed so much.

I stayed in Berlin just long enough to give a performance in the Bluethner Saal. The real goal of my vacation was my favorite big city—Paris. Before leaving for the French capital, I decided to go to Hamburg for a visit with mother. I was now in a much happier frame of mind. Ever since the train bearing me westward had crossed the Red frontier into Poland, my spirit experienced a wonderful lift, almost as if some oppressive physical weight had been lifted from my shoulders. I believe a similar sensation was experienced by every foreign visitor to the USSR during those years when the dreaded GPU, knocking on the door in the middle of the night, spread cold terror into the hearts of the people. Unless one has lived in an atmosphere of this kind, one does not really appreciate the meaning of the word *freedom*.

I arrived in the town of my birth in the last week of February. The train had been delayed because of a heavy snowfall. Over the door of mother's apartment, which she shared with my half-sister, hung a garland of evergreens; in the center was a big "Welcome" sign. "How late you are! Mother has been frantic!" my sister greeted me exactly as if she had seen me the day before, rather than thirteen years ago. A family gathering greeted me joyously when I entered the sitting room. They had been waiting for me with coffee and cakes since early afternoon.

The old familiar mahogany table presented a pretty picture with the lace cloth, a vase of roses and carnations in the center, and mother's best white, black, and gold china.

The tall green-tiled stove in the corner gave off a pleasant warmth. Every now and then someone would put a little more wood on the fire, for the snow continued to fall and the night grew colder. But in the *gute Stube* we made ourselves cozy, enjoying a late supper in the Hamburg manner with cold cuts, smoked fish, dark and white bread, and beer. This evoked childhood memories.

That night I lay down under a mountain of goosedown covers in the old mahogany bed where I was born and my father had died. For an instant I had the strange sensation that I had never left home. There was the same light from a street lamp, filtering through the lace curtains, sketching a soft pattern on the ceiling, that I had seen as a child before going to sleep. Although this was a different apartment from the one I knew in childhood—much more modern, less gloomy, and in a more attractive section of town, on a street called Pappelallee—nothing important had really changed. Only I had changed. For me this represented the old, narrow horizon. Like a visitor from a distant star, I could never feel at home in this small world again.

I tossed about thinking of these things in a restless state of mind, unable to sleep, when mother whispered to me, "Irma, my child, are you still awake?" And I answered as of old, "Yes, Mama."

In my mind's eye mother had not changed a bit since my childhood days, except that her hair was now snowy white. She had given birth to me at the age of forty-five, and I had no recollection of her as a young woman. She had always been my dear old mother. Seeing I lay awake, she raised her voice.

"You know what I was thinking? Tomorrow is your birthday and . . . and . . . this is something I have never told you. But when you were born, I suffered such pain. I had no doctor, only a midwife, and that dreadful pain lasted through the night. I thought I would not be able to stand it longer when—just as the sun was rising and cast a reddish glow over the room—you were born. And oh, my Irma, how happy I felt to hold you in my arms!"

In the dark room, lying in the bed beside me, she reached over and grasped my hand. I heard her wail as if still in labor, "My child, if I had only known! Oh God! If I had only known I would see so little of you in my life—I would have never let you go!"

And then I knew. In that heart-rending cry lay mother's tragedy. And there was nothing in the world I could do about it.

The few weeks I spent with mother passed swiftly and pleasantly for both of us. I left her in a cheerful frame of mind. We made plans for taking a trip together next summer during my vacation. Now that I could earn my own living, I could lend her a little financial support. I asked her, "Where would you most like to go?" She said, "As long as I can remember, I have always wanted to sail down the Rhine. Do you think we could really make that journey together? That would be so wonderful! At the same time we could visit my brother Ehrich, the uncle you have never seen, in München-Gladbach." I assured her that she could plan for this trip next summer even if, for some reason, I would be unable to join her.

The day of my departure for Paris, the train was delayed for an hour. She saw me off, and we repaired to the station buffet for a cup of coffee. She continued to chat animatedly about the coming event that would fulfill a lifelong wish. Then, inevitably, the moment came to say goodbye. It was that same station where so long ago in the winter of 1905, we had said goodbye. And suddenly when I heard the shrill blast of the train whistle it all came back to my mind so poignantly; how she had clung to my hand walking to the end of the platform and then watched the train depart with tears streaming down her face. And now I had a sudden terrible premonition that this was our last farewell.

Before the train started to move, mother turned away and holding on to the bannister groped her way slowly up the steps. I watched her black-clad figure until it was gone and then I collapsed in my compartment overcome with sobs I could not control.

Several days later, in Paris, I received a letter from her:

My dear, dear Irma:

I got your telegram in the evening and I am glad that you arrived safely. After all the excitement of departure and the long trip, you must have been very tired. I too quickly drove home and went to bed and stayed there for a few days' rest. Yesterday, Friday, Marie and I rearranged the rooms and were delighted how inviting the new furniture looks. And I regretted that you, the generous donor, could not be there to see it.

I hope that you enjoyed your stay with me and that everything made a favorable impression on you, dear. I wanted so much to make things even more *gemütlich* and pleasant but with all the visiting back and forth and the awfully cold weather it would have been too much of an exertion for me. Next time you come for a visit with us we shall pass quieter and happier hours by ourselves.

Everybody here at home sends their best wishes for a pleasant trip back to Moscow. I wish you all the luck and good health. Please give my regards to Isadora and greetings to all the dear children of your school. The photos we took, unfortunately, did not come out; only one of me, too bad. I wanted so much to have a picture of us together. Happy journey, dear Irma, and a thousand kisses from your loving

                                        Mama

The journey down the Rhine we planned together could not be realized. My work in Russia kept me tied down and too busy to join her. But she and my half-sister Marie visited with the relatives for a month or more. She wrote me from München-Gladbach:

> We have been most hospitably received here by our relatives. They have shown us a lot of the town and its surroundings. The many industries, the tri-centenary festival, fairs, parades, etc. Also they have here a beautiful theatre with a big restaurant situated in a park among a parterre of roses. You ought to give a performance there sometime and show the townspeople what real dancing is! They simply have no conception of it.
>
> We also visited Düsseldorf and saw the "Gesolei" exhibition which was most instructive and interesting. We dined in the open on the Rhine embankment and in the evening saw the big bridge, the town and the entire exhibition illuminated. It was beautiful!
>
> Our relatives have entertained us splendidly. Young Willi owns a car and he sped us along the Rennbahn at terrific speed. Such fun! In August, Marie and I took the long-awaited trip down the river Rhine in a cabin steamer, food and everything included. We sailed between mountains, ruins, and castles down to Ruedesheim, where we saw the National Monument and the wonderful vineyards. On our way back, near Coblentz, we had to wait a long time in order to pass, because the French are building a bridge across the river, on to Cologne.
>
> I admired the "Koelnischer Dom" so very much I did not want to leave. I felt like looking at and admiring the beautiful interior of the cathedral and the tall spires over and over again. Tomorrow at ten o'clock we return to Hamburg. Uncle and his family send greetings, and Marie and I send our dearest love to you.
>
> Mama

Still spry at seventy-one, though in delicate health, she once showed me that she too could dance the foxtrot. I expected her to go on living for at least another decade. But providence decided otherwise. Three years later when the end came, I happened to be thousands of miles distant, unable to reach her in time. My half-sister Anna, writing to me about the funeral, which took place in the famous Ohlsdorf cemetery, the most beautiful in Germany, told me that on top of my mother's coffin was a large wreath tied with a lilac ribbon on which my name was engraved in gold, with an inscription saying, "From her only daughter, absent in Moscow." And so it had been most of her life.

❧17❧

Plough the Ground, Sow the Seed

"WHERE is Saturn?" Isadora wailed in her letter to me from
Samara. She was engaged on a tour of the Volga district, with
Mark Metchick, her pianist, and Zinoviev, her manager. The
trio went from misfortune to catastrophe. If, as the astrologers
believe, the planet Saturn stands for delay and death, then it
must indeed have loomed large in her horoscope at that period.
The evil planet must have foreshadowed the tragic end of her
existence, for within the short space of three years my foster
mother too was dead.

We leave this Volga, which I prefer to remember from a distance. No public, no comprehension—nothing. Boats frightfully
crowded with screaming children and chattering women. Three
in a cabin, second class. Every corner taken in first. I sat on deck
all night and enjoyed *some* quiet hours of moonlit beauty, quite
alone. But the rest—nightmare!

We leave tonight for Orenburg. No news of curtains. Telegraph and inquire for them. Then to Tashkent. Send me books
and papers and write me news. How is the divine Comrade
Podvowsky?

This journey is a Calvary. Heat terrific, almost dead. . . .
How do things progress? Much love to you and love to the
children.

> Yours, in unholy martyrdom,
> Poor Isadora

Hell of a life anyway.

Next she wrote from Orenburg, a small town situated in the
southern Urals, where those lovely gossamer Orenburg shawls
are made:

Dearest Irma:

We sent you letters and three telegrams without answer. Just received word the curtains arrived only today in Kazan! ! ! Too late to take them to Tashkent. We leave at six tomorrow. Heaven knows for what, but keep hoping. Have about fifty kopeks in the *caisse*. *Please* telegraph and write me to Tashkent. One feels so cut off from the world and all these towns so *small*, ruined and God forlorn. I am almost at the last gasp. Dancing in white lights without décors. The public understands nothing at all.

Today I visited the children's colony and gave them a dancing lesson. Their life and enthusiasm is touching—all orphans. . . .

Have found no woman and no help at the theatre—very trying. Well, love to you. For Heaven's sake telegraph me news. With all good wishes and love to the children,

Isadora

Samarkand, the end of June, 1924.

Dearest Irma:

We go from one catastrophe to another. Arrived in Tashkent without a kopek. Found theatre full of Geltzer, Hotel full of Geltzer, whole town occupied. We had to go to an awful hotel where they demanded *"dingy"* in advance, and, failing, would not even give us a samovar. We wandered round the town *without even a cup of tea* all day. In the evening we went to see Geltzer dance to a packed house! After a second hungry day Zinoviev pawned his valise with two suits for just enough to come here. And who do you think he pawned it to? Why, Kalovsky, who is now Geltzer's official husband.

We arrived here also without a kopek. The baggage went by mistake to another station. However, here is no Geltzer, it is more hopeful. I dance here Thursday, but it seems, though very beautiful, only a big village. So Heaven knows what will be the result or whether we will be able to leave! ! !

I feel a bit dilapidated. Metchick is gone in a hopeless melancholy and even Zinoviev has lost his sweet smiling nonchalance.

The country here is divine, fruits and trees and all like a garden—very hot but lovely. But it's a terrible sensation to *walk* about without a penny. Kiev was a prosperous exploit in comparison. The Tovarish that brings this note saved our lives by giving us his room and sleeping in his private car. So be very nice to him. . . .

There are marvelous things here to buy, but alas! The land seems a veritable paradise—for the natives. The whites don't understand how to live here.

Well, we're hoping for better luck. So far the tour is a tragedy. Why did we leave Friday the 13th? Please send me news and papers if possible, I don't know what is going to happen next. At any rate, I've grown very thin. Think of the lovely meals we ate at Kiev!!! Much love to you.

In turn, I told her of the difficulties I encountered, of a different nature—an ideological one. I came frequently in touch with the Commissar of Physical Culture, Comrade Podvowsky, who in the early days of the Revolution had inspired the Red Army. He often criticized what he termed the too aesthetic side of our dance. He wanted the pupils of our Moscow school to strut about in imitation of his athletes, like young warriors shouting, "Death to speculators! Death to parasites! We are the new free army of the earth!"

Needless to say, I did not see eye to eye with him. It all reminded me of that other fanatic and his *Körperkultur* and Racial Hygiene ideology—Max Merz. Being myself primarily an artist, I disliked placing too much emphasis on the physical side of our ephemeral art. In her lessons to her pupils, Isadora invariably emphasized the spiritual approach. When I wrote to her about this, asking for guidance, she replied:

Tashkent, July 10th, 1924

Dearest Irma:

Thank you very much for your very beautiful letter. I can quite understand how you feel. Blazing sun and prize-fighters are far from my vision of a Ninth Symphony (Beethoven) to be danced in a golden light of the intellectual radiance. But probably you are digging the foundations on which the future columns will stand. At any rate, if it is only to take off these horrible clothes and give the children of the new world red tunics, it is a great work. Go on with it. Surely when the government sees that this new dance has the sympathy of the working people, it will do something for the school. As for Podvowsky's ideas of dance— our dance will sweep them away, as it sweeps everything that stands in its road.

The *tournée* is a continual catastrophe. We arrived again from Samarkand without a kopek. Again no hotel. Spent two days wandering round the streets very hungry. Zeno and Metchick slept in the theatre. I, next door in a little house without water or toilet. Finally we found rooms in this fearful hotel over-run with vermin. We are so bitten, as to appear to have some sort of illness.

Yesterday Zeno arranged on percentage an evening for the students, and they advanced ten "*tchervonetz*," so we went to a restaurant and ate, the first time in three days. The theatre is engaged. The first performance can only be given next Wednesday. Heaven knows what we will do until then. I only hope we can make enough for the train.

The country is marvelous. I have never seen flowers and fruit in such abundance. In Samarkand we saw the old temple, composed of Chinese and Persian and Arab culture; wonderful mosaics. And I visited the tomb of Tamerlaine and the old Sartian town. If one had money there are ravishing scarves and silks— but *hèlas!!!*

All this discomfort and worry has made us all ill. Poor Metchick looks dying. We arrived early in the morning and had to sit all day on park benches with nothing to eat. It's a horrid sensation. But this is a primitive, wild place, and anything can happen to one. It's the sort of place to come with Lohengrin [Singer] and his millions; very like Egypt. The heat is forty degrees more in the shade and flies, bugs, mosquitoes make life unbearable.

The little photos are amusing. Try and send me some good ones of you and the children.

Courage; it's a long way, but light is ahead. My art was the flower of an epoch, but that epoch is dead and Europe is the past.

These red tunicked kids are the future. So it is fine to work for them. Plough the ground, sow the seed and prepare for the next generation that will express the new world. What else is there to do? . . .

Love to the children. All my love to you. You are my only disciple and with you I see the Future. It is *there*—and we will dance the *Ninth Symphony* yet. With love.

Isadora

"Plough the ground, sow the seed . . . what else is there to do?" she said. I wondered. This may have been the answer for a disillusioned, middle-aged woman, jaded with life in general. But was it the right answer for a young girl, eagerly standing on the threshold of life? My art and my work could not, for me, be all-encompassing as yet. As any normal young woman would, I too dreamed of being able to find some day another chance at happiness of the sort that culminates in marriage and raising a family. Whenever a young man paid attention to me and my foster mother saw me reciprocate, I was—in her eyes—as good as married. Once she even went so far as to tell Walter Duranty, the American correspondent in Moscow, that I had married. Without first checking at the source, he cabled the "news" to his paper.

No, my plans for the future—even if the right man had come along at that time (which, incidentally, he didn't)—excluded any marriage to a Soviet citizen. I had no intention whatsoever of committing such a fatal mistake. The very thought of any children of mine being born under a dictatorship and growing up as Communist slaves filled me with revulsion.

In this sad world of ours, human beings are constantly forced to make certain sacrifices at one time or another. And I fully realized that this was the one I had been called upon to make, as long as my work kept me chained to the land of the Soviets. I therefore determined to put all personal dreams behind me for the present, and devote all my energies and interests to the furtherance of my career.

My immediate concern had to do with my foster mother: to bring her safely back from her disastrous tour and, if possible, find her a more lucrative engagement, since we had to dance in order to eat. A couple of entrepreneurs offered her a tour of Germany. I immediately wrote her the good news, for so it appeared to be then, since nothing could turn out worse than the tour she had just made. She wrote:

> Volga and Turkestan are countries to be avoided. We came here because Zeno has an idiot for an advance man, who telegraphed us that prospects here were "brilliant." He must have been hired by the ballet to bring us to ruin. When you have an inspiration to save us, for heaven's sake act on it for it is the last moment.

Ekaterinberg, 4/8/24

Dearest Irma:

The moment I received your letter I sent you a forty word telegram expressing my willingness to *sign at once,* and travel anywhere away from here!!! I still await anxiously the answer. You have no idea what a living nightmare is until you see this town. Perhaps the killing here of a *certain* family in a cellar has cast a sort of Edgar Allen Poe gloom over the place—or perhaps it was always like that. The melancholy church bells ring every hour, fearful to hear. When you go in the streets the *gitan* yells *prava* or *lieva* and points his gun at you. No one seems to have any sense of humor whatever.

The head of the communists said, "How could Metchick play such disgusting music as Liszt or Wagner!!!" Another said: "I did not at all understand the *Internationale!!!*"

Our two performances were a *foure noire* and, as usual, we are stranded and don't know where to go. There is no restaurant here, only "common eating houses," and no coiffeur. The only remaining fossil of that name, while burning my hair off with trembling fingers, assured me there was not a *dama* left here, they shot 'em *all.*

We saw the house and the cellar where they shot a "certain"

family. Its psychosis seems to pervade the atmosphere. You can't imagine anything more fearful. . . . In fact this town is as near Hell as anything I have ever met.

Your letter sounds too good to be true. Telegraph us some *dingy* and I will come at once to Moscow and sign, sign, sign. . . .

With love to you,

Isadora

Poor Isadora returned from her *tournée* more dead than alive. A season later I too, with my group of dancers, covered substantially the identical ground under more favorable circumstances. Ilya Schneider's good management and improved organization helped turn our undertaking into a financial and artistic success.

While I was absent on my vacation in France and Germany, Isadora had taught the children a series of new dances executed to songs of the Revolution and to folk songs. In all of these the children both sang and danced in chorus, and I too took part, eventually adding several numbers of my own choreography, such as the tryptich called "Famine-Labor-Harvest"; and a charming group of songs by Gretchaninoff, which always brought to mind that memorable performance at Carnegie Hall when the composer himself played the accompaniment. Whenever they were performed, these dances invariably called forth an enthusiastic reception. Apropos of these "Songs in Movement" Isadora said: "I believe that my school will create a new art or show the way towards it. Only the new generation will be able to express the new world and find new genius and new ideas."

That fall, while preparing for her departure to Berlin, my foster mother and I engaged in a long discussion about our work. She suddenly said, "Do you remember the little dance you composed in Grunewald called the 'Poor Orphan Child'?"

When she asked me to dance it for her, I laughed and told her I could not remember all of it. "But I do!" she said, and surprised me no end by getting up and dancing it, movement for movement, making the same simple, childish gestures I had made. It gave me a strange turn to see so great an artist as Isadora Duncan dance in all seriousness my first childhood attempt at choreography. I was really touched. That called forth my inquiry as to how she came to choose me for a pupil that fateful day in Hamburg nearly two decades ago, and her surprising answer that it had been because of Gordon Craig. It suddenly illuminated so many things that occurred in my early school days and her favoritism toward me from the beginning.

"Then you yourself found me not particularly promising?" I asked. She looked at me fondly and said, "The moment I saw you raise your arms with such childish fervor, I knew you had something. I have always considered you and Lisa to be my most talented pupils. You must often have noticed by my expression and my tears that I found your dancing very beautiful. As I told you last summer when we danced together in Kiev and I watched you do the 'Marche Militaire'—I could not have done it much better."

"This is praise from Sir Hubert," I jokingly remarked to cover my emotion, for she seldom spoke this way to me about my dancing. "No, it is the simple truth," she said.

I had retired to my own room after this conversation and left her to pack her things for her forthcoming trip. Then, very softly, I heard a knock on my door. Isadora entered like a shy little girl, saying in a wistful voice, "Isn't it remarkable that through all the vicissitudes of life and considering all the things I ever owned that have been lost, this"—and she stroked gently the piece of rose and purple silk cradled in her arms like a baby— "this should have survived."

I looked closer and recognized one of her first dance costumes—the one I remembered so well when I saw her dance for the first time on the stage. My favorite—the tunic of "Angel Playing the Viol." She came closer and said, "Here, I want you to have it in remembrance of me"; and she handed it over as carefully and lovingly as if it were indeed a child. A rush of memories from Grunewald—the picture of my guardian angel over my *Himmelbett*—brought tears to my eyes. Too moved to speak, I contemplated the tunic as one regards a religious object. Wanting to thank her, I raised my eyes, but she had quietly disappeared.

Later that night, when we were alone and saddened by her remembrance of the past and her impending departure, she confessed to me that she often thought of committing suicide. "If I only knew a way that would not be too painful, I would not hesitate." And she continued in this same melancholy mood, "Please, don't ever grieve at my going. Promise to bury me in my old red tunic in which I have danced all my revolutionary dances, and give me a real Irish wake. Sing, and dance, and drink, and give thanks for my blessed release from the constant pain gnawing at my poor heart."

The next day was a Sunday, and she gave her farewell performance at the Bolshoi Theatre. All of us—including the five hundred red-tunicked children from the stadium—took part in the grand finale, the "Internationale." With me, as usual, leading the children, we wound in a snakelike pattern back and forth until we reached the footlights. Then we broke the pattern to form three concentric circles around Isadora, who stood in the center like a flame with her red hair and red shawl. Then, with hands raised high, we intoned the final triumphant crescendoing stanza. The audience, of four thousand Young Pioneers and Communist youth, who had been invited by Madame Kalenina (wife of the Soviet President) to see us dance, gave Isadora and her school a thunderous ovation.

That night there was no thought of going to bed, as Isadora's plane for Berlin was to leave at dawn. She thought she ought not to leave now that the President's wife and other Communist leaders had taken an active interest. She felt that something would surely come of this, and if there seemed to be any chance of the government's really doing what they originally promised to do, she would return immediately.

At dawn, at the Trotsky air field, I saw her off. Neither of us realized that she was leaving Russia for the last time; that from now on the work we had begun together in that country would be continued by myself alone.

18

If You Will Be Faithful

By no stretch of the imagination could anyone claim that my existence in Moscow was entertaining. The social amenities were reduced to zero. In this impoverished country, few people—apart from the ruling clique and the foreign embassies—could obtain the products necessary to entertain. I had to rely on my own efforts to find a small measure of distraction, and what I found was not nearly enough to satisfy a fairly energetic young woman unaccustomed to living alone among strangers. For that is what I did in the midst of a teeming institution ever since Isadora left. The few contacts I had made in Moscow with Americans were mostly of a transient nature, people such as Averell Harriman, who later became Governor of New York, but was in 1922 connected with the Hoover Commission, or my old friend Max Eastman whom I met only once. Then there was a memorable evening when Walter Duranty brought the world champion of chess, Capablanca, around for supper after winning the game. I met a number of foreign journalists among whom I became well aquainted with Eugene Lyons and his attractive young wife, then on his first assignment to Russia. They wanted to leave their baby daughter with me at the school but she was too young to be accepted. And in 1927, most outstanding of American correspondents, Dorothy Thompson, whom I met through my good friends the Hoppers. Dorothy was then soon to marry the famous American novelist Sinclair Lewis. She invited me to her engagement party but I could unfortunately not attend. On November 25, 1927, she wrote to "Red," as all his intimates called Sinclair, from Moscow, and mentioned a

visit to my school with the Hoppers. "Today is Thanksgiving,"
she said, spending the evening with the Hoppers. "After dinner,
an' there was a turkey, we went to Irma Duncan's and saw fair
maidens swathed in scarlet dance the Internationale." In her
book *The New Russia* she afterwards published, she wrote in
the chapter of First Impressions:

> Years ago Isadora Duncan came out of the west to tell the
> Russian ballet that all this artificial toe-stepping was out of date.
> . . . And one of her pupils and adopted daughters, Irma Dun-
> can, in her studio in a former palace, still teaches the children of
> the proletarians to throw their arms earthward from whence all
> good comes and revel in the free, untrammeled expression of their
> revolutionary souls.

My daily existence had little of interest to offer me. Shops were
bare; moving picture theatres nonexistent; the fashion world
dead and buried; balls and parties unheard of. What was there
for a young girl to do in search of fun and amusements?

As far as my tastes go, once I'd seen the Bolshoi Ballet I had
had it. I frequently attended the opera, concerts, and the theatres during the season. I could, however, get small enjoyment
from the plays—mostly classics—until my Russian improved.
My usual day started with a late breakfast, brought to me on a
tray by my personal maid Ephrosinia, called Frossia for short.
I ate all my meals in my room; in front of the fireplace in winter, in front of the open window looking out on the courtyard
in the warmer seasons. I would dress and take my daily outing,
snow or sunshine. I preferred riding to walking; dancing as
much as I did, I obtained sufficient exercise.

At the corner of Pretchistenka and Myortvy Pereoulok, or
Dead Alley (so named in time of the big plague), stood a
horse-drawn carriage or, in winter, a sleigh. The *izvozchik*,
Piotr—in a half-somnolent state, patiently waiting for his steady
client—would suddenly spring into action the instant I opened
the heavy oak door and stepped into the street. I hardly needed
to give directions. He knew my initial stop was at Okhotny Riad

to do some shopping for my dinner. The Hunter's Row had the best game in town. I would select a grouse, perhaps, or a snow chicken, with the customary sour cream to roast it in, and whatever fresh vegetables and fruit could be had—mostly cabbage, onions, and beets, and those tart little apples, yellow and red, called *Antonovka*. From there I continued via the Theatre Square to the Petrovka, where I knew a pastry shop that made excellent little *pirozhnye*, those cream-filled cakes the Russians love. In those youthful days I had no reason to watch my weight, which always remained the same. And of course my purchases were never complete without Malosol caviar, smoked salmon and that other tasty little Russian fish, smoked *kilki*. Sometimes, if I was fortunate enough, I would discover a dusty bottle of Abrao Durceaux, that extremely potable native champagne of pre-Revolutionary vintage, much enjoyed by the former tsars.

On my way back over the Arbat, a commercial center, I would stop for an appointment with my hairdresser or continue on to the Sofika, where a very good tailor would make me a dress copied from one I had, or a coat to order. I also frequently stopped at the Kusnetzky Most in the hope of finding something to read in English, French, or German, at the only bookstore open to customers. Usually I returned empty-handed, for books in foreign languages, even second hand, were rarer than hen's teeth. By the beginning of 1925, however, conditions had improved sufficiently for people to purchase these things.

At home, I would hand my groceries to Pasha, our cook, who ordinarily did all right with them, except once when I brought back that very rare vegetable, asparagus. She apparently had never cooked it before and served up the stalks without the heads.

Every afternoon I held my dancing classes. First the younger, or beginners group, followed by my more advanced students. Teaching is more tiring than performing, and I always welcomed the sight of the tall brass samovar, hissing a column of steam to the ceiling, that Frossia had ready for me; with a pot of that good black China tea (the best in the world), which the Russians drink out of glasses with lemon and sugar nibbled on the side.

The absence of reading material in a language I could understand turned out to be a great nuisance. But according to Emerson's law of compensation, there is a benefit to be derived from every bad situation. Forced to read Russian, I made all the better progress. And then there was always Vera Ilynishna, or some other friend, to drop in and chat with me in that difficult language till I mastered it.

On big holidays, such as Easter or Christmas, I attended the services at a small, rose-colored church at the bottom of the hill near Pretchistenka Gate, now vanished from the Moscow scene. In this way, I managed to find some small distractions. Performances and tours came as a welcome relief from the boredom and monotony of existence among the Soviets.

With Isadora's departure, I started once more to be independently active on the stage, a venture that had been impossible while she remained in charge of artistic matters. I slowly came to the realization that if I wanted to make a name for myself in Russia, it was now or never. Thus began the professional tours I made the length and breadth of that vast land. In the end, I was giving a hundred performances a year.

Isadora, in the interval since her departure and subsequent arrival in Nice, had suffered continuous catastrophes. Her Berlin engagement turned into a complete fiasco. She repeatedly sent me letters asking for help. But since all my mail had to be forwarded while I was in the Volga district, her letters reached me too late. By the time I could answer, Isadora had left Germany and settled in the south of France. She wrote me from Paris in February of 1925, when she had finally obtained some help from friends:

Dearest Irma:

I have not had the courage to write, I have been going through sad, fearful experiences. At last I arrived here. I am hardly alive, just gasping. Now I have some faint hope on the horizon, but nothing is sure yet. I was offered by the Chicago *Tribune* a sum for my "memoirs" . . .

For three months they refused me a visa to come to Paris. At last here I am. For Heaven's sake write to me. If you could only send me good photos of the school, I am sure I could raise funds for you. But people hardly believe there is a school. Write to me. Tell me what hope is there for the school? Will the house remain? Is anything stable, or is it a quicksand? My only hope of funds at this moment is the Memoirs. . . .

If I receive the $20,000 promised, I will either come to Moscow in the spring with *money*, or if you think Moscow hopeless, you can join me in London with sixteen pupils. But *reflect well* which will be best.

I am much worried about Margot, who, I have just heard by telephone, is in a hospital here very ill. I will go and see her tomorrow, but Christine should have told me sooner. . . .

Dearest Irma, I was just writing the above when they suddenly telephoned me that Margot was dying. I took a taxi and rushed to the hospital but *too late*. It all seems so unhappy and miserable. I am ill but will write soon. . . .

Unbeknownst to Isadora, Gordon Craig took the initiative to appeal to Paris Singer for help in this emergency. Singer, who was at the time in Florida, wrote from Palm Beach to Craig: "Although I did not hear of the trouble in Berlin I did hear when little Margot died in Paris and I immediately telegraphed my agent to supply our friend with all necessary funds without letting her know the source. Strange to say this was exactly your idea."

Her motto, she said, was *Sans limites*, struggling along to earn a living and never relinquishing her dream of a school for a thousand children. As if the one we had in Moscow, housing half a hundred, was not enough of a headache! I explained to her the endless difficulties I ran into trying to keep this establishment going. The government, so far, had not contributed a sou. My performances in the provinces kept the school func-

tioning; otherwise we would have no other alternative but
to close up shop. She wrote from Nice on the last day of March:

> I have just received your letter; poor darling, it sounds awful.
> By now you have my last letter and you know that if I haven't
> written it is because I have been having such a *hell* of a time
> that I really felt ashamed to send you one wail after another.
>
> Nobody realized it, but poor little Margot's death was the
> finishing touch. I simply almost gave up entirely. I am only just
> recovering from the ghastly cruelty and terror of the whole
> thing. I confess—I can't understand—the whole scheme of
> things is *too* unbearable.
>
> Any reports that I have spoken against the Soviet Gov't are
> *absolutely false,* and unfounded. . . .
>
> A friend took a studio for me here. It is a perfect gem. A little
> theatre twice as big as the Rue de la Pompe with a stage, foot-
> lights, etc. If we could arrange for you to come here with sixteen
> of the most talented children, we might succeed in saving them.
> I tried through the Soviet Embassy in Paris to have the school
> brought in the Russian Dept. of the Decorative Arts Exposition,
> but without success. Have you seen Tovarish Kalenina? Can
> nothing be done?
>
> The world is a sickening place. I am living from hand to
> mouth. My *friends* have all deserted me. The joke of the whole
> thing is that it is current gossip that I receive vast sums of money
> from the Soviets. Isn't that beautiful? I am relying on money
> that should come from Gordieff to pay for the studio. I think it
> would be at least a *refuge* at the last extremity. It would be a good
> idea, if all else fails, that you come here and perhaps together we
> may find some way out. But unless the Soviet Gov't will help, I
> think it is about hopeless for the school in Moscow. But you
> know, being a bit prophetic, I sensed as much when I was last
> there. . . . Ask Ilya to write and answer the following ques-
> tions: What does he advise? Has he any hopes for this summer
> from Podvowsky or others? Would my return make things better
> or worse? . . .
>
> If we are to die, better arrange a meeting and die together. At
> the last extremity, come here. You can sleep in the studio, bathe

in the sea and we will always find a meal. All my love. I kiss you
a thousand times and the poor, dear children.

Love,
Isadora

It was quite impossible to obtain permission for the children
to leave Russia. The authorities had even tried to hinder me
from taking them periodically on tour inside the country, though
we generally made the extensive trips during the summer vacation. Only because I put up a terrific fight—going straight over
the heads of the minor officials to Lunacharsky himself, who always was in my corner—was I allowed to continue. Nobody
seemed to be able to understand that these performances constituted our sole support. For this reason another of Isadora's
schemes fell through. But she persisted in her grandiose schemes
and when nothing came of them told a friend:

> I would have wished to devote myself entirely, creating a mag-
> nificent social center, instead of little troups which, by the force
> of circumstances, degenerate into theatrical groups, as in Mos-
> cow. The principal thing, after all, is to do *something*, to make a
> beginning. Better the Moscow school with all its faults than
> nothing at all.

I fully agreed with her last statement. That is the reason I
too persisted in my small way to keep the enterprise, founded
under such difficulties and involving so may sacrifices, functioning by any and all means. I wrote and told her so. Her answer
reached me in Moscow, where I continued to direct the institution dedicated to the dance as she envisioned it, though local
forces not in sympathy with our ideology had already started
to undermine it.

Nice, January 27, 1926

Dearest Irma:

Thank you for your letter. I only received it today. I wish you
would try and write oftener, if only a line.

I was terribly shocked about Sergei's death [Essenine had committed suicide], but I wept and sobbed so many hours about him that it seems he had already exhausted any human capacity for suffering. Myself, I'm having an epoch of such continual calamity that I am often tempted to follow his example, only I will walk into the *sea*. Now in case I *don't* do that, here is a plan for the future.

I have here a *wonderful* studio which I have not been able to use. First no carpet, then no stove, then no piano. Now I have carpet, stove, piano, thanks to dear Augustin, who gradually sent me funds to get these things and to keep the studio. I have taken a small apartment next to the studio, with kitchen and bath. My plan is that you should come here on a visit as soon as possible, if you can arrange to absent yourself. We could start here *a paying school* à la Elizabeth, and take pupils from America to board, etc. I have a very good woman to look out for the kitchen. Food is *cheap*, vegetables plenty. You could bring one or two of the older girls as co-teachers. By spending six months here and six months in Moscow we could join the ideal and the material.

Now I have a studio three times as big as Rue de la Pompe with the stage and the apartment *paid* until April 15th, but I'm sitting here without a cent or without a soul to help me. If you could come and survey the situation, there is a possibility of making a big school on business basis.

Here is ideal climate. The hills back of the studio are covered with flowers and everything is wonderfully cheap. Yesterday I ate fresh asparagus and little artichokes. I have become a vegetarian like Raymond, and have gone back to my simple dresses of Grunewald, and *sandals* and bare feet. The little time I spent in Paris, I realized that life there was finished with silk stockings at 75 francs a pair.

I see a future in the combining of this studio as a practical money-making affair and Moscow as Ideal and Art. But it has cost me the most heart-breaking effort to keep the studio and if something is not done before April 15th, I'm afraid I will lose it. . . .

No one else on God's earth is interested. Only you and I, and that's all. Since my return I have been treated as a "Communist

Sympathizer," and everything is impossible. But in spite of that, if we open here a big paying school I am sure it will be a success. The studio has a beautiful *emerald green* carpet and the only time in my life I have a studio square and large enough. The apartment has a terrace on the sea, where sixteen or twenty people can sit at table. The autobus and tramway pass the door to the heart of Nice, reach Massena and Casino in five minutes. Also the Riviera is becoming more and more a summer resort.

Please answer this letter at once, dear Irma, and see if, with what I have here as a foundation, we can't create a practical money-making school. For I see at the present epoch that it is either *that* or *suicide*. One can't continue to live on *nothing*. I suggest that also Augustin could come over in the summer and play in the theatre, which has real scenery and footlights, and there is a large English colony here in the summer.

I hope you will appreciate my bull-dog tenacity in hanging on to this studio as I appreciate yours in hanging on to the school. And together we will accomplish something yet. Remember you are the *only* pupil of mine who has understood what I am trying to do in this world. And you are the only one who cares whether myself or our work lives or dies, and it may be that the understanding of *one* will save *all*.

Can't you possibly manage to send me some pictures of the children? Often I could make propaganda and obtain help for you if I had photos. Do try and have some taken, and if you cannot, send me at least some copies of what you have. Also I would appreciate if you would let me have the dates of your *tournées* and programs. Some one told me you were all on the Volga. I knew nothing of it.

Dear Irma, if you will be faithful I still feel we may arise and conquer the earth and knock all these sham schools and sham disciples to smash. But the time is going and I am like a wrecked mariner on a desert island, yelling for help.

I am feeling very lonely and homesick. I am here quite *alone*. Only the little Russian woman who cooks, etc. When you get this letter, do make an effort and come. I am *sure* we can arrange something. I can get the opera house and orchestra in

Marseilles for a series of festival performances, if you could bring twelve of the oldest pupils (children under twelve are no longer allowed on the stage in France).

I press you to my heart, dear Irma. Let us hope for the future.

Isadora

This letter left me in a terrible quandary. Torn between my love and loyalty to her on the one hand, and my work and future career mapped out in Russia on the other, what was I to do? Such a division of my labors as she outlined in her letter was impractical. Since she relied entirely on my help, either one school or the other would suffer because of my absence. I have often asked myself in retrospect: By deciding ruthlessly to tear up the roots in Moscow and throw in my lot with her—since I could not do both—could I have been in a position to prevent her tragic, premature demise? I doubt it, for fate has a relentless way of catching up with its victim marked for death.

For me personally, the idea of spending the rest of my life on the sunny Riviera in my beloved France had tremendous appeal. There I would find all the amenities of existence in a cultured, civilized manner of living, including all the many little luxuries, so dear to a feminine heart, that I was completely deprived of now. And perhaps I would have done so, except that I found myself too deeply involved with the present. For over a year, ever since our unprecedented, enthusiastic reception by the public on our Volga tour, we had planned a similar undertaking for Siberia. Under no circumstances could I cancel it now. There were a host of other people involved in the successful outcome of it. And most important of all, there was the ever increasing number of pupils in the school, who were dependent on my artistic efforts.

I was immensely relieved to hear from Isadora's next letters that conditions seemed to improve by degrees. She arranged for some *intime* performances in the studio she had discovered in the California district of Nice, near the Promenade des Anglais.

April 7, 1926

The Good Friday performance was a great success. A hundred tickets were sold at hundred francs a ticket and great *stimmung* and excitement. The studio was lovely with alabaster lamps, candles, incense, heaps of white lilies and lilacs. Quite like the Archangel's times. Of course it is the end of the season. If we only had the money to open sooner we would have made a fortune. I have hopes of building a theatre here in a year or two. A Bayreuth by the Sea.

"Lohengrin" is coming to his villa here in May. Why not come with sixteen children; we can always make their board. And think of swimming in the lovely blue sea every morning. Please write soon. All my love to you.   Love,
                                                      Isadora

Hotel Lutetia, Paris
June 15, 1926

Dearest Irma:

I was so glad to receive your letter with the program. Please send me a line often. I have been seeing Comrade Rakowsky about a plan to bring you with some of the children of the school to Paris to make a great manifestation at the Trocadéro. They are very enthusiastic about the idea, but always the same cry: "No Money."

I still keep the studio in Nice, but if something doesn't turn up before July 15th, rent day, I'm afraid I will lose it. Did you receive programs, clippings, etc.? I have made a great struggle (here), but absolutely no one to help me. Every one takes a little piece of my idea and runs off with it to sell it. . . . It's a silly world.

Do write and tell me if I can manage to be with you this summer. *Where* will I find you and when?

She would have found us that summer rusticating on a pleasant *imenie*, the country seat of some former aristocrat, confiscated during the Revolution and plundered of everything but the four walls and roof. Situated about fifty versts from Moscow, it had a large park and a river close by. The latter was an absolute necessity for bathing, and as a source of water; for the house had no plumbing whatever, and no gas or electricity. Isadora, I'm afraid, would not have stayed there for more than a day. Knowing her habits and her dislike of living in the country (she claimed, "It always rained, and nothing could be more boring, I much prefer the seashore anytime!"), I knew she would have no part of it. The name of our *imenie* was "Roumiantsev." Few foreigners ever penetrated into this part of the provinces, so very Russian in character and completely unspoiled.

At the end of June, when the bushes were in bloom and the shiny buttercups had pushed their yellow faces high above the meadow grass, we would start our yearly trek to the country. Two truckloads of furniture and kitchen utensils preceded us. With them went Pasha, the cook, and the two maids Masha and Dasha, dressed like country *babas*, in long, straight shifts and bare feet, and with white kerchiefs tied over their heads. Under the supervision of our ruddy-cheeked housekeeper, a huge dragon of a woman by the name of Alexandra Edmundnovna, the house was primitively furnished with bare necessities to welcome us by nightfall.

The local farmers, wearing shoes made of birch bark and —at that period—not yet collectivized, sold us their produce. So did the brown-robed monks of the nearby monastery, "New Jerusalem," where they spent their days hoeing the garden, while we spent ours swimming, hiking, and dancing. At the end of each active day, everybody retired by candlelight the moment the sun had set, which meant getting up with the first crow of the cock in the barnyard. Thus the children gained health, storing it up for the long, dark winters in town. They happily whiled away their spare time gathering *maliny* or other berries, and the superlative Russian white mushrooms that are cooked in sour cream with onions and taste as good as anything I have ever eaten. Watched over tenderly by their academic instructor Anna Vasilievna, and the nurse Elisaveta Gregorievna, the children grew stronger every day and led as happy a life as it was in our power to provide for them.

Country existence presents not much of a problem when the weather is cooperative, but woe when it starts to rain. Unfortunately, that summer we had an unusually prolonged spell of wet weather. I remember standing forlornly in the former owner's library, bewailing the empty bookshelves hidden behind grilled doors. If only I could find a book to read! Watching the continuous downpour night and day for more than a week, I had half a mind to emulate Isadora and do what she would have done under the same circumstances: pack up and return to Moscow; to my comfortable room on the Pretchistenka, where I enjoyed the luxury of a real bathroom to myself, and electric light, and whatever summer amusements could be had in town. But that would have set a bad example for the rest of the school. So I remained drenched, not merely in this deluge but in utter boredom.

One afternoon, during a momentary respite from the maddening drizzle, I donned my mackintosh and went for a stroll in the park. I came by chance on a weather-beaten old barn I hadn't noticed before. Out of sheer ennui, I climbed the narrow, rickety ladder leading to the hayloft. The wild, hysterical cackle of hens, disturbed from their roost, greeted me. I was about to beat a hasty retreat when, out of the corner of my eye, I noticed a piece of white paper sticking out of what I imagined to be a heap of chicken manure. I looked closer, and to my utter bewilderment discovered the "heap" to be an enormous cache of books, which the chickens had used for a roost. And, wonder upon wonders! they were foreign books! French, German, and, Heaven be praised! English books galore of the Tauchnitz editions! Almost as hysterical as the hens, I gathered in my arms as many of these precious tomes as I could, and ran back to the house to get help in cleaning up the filthy mess, so the treasures could be rescued and restored to the former owner's library. Forgetting the rain, I curled up on my bed and spent the rest of the summer reveling in Trollope, Mrs. Humphry Ward, and Baroness Orczy novels—a Lucullan mental feast after a literary famine of more than five years.

So reluctant was I to abandon this feast that when Ilya Schneider, our business manager, informed me that everything was ready to start our Siberian tour, I almost felt inclined to call the whole thing off. All I wanted was to be left in peace with my hoard of books, more precious to me at that moment than my career. I could not take them with me, since they were not my property, and so had to abandon them to their fate. I retained only a few as souvenirs. Years later, in America, I met their owner, Colonel Serge Cheremeteff—but by that time the books were long gone.

❖19❖

To China and Back

WHEN I set out in August with a company of nineteen on my transcontinental Russian tour, I had the unusual privilege of being the sole foreign artist performing in the USSR. Other American artists did not penetrate that Communist country for many years; not, in fact, until after Franklin D. Roosevelt recognized the Soviet Union officially in 1935. I had the entire field to myself now that my foster mother had left. During the three previous years I had occasionally appeared in public at the head of my group of dancers, and we could already point with pride to the slow but steady growth of our popularity.

Every recital was preceded by a short talk delivered by Schneider, stating our aims and explaining what the true dance should be and do for the physical education of children. I offered the common people everywhere, whether in the more civilized centers or in the humble backwoods settlements, the very best I could achieve in my dance to the finest music, both flawlessly executed in a sure, professional manner. The newspaper reviews constitute a record of our combined achievement in this effort to bring beauty, art, and culture to the downtrodden Soviet masses, and tell to what extent we succeeded in giving them the aesthetic values they so craved. A number of short excerpts from reviews that appeared in some of the provincial towns where we appeared may give an indication of how much the Russian public enjoyed and appreciated our combined efforts.

Tomsk
To write about Irma Duncan's performance in simple prose is impossible. In order to do it justice and describe this unusually

273

inspiring dance recital accurately one needs to express it in poetry.
A beautiful poem set to music. This is an amazing spectacle!

Voronish

Something new, something extraordinarily powerful and direct,
is the dancing of Irma Duncan and her dancers. We are used to
the ballet, we are accustomed to see physical culture parades but
we have never seen anything like the Duncan Dancers. An unforgettable spectacle. Every single dance they performed was
beautiful. The two impressive marches by Schubert, the Elegiac
and the Warrior one, will linger long in the memory.

Baku

The performance of Irma Duncan brought us an evening of
sheer beauty. Baku never witnessed such a wonderful sight. She
is a distinguished artist and danced marvelously, especially her
"Moment Musical" called forth rapture from the audience and a
storm of applause.

Tiflis

In the effervescent, intoxicating waltzes with their free-flowing
motions, Irma Duncan and her dancers carry the spectator away
beyond the limits of the stage to green meadows . . . reviving
for us the pastoral paintings of Watteau. Irma, the leader of the
group, creates miracles of inventiveness in her war-like dances
full of power and ecstasy. From this mighty portrayal to the
tender, delicate fluttering of a butterfly in the sunlight, lies the
immeasurable diapason of a great artist. In the revolutionary
dances Irma reaches an extraordinary power of expression.

Irkutsk

When one reads the enthusiastic reviews of the many newspapers about Irma Duncan, and when one sees her perform, one
involuntarily asks oneself: in what lies her greatness? With what
means does she achieve such astounding beauty? How does she
have such a powerful influence over the audience? Her strength
of expression resides in the amazing eloquence and conviction of
her movements, and that is achieved entirely through her great
musicianship and by being the master of her art.

Chita

We were in great anticipation. We all had heard so much about Duncan and so seldom saw her art. So let us go and see Irma, the public said. As soon as the curtain rose a deathly silence and hushed expectancy fell over the audience. At last she appears. Whoever said about architecture that it is rigid music, here was music made visible in sublime motion. The lines of the body, the hands, the lines of every fold in the long, gray tunic expressed sorrow in the Elegiac March. This was not ordinary dancing, this was great art . . . To watch Irma Duncan dance one sharply realizes how much we are still shackled by our cultural inheritance of the past. The Duncan performance is no ordinary theatrical spectacle but a step forward into a new culture. Not for us but for our children in this particular field there open new and immeasurable horizons.

Krasnoyarsk

In one of his articles "The West and We," Trotsky, with a certain irony, recalls a literary critic's remark during the dark epoch of Tsarism after seeing Isadora Duncan dance. He was so enchanted he could only write: "It is worth living!" Of course in these days there is much else for us to live for. But Irma Duncan and all her youthful dancers can truly claim, IT IS WORTH LIVING, if we can create such harmony and beauty in our art.

And so we danced our way through Siberia. Omsk, Tomsk, Irkutsk, Chita via Transbaikalia, on to Khabarovsk and Vladivostok, reaping the harvest of the seed I had sown.

In Moyssei Borissovich Shein, from the Moscow Conservatory, we acquired a very fine pianist. The romantic-looking type of musician, dark-haired, tall, and slender; he added distinction to our dance concerts by always appearing in white tie and formal dress. This was something that impressed the audience everywhere—especially in the hinterlands, where most of the men could barely afford to own a suit. Clothes as well as all other commodities, taken for granted elsewhere, were unavailable to the majority of the populace.

I recall a funny incident that shows how threadbare the average citizen's wardrobe was. It happened in Blagovyeshchensk on the left bank of the Amur River. On the right bank was Manchuria, where freedom then prevailed and anything could be bought in the stores of the small Chinese town. In those days, Russian citizens could obtain a permit to cross the river and buy anything they liked, providing they could wear it on their persons. All the men in our party used this opportunity to replenish their tattered wardrobes. Early one morning they rowed over in a boat dressed only in shirtsleeves (though the day was cold), old pants, torn shoes, and no hats. When they returned at dusk, they all sported new fedora hats, gloves, half a dozen of everything starting with underwear; two suits fitted one on top of the other, a half-dozen socks on each foot, and a pair of shiny new shoes. They could barely maneuver in the clumsy get-ups. Their strategy to outwit the frontier guards was so obvious that even the latter had to laugh, but they got such a kick out of it that they closed an eye and let the men pass. Otherwise they would have had to pay a heavy fine; or worse, suffer imprisonment. But for the sake of some decent clothes to wear, they would have gladly risked almost anything short of death.

We had a few warm days left in Vladivostok before the winter set in, and I used to drive to the shore and gaze out across the Pacific toward America. California, I knew, lay straight ahead. How I longed to be back there again! Of the other Duncan girls, only Theresa lived over there—and Temple, who was married and made her home in New York. With Lisa in France and Anna Lord knew where, how widely we were scattered! With the cessation of all correspondence, we had completely lost track of each other. I liked to have a look at the Pacific as often as possible, not knowing when I would visit the Far East again, and believing that my tour had come to an end, with the return trip to Moscow next on our schedule.

My manager told me that in the old tsarist days, a theatrical tour through Siberia invariably ended in Harbin, now no longer Russian territory. It was still largely populated by Russians, though under Japanese occupation, and we decided to make a try for it. This meant obtaining exit visas and passports from the Soviets. We doubted very much we would receive them, although the authorities occasionally permitted theatrical groups to cross the frontier, in spite of the chance of their defecting. To our pleasant surprise, the authorities let us go.

I never saw such elation among the members of my troupe. They had no intention of defecting; they simply longed to breathe a little free air and come in close touch with the outside world, so long kept away from them. We stayed for two weeks, giving a show nearly every day. At the termination of our engagement, the Harbin paper noted:

> The performance of Irma Duncan and her dancers was a real triumph. The house was sold out to standing room only. Loud applause after each number greeted the artists and at the end the dancers received a standing ovation.
>
> Each time Irma Duncan appears on the stage she is different. Now she is joyful, then again she is proud, a flaming spirit calling to the oppressed masses to rise and throw away their bonds. And again she demonstrates her creative versatility in the interpretation of Chopin's Funeral March and the Berceuse, where she gives us the picture of a tender-visaged mother bending over the cradle of a child. One superbly moving impersonation succeeds another. A scarf, a tunic and a mantle, those are the only props with the aid of which she creates her beautiful art. She is as true as only a fanatic can be to the ideals of her foster mother. Isadora's work is embodied in Irma.

When the time came to depart, I was most reluctant to leave. China exerted a strange fascination over me. Peking was a city I had always wanted to visit. Now, only thirty hours away, how could I resist? Our exit permit included only Harbin, but that didn't worry me. The question that did worry me was how we would be received in China without advance booking. I decided to take a big gamble.

I gave the order to proceed, though neither I nor my managers knew anything about theatrical or any other conditions in China.

I can't remember when I had been more thrilled to enter a foreign city (short of my initial arrival in Paris) than when, on a beautiful October day, I first saw the enormous walls encircling Peking. Quickly settled at the Wagon-Lit Hotel, I was impatient to go sightseeing. Transportation was by ricksha, and I confess to a few embarrassed moments before I could accustom myself to being drawn about, not by horse or by motor, but by another human being.

It must be remembered that this was in the era of extra-territoriality. Foreigners lived in their own concessions and never mixed with the natives. Theatres were situated there, and only a select number of high-ranking Chinese ever attended them. For that reason, although I danced in several cities, I never really performed for the Chinese themselves. As far as our concert tour was concerned, it did not take place in China proper, but only in the foreign concessions—English, French, Japanese, or those of other occupying nations. Because of this curious circumstance, it is not surprising to come across an article written by a Britisher under the pseudonym of Argus, who reviewed our show in Tientsin, which was largely colonized by the English. He wrote:

A hit! A very palpable hit, as was observed by Hamlet. Not the most Philistinic would contradict the statement that Irma Duncan held the audience at the Empire Theatre last night in her graceful hand. The writer was acquainted with Isadora Duncan, the founder of the Duncan school of dancing, on her first visit to London about twenty-five years ago, when she gave her initial recital at the New Gallery and no less a person than the musical critic of "The Times," the great Fuller Maitland, played accompaniments on the harpsichord to her interpretations of the classics.

In those days her views on dancing were an innovation and contrary to all the old ideas. Like Wagner, she met with opposition and cheap ridicule. Since then she has conquered the world. And all dance recitals nowadays are more or less either Duncanesque or influenced by her teachings. Within the year we have witnessed the work of many dancers of high repute and the greatest executive ability, but the Duncan Dancers stand alone.

In the first part of the programme the audience were charmed by the portrayals of Irma Duncan and Mr. Shein, who is her companion in presenting "Chopiniana." If the great Polish master could have witnessed this delightful materialization of his work, he would have been happy that he had inspired such exquisite poetry in motion. . . .

Mr. Shein, the pianist, is of a rank which does not frequently favor Tientsin. He has a delicacy of touch and a technique not excelled by many celebrities and the sympathy of all those musically inclined went out to him last night.

Princess Der Ling, onetime lady-in-waiting to Tzu-Hsi, Dowager Empress of China, was the first Chinese person of consequence whom I met. She came to see me backstage at the Apollo Theatre in the Legation Quarter in Peking. Educated abroad—her father was once Chinese minister to France—she spoke perfect English. After we had been introduced, she said, "You know, I was a pupil of Isadora Duncan years ago." I couldn't refrain from smiling and saying doubtfully, "Really?" —for many people have claimed this and still do, though they did no more than shake hands with her.

The Princess continued, "It was in 1902. My sister and I attended her classes in Paris. That was long before she attained fame as a dancer."

Then I remembered what Mary Sturges had told me. They must both have attended Isadora's studio in the Avenue de Villiars, where she opened classes for paying students soon after her arrival in Paris. However, they were of short duration and conducted with no thought of training professional dancers. But China was the last place I would have expected to find a former pupil of Isadora!

Peking—with its monuments of former grandeur under the Mandarin rule, such as the "Forbidden City"; the famed "Temple of Heaven," entirely carved of white stone; and the vast expanse of gardens and low buildings with the peculiar, glazed, upturned roofs in the bright yellow and blues of Chinese architecture—is the most Chinese of all the cities I saw in that country. Taking advantage of the splendid autumn weather, we made several excursions to the Empress' summer palace, which was shaped like a houseboat, floating in the center of a lake. We also visited the western hills where the last remains of the first president of the Chinese Republic, Sun Yat-sen, had temporarily been laid to rest, high up in a tower overlooking the whole countryside.

Before leaving Peking, I must mention the mysterious character who daily ensconced himself in the same armchair in a dark corner of the big lobby of the Wagon-Lit Hotel. Every time I appeared around tea time, he was there. He pretended to read a newspaper but actually kept peeping over the edge and staring at me. I thought I had made a new conquest, it was most intriguing. At last he summoned up enough courage to send his card over to me and requested an interview. He had a very important matter to discuss with me, involving big profits. I sent my manager over to talk to him. The mysterious stranger turned out to be a White Russian officer of Denikin's former army, now obviously living by his wits alone. He made me the most amazing offer, one that really astonished me.

Before I tell what it was, I must mention here that Peking and most of the Manchurian provinces were then held by that most bloodthirsty of all warlords, the erstwhile bandit Chang-Tso-lin. His son, commander of one of his father's armies, was a notorious good-for-nothing. His feats as a gambler, woman-chaser and rapist, his numerous orgies had made sensational

news in the foreign press. Well, hearing of our successful performances in Peking, it pleased this unspeakable scoundrel to
invite us to his army camp to dance for him and his soldiers.
Naturally, I refused point-blank. The Russian intermediary
pleaded with me, almost threatening me with dire results if I
persisted in my refusal. He assured us we would be treated with
respect and like royalty strictly guarded and protected. A special train with sleeping cars and dining saloon would take us
there and back. And, most important, a huge sum of money
would be paid in advance.

Finding ourselves practically penniless at that period, it
perhaps seemed folly not to accept this lucrative offer. It all
looked very suspicious to me and of course I had my great
responsibility vis-à-vis my young charges to consider. As luck
would have it, that same afternoon a young secretary of the
American Legation in Peking called on me. He instantly informed me that they knew all about that offer from Chang-
Tso-lin's son, and earnestly warned me not to accept his offer no
matter how much money he was ready to pay me. I hastily assured him I had already definitely made up my mind to have
nothing to do with this extraordinary scheme. He seemed much
relieved. I was quite touched that the American Legation should
take the trouble to warn me and profess such a personal interest in me since at that time I was not yet a citizen of the United
States and therefore not entitled to their protection. I thanked
him warmly and felt much comforted to know I had invisible
friends in these dangerous surroundings and times.

In Tientsin, an American impresario offered me a contract
for Japan. I had originally intended to penetrate no farther
into China than the Celestial City. But once there, I could not
resist continuing south to discover what the rest of Cathay
looked like. Therefore the offer from the impresario came most
opportunely. Without a definite contract, it would have been
risky to stretch our lifeline to Russia too far.

The day we arrived in Shanghai, misfortune befell us. First, the Japanese Emperor died, and the tour was promptly canceled. That left us in grave financial straits, since we counted on the tour for new funds. Second, having no advance agent, we were unable to find a vacant theatre in any of the concessions other than the Japanese quarter, which was shunned by all the foreigners, on whom we relied exclusively for our audience. It was a sort of pariah among concessions, something we could not possibly have anticipated. We danced for a couple of weeks to small crowds, consisting only of Japanese, at less than popular prices—not enough to defray our expenses. The situation, especially around Christmas time, became alarming. I saw myself forced to ask for a loan. Ilya unearthed a Russian Jew who acted as money lender in the Japanese concession, where we then lived to save money. I hated to do it. But living was expensive in Shanghai, that teeming city on the Whangpoo River by the Yellow Sea, with its strange admixture of Oriental and European cultures. We continued to hope for a good break to set us on our feet again. None appeared, and the Shanghai Shylock demanded payment. The alternative was to have me thrown into prison, which would have meant a Chinese prison. This horrible fate was imminent when a policeman, accompanied by Shylock, came to my lodgings to arrest me.

Not knowing how to escape this dreadful predicament, I sat hopeless and forlorn in my locked and bolted room, while a ferocious fracas went on outside. All the men in my company tried to prevent the arresting officer from reaching my door. Frightened, I jumped from my chair and ran to a closet to hide when I heard a loud knock at my door. Careful inquiry revealed that a Soviet Embassy secretary desired to speak to me. I opened the door.

"What is that awful noise downstairs?" he asked on entering. "I could barely get by several fellows at grips with each other, while an English bobby tried unsuccessfully to tear them apart."

"Those are my friends trying to save my life. Somebody is out to get my blood," I said with a laugh, trying to seem flippant and unconcerned. The last thing I wanted the Soviets to know was my financial dilemma.

"May I ask how large a sum you owe?" he asked casually, surprising me no end. How did he know? I told him, and without further ado he reached for his wallet and presented me with the exact amount. I was speechless, and so terribly relieved I could have kissed him. He, or rather the Soviet Embassy (which knows all, sees all, and hears all), had literally saved my life. He further passed on the information that the Embassy had wired to Moscow for sufficient funds to bring me and my whole company safely home. After the tumult and the shouting below had died, with the fortuitous repayment of the debt, he invited us all to a New Year's party at the Embassy.

I had corresponded with no one since leaving Moscow. No news of Isadora had reached me. I made use of the Christmas holidays to write letters to both my mother and foster mother. The latter passed the time between the Hotel Lutetia in Paris and her studio in Nice, preparing her memoirs for publication. Since no further communications passed between us, I discovered only years later that my journey to China had simply infuriated her. She went so far in her anger as to tell friends that I was a "bandit" who had "absconded with her school"—a statement bordering on madness. She wrote a formal letter of protest to some Soviet official complaining that when she received my news it was:

> The first word I have heard from the school for *six months,* and the first knowledge I have had that they are in China. I wish to protest that this school which I formed at the sacrifice of my fortune and person, and for which I had become naturally boycotted by all my former friends and audiences in Europe, should be allowed to pass from my control and into the hands of private speculation. Those sacrifices that I made, I made gladly for the cause of the people; but when it comes to the exploitation of my work by a private organization without so much as asking my advice—I must protest!
> This is an exploitation of my art which I would not have

expected, considering the primary object of my visit to Russia was to escape from just such exploitation of Art, which Soviet Russia condemned Europe for in 1921.

"Private speculation?" "Exploitation of my work?" Was she talking about me? I too had formed the school at the sacrifice of my future and person and fortune, since I received not a penny for my work. And besides, from the opening in 1921 until that Christmas of 1926, I had done all the work with the children, Isadora being absent from the school 75 per cent of the time. For some reason known only to her, it was all right for me to perform in France with sixteen pupils from the school, but not in China. In the former instance, it would have been "for the cause of the people"; in the latter, she considered it a dreadful "exploitation" of her work. These contradictions in terms remained incomprehensible to me. Was I doing anything wrong?

At the Embassy party to celebrate New Year's day in Shanghai, all the children—ranging in age from ten to sixteen—were given presents. I too received a pair of handsome black cloisonné vases filled with poinsettias, which, now holding other flowers, grace my mantelpiece to this day. Among the guests were foreign correspondents, who had come to China to cover the civil war then raging in the interior. In Peking I had already become familiar with the name of Chang Tso-lin, a mighty war lord, and here in Shanghai the name of Chiang Kai-shek was much in the news. Without realizing it—for I shied away from politics—I had arrived at a crucial moment in the revolutionary history of that country, in which I was to become unwittingly embroiled to a minor extent. No one in the rest of the world, except Soviet Russia, paid much attention to what was going on in China. The American papers were concerned only with domestic affairs.

The Chinese Revolution, which had started twenty years earlier under the leadership of the great Sun Yat-sen (who had been proclaimed president in 1911) was about to enter a second stage. The Bolsheviks, continuously on the prowl for further acquisitions to their own cause, had given Sun Yat-sen money and munitions, and also military and political advisers. When Sun Yat-sen died in 1924, the revolutionary movement continued to grow. The various war lords, who governed China according to a feudal system, opposed it to a man. The Canton armies of the Kuomintang (People's Party), inspired by Sun Yat-sen, were then sweeping down the Yangtze-Kiang under the leadership of Chiang Kai-shek, and had recently taken Hankow, soon to be followed by Nanking and Shanghai. Anti-foreign feeling had been aroused among the armies, and all foreigners were advised to settle on the coast near Shanghai or Tientsin. The political adviser the Russians sent to the Kuomintang was an aquaintance of mine, Michael Borodin.

The young, victorious commander-in-chief, Chiang Kai-shek, even then engaged in certain maneuvres to further his own ambition (which eventually culminated in making him president), was trying to break with the left wing of the Kuomintang, which was largely under Russian influence. Word had reached the Soviet Embassy at this time that a critical situation had developed with respect to the Kuomintang.

During the New Year's reception the Soviet Ambassador asked me to step into his private office for a moment. He had something important to say to me.

"I have received official notice from Narkompross [People's Commissariat of Education] in Moscow that you are to return immediately to Russia," he informed me, when we were seated at his desk. I had no knowledge then of Isadora's protest, and could not guess that she had a hand in this. I retorted, "That suits me fine. Shall we be leaving at once?"

The Soviet Ambassador (I have forgotten his name) regarded me for a minute in silence. Then he leaned far across his desk and said in a hushed voice, "No, I don't want you to leave yet for Moscow."

Intrigued by his conspiratorial tone, I raised my eyebrows

and asked for an explanation. In the same hushed tones he added, "My staff and I have come to the unanimous conclusion that you and your company should proceed to Hankow instead."

"Hankow?" I cried in alarm. "Isn't that the place where a wave of anti-foreign agitation has broken out, with foreigners being killed right and left?"

"That is true," he admitted and raised a forefinger, quickly adding, "but not Russians!"

How the enraged Chinese could tell the difference in nationality or bother to find out before slaughtering anyone, I couldn't imagine. I showed no enthusiasm for the idea of leaving safe Shanghai and venturing forth into the front battle lines, and told him so. He calmed my fears by explaining that the Borodins would look after us and protect us and not to worry on that account. Things were actually not so bad. "The people will welcome some diversion, and your performance will, I am sure, give them new hope and inspiration."

He was so insistent that I got the impression this was more of an order than a request. "How shall we get there?" I asked, still not sure if this was the right thing for us to do. "We are completely broke."

"You can use the money Lunacharsky forwarded for your return trip."

"Isn't that going against official orders?" I asked, surprised that he should even suggest such a thing, and unwilling to get myself into trouble with the authorities in Moscow.

"Leave the rest to us," he assured me. "I shall give the necessary explanation when the time comes. The important thing is—will you consent to go?" I remained silent, thinking of the enormous responsibility involved. It wasn't just myself I had to consider, but all my company.

"Of course you are not forced to go. If you are afraid . . . we will understand. This is only a suggestion on our part," he said.

Adventure is in my blood, and I had no actual fear for

myself to see a bit of history in the making. I hesitated only because of the girls. "Will they be safe?" I inquired.

"The enemy has not yet reached the river, and although the voyage to Hankow may not be too comfortable, there is nothing to fear. Once you reach the Wuhan province upstream, the Borodins and Chiang Kai-shek with his victorious army will receive you with open arms. They are well supplied with everything and will give you a good time."

"In that case, as long as I have your official assurance all will be well with us," I said, "we shall go on to Hankow." One is young only once and at that period of life seldom reckons with the consequences. I asked him when he wished us to depart.

"Tomorrow. The sooner you get there the better. A Japanese streamer is about to sail for Hankow. It will take only three days."

What he did not communicate to me, so as not to alarm us unduly, was the fact that the enemy army of the northern war lord Chang Tso-lin, more ferocious even than the southern army, was momentarily expected to capture Nanking. The Soviets purposely left me in the dark, because they were anxious—for reasons of their own—that we should make contact with the Borodins. The Soviet Embassy saw in our dancers a providential means of extending a friendly gesture to Chiang Kai-shek. In other words, they tried to use us as propaganda to help smooth the ruffled feathers of the Chinese-Russian entente.

The parting words of the young secretary of the legation, who once came to my rescue and who now saw us off, were, "You don't know how courageous you are to undertake this journey. If I were in your place, I don't think I would have done the same."

This remark hardly helped to put my mind at ease. I somehow sensed that my small bark, having so far navigated safely, was about to encounter the ground swells of much deeper water.

Traveling native style in China is quite an experience. It is not one that I would ever care to repeat. In order to save money, our manager had bought third-class accommodation for all of us. We slept on hard bunks in cabins of our own, but meals were another matter. There was no dining room. We were obliged to squat, Chinese style, on the bare floor. The food was served in porcelain cups with chopsticks. This would not have been too bad, since one can adopt native customs temporarily. It was instructive and might have been fun—*but*—there were grave reasons for shunning these meals served on the floor outside the cabins. That same place was also used by the native passengers for other and more private purposes, as unconcernedly as if they were animals.

I rushed in shocked protest to the Japanese captain of the ship, asking permission for me and my company to eat in the first-class dining saloon and paying for the privilege, but he refused. What to do? I first thought of mutiny, by simply taking over the dining saloon and staying there to the end of the trip. I consulted with Elisaveta Gregorievna, who told me of a supply of baked beans she had taken along, just in case. That solved the problem. For three days, three times a day, we all ate cold beans, right out of the cans, in our own cabins. We never traveled without tea and a couple of samovars; thus we had enough to drink. The girls spent most of the time playing on deck, but I never left my cabin. Frossia, my maid, took care of all my wants. I invariably traveled with my own bedding, wash basins, buckets, pitcher, etc., as well as linen and mosquito netting. These were things one could not do without, considering the primitive state of lodgings in all of Russia outside of the larger cities. Fortunately, most places had public baths. In this way, we kept clean and free of disease, despite the ravages of typhoid fever and cholera rampant in certain areas. Though none of us had been especially inoculated, our group suffered no serious illness all the years we toured together. Whenever one of the children complained of feeling sick, Elisaveta Gregorievna employed but one remedy—castor oil. This, she insisted, cured everything, and it worked wonders; but here in China, under these unbelievably filthy conditions, I feared the very worst.

From my cabin window, I watched the scenery along the largest river in China. We passed Nanking safely. Soon thereafter the river narrowed and the mountains appeared in fan-shape form—a view made familiar through Chinese art, which has a character and charm all its own. We had come about six hundred miles upstream when, in the second week of January 1927, with the civil war about to reach a climax, we landed in Hankow, the most important commercial center in the midlands.

The day was sunny and warm. The children stood lined up on deck in their school outfits, with their overcoats cut in military style resembling the Red Army uniform. I too came out of my seclusion below deck, glad to see the sun and inhale some fresh air. As the boat approached the landing stage, I noticed two ladies, both dressed in Chinese garb—although one was a foreigner—standing on the dock and waving at us. The foreign woman, in her forties, very short and rather squat-looking in her gray Chinese dress reaching to the ankles, called out in Russian, "Hello, I'm Fanny Borodin. Welcome to Hankow!"

Borodin was not her real name. Both she and her husband, whom I had met before, came from Chicago, where he had taught school. Delighted to be able to speak to an American woman again, I said some words in English, upon which she quickly shushed me, saying in Russian, "Please don't speak English in public! Do you see that building full of bullet holes?" and she pointed to a warehouse nearby. "That is where they shot every man, woman, and child of the English colony, who had barricaded themselves there last week. So, please, be very careful. It's all right to speak Russian."

She introduced me to her companion, a Chinese lady of very delicate proportions and a charming face. It turned out to be the Martha Washington of revolutionary China, none other than the widow of the first president, Sun Yat-sen. Soong Ching-ling is the sister of the present Madame Chiang Kai-shek. She handed me a bouquet of flowers and whispered a few words of greeting in English, for, like her more famous sister, she was educated in America.

Fanny Borodin informed me that, besides her own family, I and my company were the only foreigners then in Hankow. That did not make me feel very much at ease. After that awful boat trip, I fully anticipated the worst. She and Madame Sun Yat-sen led me to a limousine in a line of other cars all prominently displaying the Kuomintang flag—an eleven-pointed white star in a field of blue. The English and French concessions appeared to be completely evacuated, and we drove through them without stopping anywhere. Presently we approached a polo field on the outskirts of the city, and I prepared myself to be housed in Chinese fashion with all the attending discomforts for a Westerner. But the limousine entered some iron gates set in a high wall and stopped in front of an impressive modern mansion.

"What do you think of it?" Mrs. Borodin, now addressing me in English, said as we mounted the stairs. "It looks brand new," I retorted, gazing about in amazement, for this was the last I had expected. "It is!" she said, and laughed. The house, she explained, was especially built for Wu Pei-fu, the big war lord of the midland provinces. "But we captured Hankow before he had a chance to occupy it, and now it is yours for the duration of your visit with us."

So saying, she conducted us into the house; and indeed all the furniture, down to the last lace doily, still had a price tag attached. We all stood there laughing. It was so marvelous to think we got there ahead of Wu Pei-fu! We moved in and took possession of this grand trophy of war, whose wraps had not yet been removed.

"I hope you will find everything to your liking, and that you will all be happy here," Madame Sun said in her gracious manner, so different from the abrupt Fanny Borodin. "This is the very best place we can offer you," she continued, leading me to the dining room that opened out onto a terrace. Her smooth dark hair, tied back into a knot at the nape of the neck, framed a pale, sensitive face with very black eyes. She spoke and moved with the stately bearing of an aristocrat; her ideas of housekeeping were those of a woman brought up in luxury. Surveying the dining room she said nonchalantly, "Instead of hiring a cook and servants, such a bother, I thought it would be ever so much more convenient to hand the whole problem of meals over to a good caterer. Don't you agree?"

The arrangement seemed perfect. The only thing that bothered me was the expense. "Are we to pay for them?" I inquired of Mrs. Borodin before she left.

"Certainly not!" she exclaimed. "All of you are the honored guests of the Kuomintang Party. Besides, Madame Sun's brother, T. V. Soong, is Finance Minister, so you can just sit back and relax; everything will work out."

I thanked them for the wonderful hospitality, and then Mrs. Borodin warned me once more about speaking English in public and told me not to worry about the isolated location. "You shall have a round-the-clock bodyguard of armed soldiers," she assured me. "We have also placed a car with chauffeur at your disposal, but don't go anywhere without taking two armed guards along!" and she warned me further, "Always be sure to display the Kuomintang flag prominently!"

Before driving back to town with Madame Sun, she gave me her telephone number and promised to return the following day. I entered the house again and noticed several white-coated waiters setting the table as for a festive dinner. There were flowers, silver, crystal, candles—and they served nothing less than a seven-course meal every time we sat down at table. What a far cry from the cold beans eaten out of a tin!

At night, when I retired to my private room and bath, all the fixtures gleaming in a brand-new state, I looked out the window and saw the bonfires lit in front of the tents the eight soldiers of our night watch had erected in back and in front of the house. My thoughts went back to all the strange events leading up to this moment. How did I ever get into a situation like this? No matter how often I had dreamed of visiting Cathay, not in my wildest imagination could I have conjured up an adventure similar to this one. What was our next move? I wondered, for almost anything was possible now. The warlike atmosphere created by the soldiers guarding our high-walled enclave brought a shiver of apprehension, for in spite of all the luxurious surroundings in which we lived, I could not forget that we were encamped in the midst of a fierce civil war whose outcome still lay in the balance. At any moment the tide might suddenly turn for the worse and engulf us all in the most ghastly disaster. All night long the spectre of Wu Pei-fu, the vanquished war lord, taking Hankow again by storm and making us his prisoners, prevented me from sleeping soundly in his house. And I wished I were a thousand miles from there. Why, oh why! had I not heeded Isadora's plea? I would now be basking in the mild Riviera sun, bathing in the blue sea, instead of facing terror and bloodshed and gruesome death from which there might be no escape.

These nightmarish thoughts vanished on the following day. We were too busy getting ready for our debut in Hankow to think of anything but the business at hand. The night of our performance in a small theatre in the former French concession, the entire route leading from the center of town was lined with soldiers. All the dignitaries from Chiang Kai-shek down would attend. We tried to give our best to our first all-Chinese audience, and they responded with great warmth. Mrs. Borodin came backstage during the intermission and said, "Your dancing is divine! It is a shame Chiang Kai-shek can't see it. He did not come."

I told her we had then failed in our mission, for this was **the reason** we were sent to Hankow. She told me to have patience; she had sent several messengers, and he might still appear. At the end of our performance she once more came to my dressing room, this time elated and excited. "He is here! He is here!" she shouted. "He just came! Now you must do the whole thing over again!"

Exhausted from my three-hour show, I pleaded with her not to insist on a repetition of the entire program, but only of the last part, composed of our revolutionary songs and dances. She agreed, and I had prepared a surprise. At the very end, after several curtain calls (for none of the audience had left and Chiang Kai-shek applauded as loudly as the rest), we all came out dressed in little coolie shirts. I displayed the Kuomintang flag, and the children sang the Kuomintang national anthem in Chinese, to the incongruous tune of "Three Blind Mice." It was a tremendous hit!

Mrs. Borodin embraced me in her enthusiasm crying, "That was wonderful! Just the right thing! You have won over Chiang Kai-shek completely. You know, all the top officials are so pleased they are going to tender all of you a nice banquet tomorrow."

Madame Sun Yat-sen called on me the next day and said, "We all think it would be so much pleasanter to hold the banquet in your honor right here in your house instead of at a formal restaurant in town. The caterers are already here, and we can spend the whole evening together, *en famille* as it were."

That evening the top officials arrived and many brought their children along. I sat at the head of the table next to the hero of the Chinese Revolution, Chiang Kai-shek, and the Foreign Minister, Eugen Chen. Madame Sun Yat-sen sat on the other end with her brother the Minister of Finance, and Michael Borodin. They made speeches and drank my health in wine, all except Chiang Kai-shek, who drank water. He also spoke no English. He just sat there and smiled. So I conversed mainly with Eugen Chen, a very cultured gentleman, educated in England, who had a good sense of humor.

For this gala occasion, I wore a Chinese costume that I had bought in Peking on Silk Street, with a large jade pendant I had bought there on Jade Street. Both the long jacket and the trousers were of red silk. The loose-sleeved jacket was richly embroidered in white, blue, and gold. I considered it most appropriate and could not resist asking Eugen Chen whether he did not agree. In his clipped Oxford accent he said, "It is of course very lovely and all that, but . . ."

"What is the matter with it? Is something wrong?" I inquired, taken aback.

"Well now, I really don't know what to say. Let me put it to you this way, my dear girl. Ah-h, suppose I had been given a banquet in Paris and turned up dressed as Louis XIV! Eh! It would be rather funny, wouldn't it? Ha, ha!"

I saw the joke when he explained that the Mandarin style had disappeared with the Manchu dynasty. To me, all Chinese clothes looked alike. Then I learned that the modern Chinese women no longer wore trousers nor tied their feet with bandages in childhood to stunt their growth. I too promised to reform and buy myself a modern Chinese dress. Only I could nowhere find one to fit me—the Chinese women are all as small as dolls.

While the Russian and Chinese children amused themselves with parlor games after dinner, I had a long conversation with Borodin. I had met him before, in the summer of 1921 shortly after our arrival in Moscow. I remembered the occasion now. It was on a day in August, after we had settled in the *dacha* in Sparrow Hills (now called Lenin Hills). Isadora and I, simply clad in white tunics and sandals, had been wandering among the trees on the wooded heights above the river. Weary of our promenade, we sat on an open grassy slope near the stream. Soon several men in a rowboat appeared around the bend; and, apparently attracted by our white-clad figures, they moored their boat and climbed the slope toward us. They must have recognized Isadora, because they asked if they could take a snapshot of her. The chief of this little band was Borodin. Tall and dark and good-looking, he seemed more cultured than the others and was the only one who spoke English. We invited them to lunch at our *dacha*. We did not have much food, but Jeanne managed to rustle up a few eggs for an omelet and fresh tomatoes for a salad; and they, used to a diet of dried fish and hard black bread, considered it a lavish meal. We had never seen Borodin again, and I certainly had not expected to run across him in the middle of China. But here he was, and he had an interesting proposition to make.

Would I, he wanted to know, consider giving up my performances at the theatre in the French concession—which was, after all, a symbol of colonialism in the eyes of any Chinese— to dance instead in the theatre in the native quarter? That was something no foreign artist had ever done. I readily consented, without giving it a second thought. The fact that for the last three months we had performed in every large city in China and not once for a purely Chinese audience, except in Hankow, was something I did not like. It did not seem fair. Why should the natives be forced to enter the hated foreign concessions in order to see the artists who came to their country?

"Bravo!" Borodin exclaimed. "You will have the distinction of being the first foreign artist to perform professionally in the Chinese quarter; outside the settlements, and in a Chinese, not European-style, theatre."

The population of Hankow was then about a million souls. And I don't think it too much of an exaggeration when I claim we must have danced for most of them! Borodin had warned me that the Chinese theatre was different from what I was accustomed to. Indeed it was! To begin with, the windows had only transparent paper to cover them, most of it torn to shreds; and cold blasts of air circulated through the auditorium, which seated several thousand people. A heating system was conspicuous by its absence. At the end of January it had started to snow, a freak of the weather this southern town had not experienced in thirty years. There was another inconvenience of a very serious sort—the theatre had no dressing rooms. The cold and the lack of dressing rooms may have been perfectly all right for the all-male Chinese performers, dressed in elaborate amounts of costume. But I and my girls needed a little privacy for disrobing and change of costumes, which consisted in the main of diaphanous scarves worn over bare limbs. Borodin made a long face when he noticed my disgust with the setup, afraid I would renege on the whole scheme. However, I decided to go through with it; which is my usual attitude when challenged.

Backstage we rigged up screens like small nooks, with braziers of hot coals inside to keep us from freezing. Even so, the cold was so severe that when the girls entered the stage singing, little spirals of steam could be seen escaping from their open mouths. No matter how energetically we moved about, our limbs seemed absolutely frozen. As for poor Moissei Borissovich, he insisted on wearing woolen gloves so he could play the rattling old upright box that no true musician would honor by the name of piano. None of us had ever experienced anything like it. We thought the extreme cold would keep the audience away. But no; they continued to pour into the theatre to full capacity at each and every show. They had, of course, nothing to worry about. The national costume is a padded suit and padded coat in which they sat, warm as toast, drinking—throughout the recital, if you please—pots of hot tea and eating sweet cakes.

The Chinese theatre also boasts of no curtain or spotlights. While dancing I am usually unaware of the audience, for I am completely wrapped up in my interpretation of the music. Here this was impossible, no matter how much I tried to concentrate. On that Oriental music box, even Chopin—played by my pianist in woolen gloves—sounded Chinese. And out in the auditorium, lit up as bright as day, I heard the noise of constant chatter and saw the tea being served, while an occasional hot towel went flying through the air from customer to towel-vendor for the purpose—of all things!—of wiping *sweat* from the brow! To cap the whole incredible performance (in which the public actu-

ally took a more prominent part than we, poor frozen dancers),
they all—thousands of them—held up their thumbs and shouted
"Ho!" instead of applauding at the end of a dance. No wonder
we were complete wrecks at the finish of our engagement, which
could have been prolonged indefinitely, because Borodin invited
the various labor groups and army units to see the show free.
A halt was called only because some army units mutinied, took
over the entire theatre, and refused to quit and make room for
others. They bivouacked there, and the riot squads had to be
called out of the barracks before they evacuated the premises.
With those fellows we had apparently made a smashing hit. The
Chinese masses had never seen Occidental performers before,
except in movies and, like shoo-fly pie, they simply couldn't "get
enough of that wonderful stuff."

But I decided *we* had had enough. And, undoubtedly leaving
in our wake uncounted new adherents of the Duncan dance
à l'Orientale, we bade farewell to our friendly hosts. But here,
too, Oriental style had to be observed. Madame Sun entertained
me at tea, presenting me with a pretty Chinese-embroidered
shawl in the Imperial color of the celestial kingdom—bright
yellow—symbolizing the heavenly orb. I still have it.

Then there was the governor of the province, who extended
us a farewell feast of thirty-five courses—all Chinese. It started
off with a hot, steaming shark-fin stew, prepared by his own
hands at the table. Seeing those bleeding pieces of fish drop into
the pot one by one had an effect the opposite of raising my
appetite. The various Oriental dishes followed one another in
slow procession, including such choice morsels as hundred-year-
old eggs that gave off enough ammonia fumes for a general gas
attack. Everything was eaten with chopsticks out of tiny, transparent porcelain bowls. This went on for hours with nothing to
drink but green tea. To my Occidental palate, these dishes were
repulsive; I could not swallow a single bit, never knowing
whether it was a slice of chow dog or worse. I raised my chopsticks dutifully and pretended to taste each course as it was set

before me, but not a wee morsel passed my lips. Finally, at the
end, the servants brought in large wooden bowls filled to over-
flowing with snow-white rice, every kernel separate, just the way
I like it. My face lit up; I smacked my lips. Starving for some
sustenance after a three-hour wait, I was about to raise my chopsticks and dig in with relish, when someone rudely kicked me
under the table.

I turned to my neighbor, Michael Borodin, and whispered,
"What's the matter?" He shook his head and whispered back,
"Don't eat it!" I turned pale, thinking it might be poisoned;
such things have happened at Oriental courts, I knew from
reading history.

"I like rice, and what's more I am starving!" I whispered,
fiercely determined to eat something at this gorgeous feast. He
reached for my arm and held onto it so I wouldn't commit a
grave breach of protocol.

"It's not proper. The host will be gravely offended if, after
a dinner of the finest Chinese food, his guests are hungry enough
to eat such common, every-coolie's-staple as rice."

"Then why do they serve it?"

"Ah, that is a curious Oriental ceremony having to do with
polite manners," he said; and as we got up from the table he
added with tongue in cheek, "Now, if you really want to show
your gratitude and appreciation of the excellent meal your kind
host has offered you, give a good, loud, resounding belch!"

"What with?" I retorted petulantly. "I haven't eaten anything."

"No matter, do it anyway. It is a great compliment. Nothing
delights a Chinese host more."

"After you, Sire," I said and laughed. "Men come before
women in China." But he too would have no part of this particular Oriental protocol. And so I rose as hungry as I had sat down
at the governor's banquet in my honor.

On the morning of departure, a large delegation of men and
women, representing different organizations, appeared at our

house on the outskirts of town, where for the last six weeks we had lived as guests of the Kuomintang government. They presented us with various painted silk scrolls and other gifts on behalf of the Chinese people. There was also a letter from the Foreign Minister:

Palace Yian-cen, Hankow
February 6, 1927

Dear Miss Duncan:

In the name of our Chinese comrades I wish to express to you and the pupils of your school, our great appreciation of the unique work and the beauty of your dancing, which you have shown us during the period of your sojourn in Hankow.

You have not only brought us a cultural form new to our people, but have also enriched our vision, and you have demonstrated that your art expresses in movement all the natural energies that create joy and beauty.

Very cordially yours,
Eugen Chen

I was grateful for their warm appreciation and felt that all of us—dancers, pianist, managers, chaperone, and maid alike—had bravely fulfilled the difficult assignment for which the Soviet government had sent us to Hankow.

~✌20✌~

Return to Moscow

FOR our voyage down the Yangtze-Kiang to Shanghai, the first
lap of our trip, we boarded a Russian boat that had come to
Hankow to take on a cargo of black tea. We made the return
trip in far greater comfort. Several Chinese friends accompanied
us, as did Mrs. Borodin, with her son Norman. She told me she
was seeing her twelve-year-old boy off in Shanghai, where we
were to take a steamer for Vladivostok. She asked me to see that
he got safely on the train there for Moscow, where he would
go back to school. I promised to do so. This seemingly simple
circumstance was to play an important part in the life of Fanny
Borodin, who was soon to make the headlines the world over.
I must here tell the story and the key part I played in that
drama, details of which have up till now not been revealed.

On our way to Shanghai, while the Chinese civil war was still
raging, we got word that the enemy army led by Chang Tso-lin
had captured Nanking. This news threw everyone aboard into a
panic. My panic was the more terrifying since I remembered my
categorical refusal to dance for his army and naturally feared
the very worst of fates from his hands in revenge. Before reaching Nanking we stopped several miles upstream to wait for
nightfall. Under the protection of a heavy February fog and
with all lights extinguished, we silently slipped past the enemy
foothold and got safely away, to our enormous relief. What
might actually have happened to any of us if we had fallen into
enemy hands can be seen by what did happen to Mrs. Borodin—
or Mrs. B. as she begged me to call her, being afraid to mention
her full name.

On her return trip to Hankow, sometime in March I believe, she was captured and turned over to Chang Tso-lin. The irate bandit wanted to strangle her on the spot, ostensibly as a spy, but was dissuaded from taking so drastic an action. After languishing in prison for months, she was finally brought to trial in the war lord's stronghold, Peking. They tried her and found her guilty. The usual punishment for that crime was beheading, but because she was a foreigner and a woman they were going to give her an aristocrat's death without spilling any blood. She was to die by either strangulation or drowning. Her defense attorney, A. I. Kantorovich, did everything in his power to free her, offering bribes right and left, all to no avail. The affidavits from Moscow in her defense proved to be mere scraps of paper as far as the Chinese court was concerned. They needed something more credible than that: an affidavit as to her reason for going to Shanghai in the first place, coming from an impartial source. Fanny immediately thought of me, but hesitated to drag me into this mess on account of my future career. The presiding judge had accepted the bribe, a big one; all he needed to release her was my affidavit. Her life depending on the outcome, they very reluctantly got in touch with me. I was then in Paris.

I had absolutely no knowledge of any of this, because the Russian papers and their system of suppressing news inimical to the Communist Party or any of its members carried nothing about Borodin's story. It came as a complete surprise. I did not hesitate to sign the affidavit proving that she had seen her son off to Russia in Shanghai. This document, which I was supposed to hand to the Chinese Ambassador in Paris, and a cable sent in my name direct to Peking, apparently effected her release. The judge acquitted her, and he, as well as Fanny Borodin, instantly vanished off the face of the earth. Chang Tso-lin flew into a rage, turning Peking upside down to find the escaped prisoner, but she remained in hiding for months before starting her homeward journey in disguise.

I saw her again in Moscow. In the interim of her imprisonment, the revolutionary movement in Hankow collapsed through a counter-revolution led by one of their generals. Madame Sun Yat-sen, Eugen Chen and his family, and Borodin scattered to the four winds. They eventually also ended up in Moscow, where I encountered them all once more, and Eugen Chen's daughter became my first Chinese pupil. Fanny Borodin told me the story of her escape, saying, "I am writing a book about my experiences. But don't worry, I won't mention your name or the important part you played in effecting my rescue. As a matter of fact, you did save my life, and I am eternally grateful. That must remain a secret between ourselves, for two reasons. You see, my husband has failed in his mission, and the government is keeping us under house arrest. We are to speak to no one and see no one. You are the only exception. And then there is your career to think of. The less said about this, the better. You understand, don't you?"

I failed to see where my personal career as an artist had anything to do with it. All I did was tell the truth as I knew it to be when asked about her whereabouts on a given date. I never saw either of them again. That chapter in the book of my life was closed.

We landed in Vladivostok at the end of February 1927. To the Russian people in those early years of Communist rule, anyone returning from abroad of his own free will, after having tasted freedom, appeared as strange and marvelous as some weird animal in the zoo. Since we had been *zagranitsa*, as they call it, the public looked at us in amazement. The local theatrical managers refused to let us slip by without cashing in on the occasion. We obtained a two-week engagement from them with a financial guarantee. That was quite an ambitious undertaking on their part, considering we had played that length of time in Vladivostok before our departure in September. But we had not reckoned with their ingenuity.

They came to me one morning and asked me whether I

would consent to an exhibition of our trophies and purchases in the foyer of the theatre. I had no objection. However, they didn't stop with our trophies and Chinese souvenirs. They persuaded me to exhibit every dress and hat and piece of silk underwear, including stockings, that I had bought; even such silly items as powder compacts, lipsticks, and perfume, of which I had brought along a considerable supply, knowing the total dearth of such commodities in Russia. I laughed out loud and exclaimed, "You must be joking!"

"*Nyet! Nyet!*" they said and assured me to the contrary.

How right they were in estimating the avid interest in foreign goods by the average citizen was proved the night of our first performance. The audience could not be torn away from the exhibit in the outer foyer, and had to be coaxed back into their seats again. I was so delighted with this opportunity of engaging in a bit of effective propaganda in reverse, by showing off the sorts of goods available to all the people on the "other side," that I gladly agreed to Schneider's suggestion that we stop over on our way home at all the larger centers—Khabarovsk, Chita, Blagovyeshchensk, Irkutsk, Krasnojarsk, Tomsk, Omsk, etc., right into Moscow. We would, as he put it in the Russian equivalent, "clean up" and return solvent. This plan was fouled up by an order from the Narkompross to come home immediately. The children, absent from school for seven months, had to make up their curriculum for that academic year. It never occurred to the wise Big Brothers in the Kremlin that the children had learned more, had gained a broader outlook on the world by traveling, than through all the Marxist-doctored books at school. But, having once more set foot on Soviet soil, we had to obey.

Stopping over for a couple of days in Khabarovsk, where we had already been booked in advance and could not break the date, I had the oddest experience. The temperature in the middle of March was down to forty below zero. The snow lay foot-high all over this city on the Amur, named after a hetman of the Cossacks. In front of my hotel the statue of the founder, Count Mouraviev-Amoursky, was invisible under his mantle of snow. Siberia, so warm in August, when the rich black earth was yielding a golden harvest on our eastward trip, now showed itself in its true colors. For this is how it looks the larger part of the year—an icy, frozen waste, unrelieved by tree or bush. This is the home of the ermine and the elusive sable. The houses are log cabins with double windows sealed against the deadly cold.

The hotel offered its guests unusual comforts and warmth. I had a big room, whose main feature of attraction in that arctic climate was the white porcelain stove reaching to the ceiling in one corner of the room, so situated that servants could easily stoke it from the corridor outside.

The hour was nearly midnight on the seventeenth of March when it happened. I had retired early after my performance; I usually liked to stay up late, being too keyed up to go to sleep. Lying stretched out on the bed in my nightgown, ready to turn off the light, I was suddenly overcome by a choking sensation. Gasping for breath, I rushed to the window for air. Because the double window was sealed tight, I had to climb up onto the sill in order to open the small ventilator that was just large enough to push my head through. At that moment Elisaveta Gregori-evna entered my room to bid me good night. When she saw me sticking my head out the window ventilator, while the tempera-ture hovered near forty below, she called out in alarm, "Why Irmushka! What is the matter with you! Are you ill?"

"I can't breathe," I gasped, and tried to inhale the icy air.

"Come right down from there, you'll catch pneumonia!" she commanded in her most professional accents as a nurse. I meekly obeyed, feeling suddenly quite normal again. But she insisted on getting a servant to inspect the stove for any possible coal fumes, which could have been dangerous. All was in order.

"I hope you are not coming down with anything serious," she said, and took my temperature. All was in order here too, and I assured her I felt fine and proved it by falling promptly to sleep.

I slept soundly until morning when a rap at my door woke me up. It was a telegram from my half-sister in Hamburg. "Mother died last night," the message said. That was all. Under these strange circumstances I learned that my dear mother had passed away. I did not associate my previous night's experience with this sad news. And I could not possibly get to Hamburg in time for her funeral.

The Trans-Siberian Railway took eight days to reach Moscow, and no plane could be had. Nothing was quite so mournful as this long railway journey. It took the traveler through limitless steppes, empty of any sign of habitation, and passed for days on end through the *taiga,* a forest wilderness, much like our Middle West in flatness only more desolate in aspect. I was glad to get off the train in Moscow. It seemed I had been gone a lifetime.

Things had changed at 20 Pretchistenka during our long absence. Living quarters being at a premium, empty space filled up automatically, like water running into a ditch. I suppose because we had gone to China, the housing authorities thought it only natural that a group of Chinese students should occupy our space while we were away. Luckily, my room was still available, but my bathroom had been appropriated, the fixtures torn out, and a row of six toilets installed instead. I was so outraged that I complained to the most important official—Lunacharsky—and he as usual came to my assistance. Within two days I had my bathroom back *intact.* We discovered that the heavy snows of winter had caved in part of the tin-covered roof and that most of the money we had sent for the upkeep of our school had gone to make repairs. The government refused to allot funds for that purpose. It looked to me like a hopeless situation. How could I ever make any real progress in this country?

The old depression took hold of me again. And on top of all this, the sad news of mother's death made me feel low in mind and spirit. I had written to my married half-sister Anna Axen—who had told me about mother—and asked her to give me all the details she could. I found her letter when I got home. She described mother's funeral and went on to say:

It all happened so fast and even for us it came quite unexpected. Only a fortnight ago mother herself walked to the hospital and the first eight days she seemed not to be very ill. She even joked with the nurses. But our dear mother had an old complaint, asthma and a weak heart, so the doctor said. At first we went to several specialists because she always complained about a pain in her throat but they could find nothing there.

On Wednesday last I visited her with my children. She was ever so glad when someone came to see her. It was then already very noticeable that her health had begun to fail. However, she talked a lot and when I came again the next day we talked about you. Once again I brought up the question of notifying you of her illness, but her express wish was that you should not be told. She would not hear of it. She repeated, as she had so often done, that you should have *no worries*. But she thought of you always and constantly nourished a great longing in her heart for her beloved daughter, Irma.

She appeared very weak on Thursday morning. She said to me: "Oh Anna, how do I come to such suffering!" . . . and then I had to open the window for her because her breath came too short. . . .

She said: "Take a chair and sit here beside me and keep quite still."

I took her hand in mine and she never let it go. We sat thus quietly for a long time, the stillness broken with an occasional moan, for mother was in her last agony.

The doctor came, and mother complained she could not swallow. He said he would fix that and gave her an injection. After that our dear mother gently breathed her last, she went to sleep never to wake again.

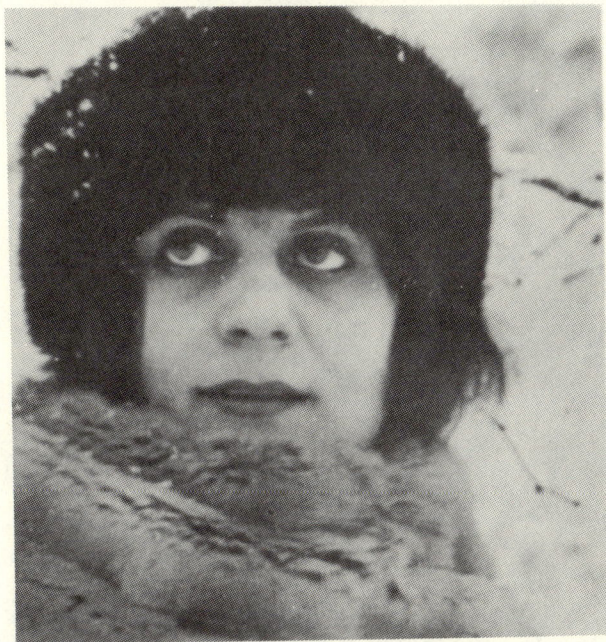

Irma Duncan in Moscow, ca. 1925.

The Isadora Duncan School, Moscow.

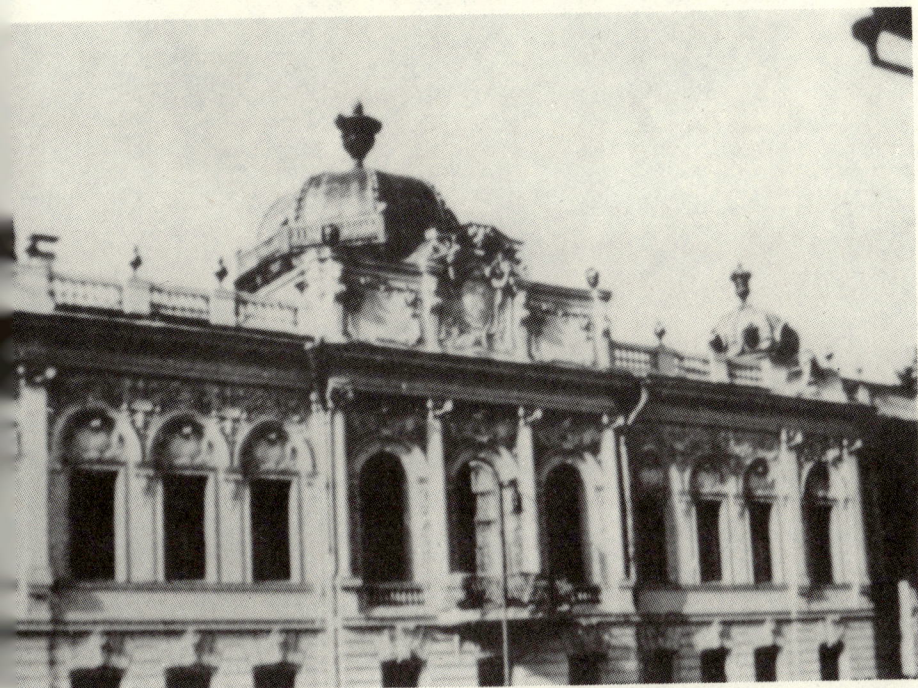

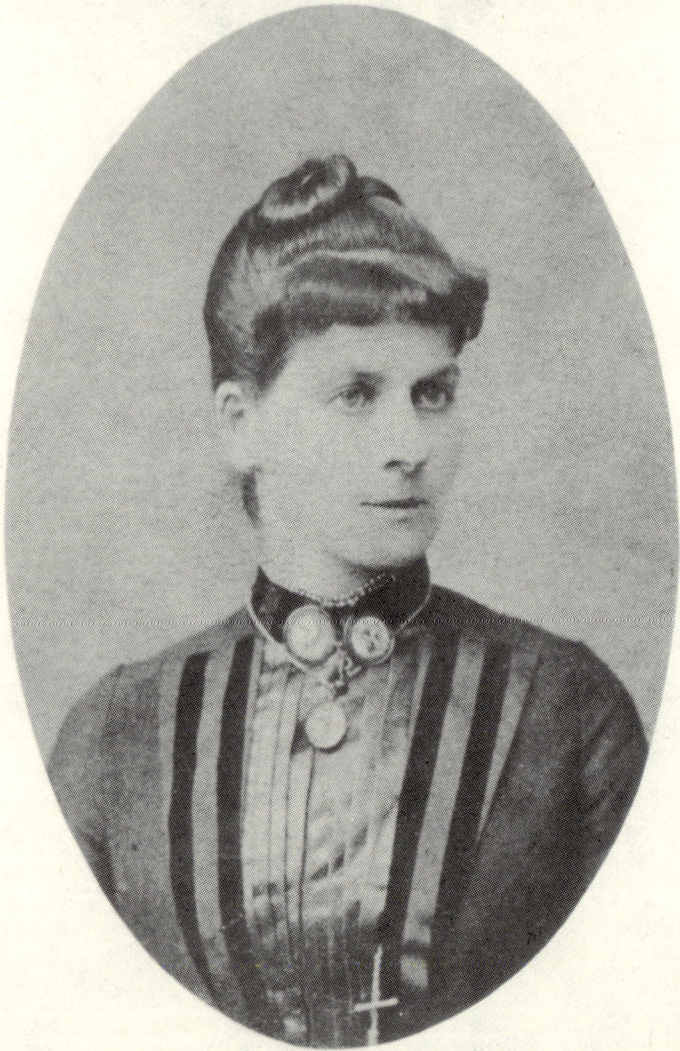

"The young woman I never knew." Irma's mother, photographed years before her marriage.

When I read the sentence "I had to open the window for her because her breath came too short," my mind instantly flashed back to that hotel room in Siberia and how I suddenly opened the small window, gasping for breath the day mother died. And then I knew it had been a premonition, for there was nothing physically the matter with me. Some strange, supernatural manifestation had taken hold of me—what is known as a psychic experience, to prepare me for the shock that was to follow. I made preparations to leave for Hamburg and settle mother's small estate. In the meantime I wrote another letter to my sister and in due course received an answer from her. She said:

I am so glad to know that you are safely back in Moscow from your long oriental tour. Here at home, we have always followed your travels on the map because this interested mother enormously. She used to subscribe to a magazine, and last winter there was much written about Siberia and China with many illustrations. She used to tell me about these countries and remark how much better she could now visualize what your surroundings looked like.

Yes, dear sister, as you mentioned in your letter, you really have lost a very devoted and self-sacrificing mother. She wept bitter tears because of her longing for you, her only child. She loved to pour her heart out to me since I too, in a way, was her child, not having known any other mother but her. I was only five years old when she came to us and took care of me after my own mother died. Her life then was not an easy one, but she always looked towards the future with optimism hoping for better days.

I often tell my own children about grandmother and her struggles in life and the cross she had to bear. And how sad that in her last years, just when things looked brighter for her, she, poor soul, had to leave us. You must have received her last letter written on her birthday February 18th, when we all spent the day together. She got so many presents and flowers and seemed so happy and gay. She even indulged in all sorts of nonsense with the children. My own little Irma had crocheted the edge of a handkerchief for her grandmother. This gave mother so much pleasure she told her: "This lovely handkerchief I'll take with me into my grave." And four weeks later she was dead. How strange life is!

I visited mother's grave when I went to Hamburg. She loved flowers. All her life some pots of cactus or geraniums filled her kitchen windows. I planted roses on her last resting place. I left everything she owned to my sisters and kept only her photograph—a picture of her taken long before I was born, of the young woman I never knew.

❧21❧

Finale

In June, as soon as my visit with my relatives had ended, I intended to go straight back to Moscow where pressing work awaited me. And if it had not been for a letter from Lisa, who was then dancing in Brussels, telling me of Isadora's performance scheduled for the end of June at the Trocadéro, I would never have seen my foster mother again. That small inner voice, which I so seldom heeded, told me quite plainly to drop everything and go to Paris. This time I obeyed. I had some curious premonition that this might be the last time Isadora would dance in public. There was no particular reason for this notion. In her forty-ninth year Isadora was still in good form—a little too stout, perhaps, but otherwise strong and healthy. She could easily count on several more years of artistic activity, sustained as she was by world-wide fame.

When I arrived in Paris, I had not the slightest idea where to find her. Our correspondence had stopped completely. Except for a wire from her when my mother died, saying, "Deepest sympathy, planning school you, me, Trocadéro," sent from Paris, I had no knowledge of her whereabouts. I stayed at a small hotel just off the Rue St. Honoré near the Elyseé Palace. The first thing I did was to consult the papers and *affiches* on the street corners, hoping to find an advertisement of the performance. There was nothing. Just by chance, strolling about in the lovely June sunshine and breathing Parisian air I had missed for so long, I ran into a friend I had not seen since leaving America. Alfred Sidès was able to tell me all about Isadora.

Since her return to Paris from Nice, a committee of friends, with Fredo Sidès as chairman, had attempted to collect funds and buy back her former residence in Neuilly when it came up for auction a second time. Madame Cécile Sartoris acted as treasurer. With the aid of the French newspaper *Comedia* and the Paris edition of the *New York Herald*, a public subscription was started, and the committee also received gifts of works of art, which were to be auctioned off to aid the fund. The idea was to turn the house into an Isadora Duncan Memorial School, where she could live for the rest of her life. Afterwards, it would be turned over to the French government, which would carry it on to perpetuate her name and ideals in the future. Unfortunately, nothing came of it. And I doubt very much that Isadora would have liked to return to that house of tragedy, haunted by the spectres of her dead children.

Fredo told me that she was living in a studio-apartment on the Rue Delambre, in the Montparnasse district. It was a duplex arrangement, with bedroom and bath opening onto a balcony overhanging the studio below. He said she had finished her memoirs, called *My Life*, and expected the book to be published in America that fall. I thanked him for all this information and told him I would see Isadora that afternoon.

On my way to see her, I stopped at the flower market in front of the Madeleine. Seeing some roses I fancied of a very delicate shade of pink, I bought the whole basketful from the astonished woman—all my arms could carry. I was dressed in brown for the reunion: a brown chiffon dress, brown straw cloche fitting tight over my head, and brown suède shoes. I had not seen Isadora for nearly three years, and I looked forward to this meeting with great joy and excitement. I had so much to tell her about my trip to China. I had no idea that she had gone so far as to make an official protest to the powers that be. I simply could not have imagined such a step on her part where I was concerned. If I had known, I would have had it out with her there and then. But since I did not know, there seemed nothing to mar the pleasure of our reunion.

She was waiting for me at the Rue Delambre. Mary Desti was there, and Isadora's friend and pianist, Victor Seroff. A long, narrow corridor with doors on only one side of it led to her studio at the very end. On opening the door, I brushed the armful of flowers inadvertently against it, and some pink rose petals scattered before me to the floor. The first words that greeted me—like Poe's raven of doom—were Mary's cry, "Ah, ça porte malheur!"

I disregarded this and presented the roses to Isadora, who embraced me joyfully. Mary's superstitious belief that scattered flowers bring bad luck had no effect on us. Isadora insisted on ordering champagne, which she could ill afford, to toast my arrival. I invited all three to have dinner with me in a little restaurant I knew in Montmartre called Madelon. It was the first time in my life that I was able to treat my foster mother to a meal. When I told her I had come expressly to see her performance, she informed me that it had been postponed till July. She begged me to stay on, but this was quite impossible. I had too many engagements booked for the summer. She wanted to know if the rumor she heard of my going to America with the pupils was correct. I told her I had thought of it.

"Then you must take me with you," she said, and added, "You really should have asked my permission to go to China with the school."

I assured her I would like nothing better than that we all go to America together. "However, when it comes to asking your permission every time I want to dance with my pupils (for they are mine too, you must know)," I told her quite bluntly, "that is out of the question!"

She gave me a startled look, for I had never been so outspoken on this particular subject. I had won my independence the hard way and had no intention of giving it up a second time.

The experience in Greece had taught me to beware of falling into another trap of vague promises. The reins of my career would remain in my own hands from now on. I spoke quite frankly; and, surprisingly enough, Isadora seemed to understand my viewpoint when I had explained.

"Remember that I kept the school functioning after you yourself had given it up for lost," I reminded her, "and without my heroic effort in the face of every obstacle there would be no school at all!"

While we were on the most important subject relating to our working together, I confided to her exactly what was on my mind in order to clear the air for future collaboration. I told her I had earned the right to an equal partnership and would tolerate no more nonsense about who was exploiting whom. I had not meant to speak so severely, but this question had nagged at me for a long time. She took it all very amiably and was in complete accord with my views. I felt relieved and glad we had this question of our relationship resolved at last. I need not have taken the trouble. Fate has a way of settling all human endeavors for good.

Much as I desired to prolong my visit with Isadora and stay for the performance in July, it could not be arranged. Time and money ran out. I had to return to Moscow. I spent a few days alone with Isadora at a hotel in Saint-Germain-en Laye, called Pavillon Henri IV. This typical French inn of the more expensive kind had been part of the château built by the monarch of that name, and Louis XIV was born there in 1638. In this old place, redolent with French history, Alexandre Dumas wrote his *Three Musketeers*. It had a magnificent view over all of Paris, and we were constantly reminded of a similar one—the one spread out before us in her school at Bellevue-sur-Seine—that short-lived dream called Dionysion. We talked of that and of what the future might bring. A heavy, sad atmosphere hung over the place, which no good French wines and food could dispel. We both sensed this and decided to motor back to Paris. I had to leave in any case.

I'll never forget that last day. In the morning, in her studio, I spoke of the Chinese theatre and the acting I had seen there. I showed her some of the curious gestures the actors make, always very large and exaggerated. She told me she had been working on Liszt's *Dante Symphony*, which inspired her to make similar gestures. She asked Seroff to play parts of it and showed them to me. Later she led me upstairs into her bedroom to show me the small trunk containing her manuscript, which she had written in longhand. Her large, flowing script filled each page with only a few sentences; hence the manuscript filled the entire trunk.

She laughed and said, "It is mostly about my love affairs. I wanted to write about my art mostly, but the publishers were not interested . . . and I needed the money desperately."

I always hated to leave Paris and, since it was a beautiful day, I proposed a little promenade along the Champs-Elysées so I could have another look at it. I then invited Isadora to lunch at Fouquet's. We sat outside in the sun and ordered from the huge menu à la carte, for that is the way she preferred to eat, even with no money in her pocket. She had ham and asparagus with holladaise sauce and brandied peaches for desert. I took the chef's special, whatever it was, for I had to count my francs, having just enough left over for my *wagon-lit* ticket to Moscow. Afterward, we taxied back to her hotel on the Rue Delambre.

Mary dropped in for a while, and some other people. In the end we remained alone. We were talking of this and that when the telephone rang. To my surprise, someone from the Soviet Embassy wanted to see me immediately. I told him to come to Isadora's studio.

"It is important that I see you alone," the man said when he arrived. His voice sounded very mysterious. I told Isadora and she disappeared upstairs into her bedroom. This was the precise moment when I was told of Fanny Borodin's plight, which was considered a state secret at the time. I sent the telegram to Peking, as the Secretary of the Soviet Embassy requested, but could not promise to deliver the letter to the Chinese Embassy the following day. My train was due to leave in half an hour. I suggested that Isadora Duncan deliver the letter in my stead. He agreed and I called to her to come down again. She was quite willing to comply. The man left and we were once more by ourselves. I recall we were sitting close together on the divan when I said, "Well, Isadora, I have to say goodbye!"

We looked at each other for a while without saying a word. And then we both broke down. We had taken leave of each other many times without shedding any tears. But this time it was different. We both must have sensed this, for we clung together as fond pupil and teacher, daughter and foster mother, and dearest of friends.

"When will we see each other again?"

"Soon, I hope."

"I'll come to Russia when I receive the money from my memoirs."

But it was never to be. I had walked only a few paces down that long corridor when she cried out, "Wait a minute!"

She disappeared into the studio for a second and came out draped in her red shawl. She stood directly under a ceiling light in flaming red as I had seen her so many times on the stage. She suddenly started to sing and dance the "Internationale" as a farewell gesture to me on my way to Russia. I joined her in the singing and the dancing, moving backward with each step till I reached the end of the corridor. Then, with the usual last flourish, we ended up in our grand finale. My last view of her was in that triumphant gesture with arms raised, head thrown back, and looking upward.

I never saw Isadora again.

·❧22·❧

Curtain

On July eighth, an eyewitness reported:

Isadora gave her last performance in the Mogador Theatre. Although it was the *saison morte* of the summer, the theatre was packed by a very distinguished audience of French and Americans. The Pasdeloup Orchestra, conducted by Albert Wolff, opened the matinee with the allegretto from Cesar Franck's Symphony. This was followed by Isadora's mighty "Redemption," to the music of the same composer. Then came the beautiful "Ave Maria" of Schubert, danced in such a way that there were those in the audience who sobbed aloud. Who will ever forget the ineffable gesture of the maternal arms cradling nothing? The pitiful tenderness and heart-breaking beauty of it? After the orchestra had played the first movement of the Unfinished Symphony of Schubert, Isadora came out again to dance the second with a more tragic profundity than ever before.

Following the intermission came the *Tannhäuser* Overature and the "Love-death" of Isolde, both danced by Isadora Duncan. At the end of her last dance the audience rose and cheered . . .

The French writer Henriette Sauret gave her impressions after the performance:

Poor great Isadora! After that performance, after the applause and the recalls, I saw her again before the blue curtains, standing between clusters of trembling flowers, making toward the orchestra leader and the musicians the sweet gesture that associated them with her triumph.

We went to congratulate her in her dressing room. She lay there, her bare feet coming out from her half-detached dress, her lovely arms holding up her tired head. Her look was heavy, her made-up red mouth was silent, and the red locks of her hair, twisted in curls like those of antique statues, fell on her shoulders like weighty stalks. She had lain down, without paying much attention, on the light costumes which she had successively worn in the course of the matinee and thrown pell-mell on the divan. And on that chaos of crumpled veils with rainbow colors she seemed to have fallen, a vanquished goddess. . . .

I do not know why, at that moment, the heart oppressed in spite of the joy she had just given us, I recalled the picture of Elizabeth of England dying on her royal carpet piled high with cushions, surrounded by courtiers and ladies of honor . . .

A month later Isadora motored to Nice with her friend Mary Desti. They spent part of the summer at Juan-les-Pins. With no money and none in sight, Mary Desti went boldly to see Paris Singer, who was spending the summer at his villa on Cap Ferrat. He agreed to offer financial help to Isadora for the time she required to work out a new program, which was to include an interpretation of the *Dante Symphony* by Liszt, parts of which she had shown me at her studio in Paris.

Isadora had taken a passionate interest, it seemed, in a small racing car, a Bugatti, and its handsome Italian driver. She wanted to buy the car from its owner, Benoit Falchetto, who also kept a garage. They made a date to go for a ride in the car and try it out on the evening of September 14. Mary had a strange premonition, she said, and begged her friend not to go out on the road that night in the little Bugatti. Nobody could stop her.

She wore her red shawl (the same one she had used on the stage) and, sitting in the low vehicle, with the driver in front and the passenger slightly behind, the end of her shawl dragged on the ground. The moment the driver started the car and raced off, that piece of her red shawl got entangled in the wire spokes of one wheel. As the shawl had been wrapped about her throat and flung over her shoulder, she was caught in it as in a vice. Her body was pulled over the side, her face crushed against the car, and her neck instantly broken. The onlookers screamed, the car stopped; they rushed to help her—but it was too late. Isadora Duncan was dead.

At that tragic moment in my life I was far, far away, giving a performance somewhere in Russia. The curtain had gone up and we were in the midst of our opening dance, a funeral march, which Isadora originally choreographed in memory of her children, and with which we usually started our program by way of dedication. Dressed in long, trailing chiffon robes of beige, the girls formed the chorus; while I, the mourning figure, danced the solo part. At the musical climax I sank to the ground in sorrow in a kneeling position, my head and arms touching the floor. I held this pose for a few bars and then slowly began to rise again. I had danced it like that I don't know how many times.

But on the night of September 14, the moment I assumed that kneeling pose with my body bent forward and my brow touching the floor, something weird came over me, and I remained frozen to the ground. As if paralyzed, I could not stir a muscle. Without knowing, I had assumed the same position in which my dear foster mother had died that night. While in the grip of this strange trance, in full view of the audience, I never lost consciousness. I commanded myself to rise and continue the dance, but my body refused to respond for several minutes, and I remained where I was until just before the end. My immobility had in no way interfered with the movements of the chorus, who went through their motions as usual.

As soon as I could move again, I finished the dance and then rushed backstage into my dressing room, where I collapsed into a chair, white and shaken. I was sure I had creeping paralysis—entirely unaware, again, that I had just experienced a psychic phenomenon. Nowadays, with the study of extrasensory perception, scientists may be able to explain what happened to me. I was at that time totally ignorant of such matters.

The news of Isadora's death was instantly flashed around

the world by radio. It had that night also reached the place where I performed. The authorities promptly sent a messenger to the theatre to notify me of the tragic event, but my manager intercepted him and would not let him come near me. He told the messenger I had a performance to give and nothing must disturb me till it was over. But my psyche had already received the message through the spiritual world. As Shakespeare said in *Hamlet,* "There are more things in heaven and earth, Horatio, than are dreamt of in your philosophy."

That night after the program, the directors of the steel plant for whose workers we had given the performance showed us all over the factory. Watching the night shift forging the steel as it came red hot out of the furnaces reminded me of Dante's inferno. And as I jumped out of the way of those glowing red bars snaking along the floor, I thought of Isadora and her interpretation of Liszt's *Symphony* and wished she could be here to see this. Most factories are dull and boring. But these steel mills, especially at night when the glow and the fantastic shadows combine to accentuate the forceful movements of the laborers—half-naked and covered with sweat—are the stuff that pure drama in motion is made of. I slept peacefully that night, my dreams colored in fantastic lights. It would be quite a while before I could slumber that soundly again.

They told me the next day, on the station platform while we waited for the train to Moscow. I refused to believe it. Isadora had often of late made attempts at suicide by walking into the sea (so the papers claimed), and I insisted it was just another sensational item about her, without foundation in fact. I wired to Lisa in Paris for the truth. When it arrived, I collapsed.

I immediately made plans to fly to the funeral. In those days in Russia, that was easier said than done. I had no trouble getting my papers without red tape. But oh, that ancient Lufthansa plane! It flew just above the tree tops in a dense fog, and when I thought I had come down in Danzig, it was actually Moscow to which we had returned. I was all alone in an eight-passenger plane on my first flight and scared to death. The engineer carried the Russian pilot off the plane in a stupor, dead drunk. After three days, I finally made the Tempelhof airfield in Berlin. I wired to Raymond Duncan to postpone the funeral for a day. He did not answer.

I might as well have taken the train and arrived in Paris sooner and at less expense to my mind, my nervous system, and my pocketbook. When I did arrive, the funeral was over. Lisa was the only one of Isadora's disciples to walk in the procession behind her coffin to the Père Lachaise cemetery, where her body was cremated and her ashes placed in a niche beside those of her children. I was heartbroken not to have been beside her for that last rite.

I arrived, sad and shaken, at Mary's apartment on the Boulevard des Capucines. She greeted me and then pressed something into my hand without saying a word. Lying in the palm of my hand was a piece of red fringe caked with blood. No need to ask what it was. The strange relic told a mute and horrible story. Tears flooded my eyes, and I wanted to be alone for a few moments. The door of the balcony stood open and I stepped outside. I paid no attention to the traffic and the noise from the street below. I was oblivious to everything that happened about me, conscious only of the "souvenir," as Mary called it, in my trembling hand. I closed my hand tight. I did not want to see again this tiny red thread—the gruesome reminder of the monstrous blow that, like an executioner, had cruelly shed Isadora's blood and snuffed out her life. By what bizarre twist of fate should this great and generous-hearted woman, who sought only to bring light and beauty into this world, suffer so horrible an end?

The top-floor apartment afforded a typical view over the roofs of the city which more than any other had been her home and where her restless self had now found its last repose. So as not to break down, I tried to think of all the wonderful moments we had shared, but only inconsequential things crowded into my memory . . . the little wooly lamb she gave me when I was a child . . . and the magic spell she cast over me when I first saw her, that foggy day in January so long ago. And it suddenly struck me by what extraordinary coincidence (or was it that?) we had met and we had parted.

We had danced together at the very beginning and danced together at the very end. Initiation and consecration. In this same year, 1927, I lost both my mothers; the one who gave me life, and the one who made that life worth while. "If something gives a value to human life," Plato said, "it is the contemplation of absolute beauty." Thanks to Isadora and the beautiful way she taught me to dance—always remembering her words: "I have given you the very secret and most holy of my art"—the prize that gives value to human life was mine.

At the news of my foster mother's death I had experienced the weird sensation of having lost the use of my limbs. And I had lost also all desire ever to dance again; as if all along I had done so only under the force and osmotic attraction of her spell, which now was broken with her death. Still, I had to carry on the torch (had she not given me that symbolic picture of Demeter and Persephone?) and continue with my work as she would wish me to do.

I had no sooner returned to Moscow than an amazing thing happened to me. After years of utter neglect, the Soviet government now sprang into action to support the work Isadora had started there in 1921. One could only come to the conclusion that they had waited for her to die. I received an official summons to attend an important conference to discuss the future of the Isadora Duncan School in Moscow. I mapped out a plan for the Ministry of Education that had occupied my mind for a long time. This consisted of incorporating the Duncan method of dancing into the curriculum of the public school system. The present institute on the Pretchistenka could be turned into a teachers' college, where future instructors could be trained. This plan was approved and fully endorsed by the Ministry. I was elated. Our dream come true at last! All the hardships and privations I had endured to bring this about seemed worth while, now that victory was in sight. And since the only true immortality we can achieve consists in the good works we leave behind us on earth, I rejoiced that I could play a small part in building this memorial to the great American whose genius had liberated the art of the dance, from which millions could now benefit. In my elation, however, I had not reckoned with the Marxist-Leninist system that regulates all artistic matters by the ukase of its cultural commissars.

It was pointed out to me that my former position as artistic director would be eliminated, and I would henceforth act merely as an instructor with the salary commensurate with that job. Everybody now associated with the institute would be replaced by Communist Party members, and I myself would have to undergo indoctrination. They did not demand that I join the Party immediately, but that would obviously have to follow if I wanted to function successfully in an entirely communistic organization. I could never embrace such an autocratic ideology. It went against my whole conception of what a free society of men should be. I had been imbued too deeply with the American, democratic principle of government. When it came to my own work, my allegiance belonged to Isadora and her ideals of physical education for children, and not those of the Communists as represented by Comrade Podvowsky. I had fought that principle all my life in the Elizabeth Duncan school under Max Merz's direction, so how could I now, in all conscience, align myself with it under the Soviets? They were determined to uproot every single spiritual aspect of our dance and turn it into simply another gymnastic for women and children. I would not assist in the murder of an art that was created for the attainment of a noble beauty in movement. People who did not believe in the human soul were out to kill the very soul of our dance, the dance as Isadora Duncan envisioned it.

In those days, the late 1920's, I was one of the small number of people from the West who knew what the Communists in Russia were doing to artists. Today, especially with the sad example of Boris Pasternak, it is common knowledge. That domination of the creative instinct in artists by the Big Brother in the Kremlin was what I had to escape. There is no place for a free-thinking artist in an enslaved society. That prophetic inner voice of mine fairly shouted at me to get out before it was too late. I had a big decision to face: remain, to see myself and my art enslaved for the price of government support, and make at least that part of Isadora's dream come true; or leave, and burn my bridges behind me, with the prospect of starting all over again in a free society. I chose the latter.

I entertained secret hopes of being able to save a remnant of my work. To that end, I entered into negotiations with Sol Hurok, the American impresario, to bring myself and my group of Russian dancers to the United States. It was difficult business to negotiate from such a great distance, since I had to labor under the stringent restrictions that govern the actions of every Soviet citizen. I was free to leave at any time. But would the government consent to release the young girls, who had worked and danced with me for seven years? With the aid of a few influential friends in the upper hierarchy, I was finally given permission to take the members of my dance troupe with me to America for a grand memorial performance in Isadora Duncan's honor. It was the first dance ensemble Hurok imported from the Soviet Union, although many have followed since. I wrote him then:

Moscow, May 27, 1928
As soon as I received your contract I started to put the enormous bureaucratic machine here in motion. First of all, I had to get official permission to take my ensemble out of Russia. Then

the contract is looked over for sufficient guarantees. . . . Last
but not least come the passports; each Soviet passport costs $10.00
and there are thirteen to be obtained. All this takes a long
time. . . .

I am sending you photos but no advertising material as it is in
Russian. It will surely be returned by the censor, as happened on
a former occasion. Kindly inform me about departure, tickets,
train connections and steamer, and opening dates.

On the eleventh of June we are giving a memorial performance for Isadora Duncan here in Moscow at the Bolshoi Theatre. Lunacharsky will speak, Stanislavsky and others, important
personages in the arts and sciences. A short film, showing Isadora
on her last trip to Nice a few days before she died, will precede
the performance of myself and my girls in Tchaikowsky's "Symphony Pathetique," with the Moscow Symphony Orchestra. I
shall send you programs and clipping afterwards.

During the summer months, before leaving for America in the
fall, I shall work and rehearse our programs. I heard through
Mrs. Augustin Duncan about the memorial festival you are planning at Madison Square Garden and I hope that something
beautiful will come of it. I will do everything in my power to
help make it so.

Since the planned memorial performance at the Bolshoi Theatre was postponed till the month of October, I employed the
intervening time touring the south of Russia. In my diary for
that year I find nothing but empty pages, mere notations of the
various places we danced—Kharkov, Kremenchug, Cherson,
Kiev, Odessa, etc., etc.

At the beginning of June, the writer Allen Ross Macdougall,
a friend of Isadora and her former secretary, came to visit me in
Moscow. We agreed to collaborate on a book about Isadora's
Russian days to complete her own memoirs, which stopped with
her arrival in Moscow in 1921. He accompanied me on our tour,
and in my free time I worked with him on the Russian part.
He was going to fill in her last years in France, having more
knowledge about them than I, since he had seen her often in

Nice and Paris at that time. He left for America before we did, hoping to get the book published in time for our performances there. He wrote me from Paris in October:

Au Café, Lundi soir,

Dear Irma:

Just a word in haste. . . . I shall sail Wednesday on the *Ile de France*. I'm just making it and very close. I shall arrive in New York about the 16th. First I shall see Dudly Field Malone, my lawyer, about the prospects of the book. Then I shall go to the Farm (Steepletop, in Austerlitz, Col. Co. N.Y.) of Edna St. Vincent Millay. She has sent me a letter of invitation. And with her I shall have time and peace to finish the book and she will help me correct and revise it. And then give me letters to the various publishers. . . .

I will do what I can in America. In the meantime you must send me the rest of the Russian material right away to the Banker's Trust, they will forward it to Miss Millay's farm. I must have it to incorporate into the revised copy. All my love and best wishes in the meantime for your successful voyage and arrival in America. I'm happy the Memorial went off so well.

Dougie

That memorial performance to Isadora, on the first of October, was my farewell to seven years' work in Soviet Russia. The newspaper *Isvestia* commented:

Isadora Duncan's whole life was devoted to beauty through the means of physical education. Before her eyes she always carried the Greek ideal. In her endeavor to find an enlarged field for her experiments she wandered from one country to another. From Germany, to France, from Greece and America to the USSR. She wasn't satisfied to work with a small quantity of children. Her goal was to see her ideas realized on a much grander scale. She wished to see an entire generation of youth educated in the spirit of her doctrine in order to re-create, if not the whole world, at least one entire country. . . .

At the Memorial performance last night Irma Duncan, her adopted daughter, appeared with the pupils of her Moscow school.

At the present time it is the only existing school preserving in its purest form the legacy of Isadora Duncan.

And as far as Irma Duncan was concerned, that legacy would remain that way for as long as she lived. In order to preserve it in its purest form, I had to find a safe haven for it to grow and flourish for the benefit of the DANCER OF THE FUTURE, a free spirit in a free body, the dancer who will not belong to one nation but to all humanity.

I left Russia hoping and praying that I would find that haven elsewhere. For when I walked out of that heavy oak door in the house on Pretchistenka, it closed behind me forever.

✺23✺

The End and a New Beginning

I ARRIVED in New York on Sunday, the twenty-third of December, 1928. For me it was a wonderful homecoming after an eight-and-a-half year absence. Something, some force, had drawn me irresistibly back to America. I came with ten of my pupils in charge of Elisaveta Gregorievna, and Maurice Sheyne (as he now Anglicized his name).* Newspaper reporters crowded in for interviews on the pier, and the newsreel cameras ground away. Friends, new and old, waited to welcome us. Coming from the slow, deliberate pace of life in Russia, we required some time to get accustomed to the pulsating, hectic atmosphere of New York, where the air is charged with electricity and the unceasing, restless traffic and noise continue unabated day and night.

"East side, west side, all around the town" was governed by dapper, uninhibited Jimmy Walker, New York's most colorful mayor. Under the influence of prohibition, a lively revival of the old-fashioned melodrama *The Black Crook* flourished in Hoboken, with bootleg beer served during the show. In sports, Gertrude Ederle filled the front pages of all the newspapers with her feat of swimming the English Channel—the first woman to do so. Herbert Hoover, who had organized the wonderful famine relief in Soviet Russia eight years earlier, had just been elected President.

We made our New York debut on December 27, at the Manhattan Opera House. I felt proud and happy to be able to show my Russian pupils to America. On that day more than

* Mikhail Sheyne, as he is presently known, former head of the Westchester Conservatory of Music, has again returned to the concert stage.

eight years before when I sailed for France, I never imagined
what my homecoming would be like. When the curtain rose and
I made my first entrance on the stage, a storm of applause
greeted me. On the following day, the reviewers had many
complimentary things to say about my work and that of my
pupils. Mary Watkins of the *New York Herald Tribune* came
to interview me at the Alamac where I was staying. She wrote:

Irma Duncan was peacefully eating her supper, that is she was
doing it as peacefully as she had been able to do anything amid
the whirl of rehearsals and complications with the immigration
authorities which have marked the few days since her arrival at
this port, when this department walked in on her quite unexpectedly. Various telephone messages had crossed at random, but
nevertheless, the interview materialized, if somewhat informally.

Miss Irma talked in a very friendly manner while consuming
a lamb chop and tea . . . the talk lasted some ten or twelve
minutes, so impressions were naturally a little hurried. But we
recorded them much as they occurred.

This dancer, one of the torchbearers of the Duncan tradition,
adopted daughter of the illustrious Isadora and now head of the
Moscow school, is a wholesome-looking young woman who said
she felt tired and harassed, but whose appearance denied her. She
has very beautiful, expressive hands, black hair, and bears a most
striking resemblance to her foster mother. On this resemblance
we commented.

"Oh, yes," she said, and her English is excellent, although she
has spoken and thought in only Russian for over eight years she
asserts. "Everyone notices it, but you will find that all the girls
. . . show a strong 'family' resemblance, it comes from thinking
the same thoughts . . . and expressing physically the same artistic ideals."

Irma's sense of harassment sprang, not unreasonably, from the
difficulties incident to extracting four of her youngest followers
from the grip of officialdom on Ellis Island. . . .

they are not the only ones who worry me, the others
being in New York, that rehearsals are only
spirits and dizzy heads. You can imagine

that coming as we did with very little preparation and in, as you might say, one jump from Moscow to Manhattan, with only a foot touching the ground briefly at Berlin, was enough to take away the breath of the seasoned traveler, not to speak of a group of emotional young Russian girls who have never been to America. And we really didn't know until the very last minute that we could actually come. That is the reason for the many rumors and counter-rumors here about the dance festival. We were not sure till we were actually on board the train and over the border, anything can happen in Soviet Russia, you know . . ." she said as a matter of familiar and accepted fact. We called on Wednesday . . . and the Duncan Memorial Festival flung wide its doors last Thursday night at the Manhattan Opera House.

Among the many dance enthusiasts who always flocked backstage to greet me were quite a few dancers who, then practically unknown, have since made names for themselves. One of my female admirers said, "I saw you leave a mere slip of a girl and here you have come back to us in beautiful, dominant womanhood. Isadora's ideal of the highest intelligence in a beautiful body has been most certainly realized in you." I considered that quite a compliment.

The reviewer of the *New York American* wrote:

A new generation of Duncan Dancers, was locally introduced to us, a company of lithe young Russian girls . . . formed this latest contingent of classic dancers to perform publicly in New York, and the shade of Isadora must have smiled benignly at the fascinating artistry of her young disciples of a second generation. . . . The spectator realized forcibly that not in her most fruitful and successful epoch did the great California dancer produce any more delightful or captivating pupils than those seen last night. . . . Irma was the leading spirit in her elfin group. The others were—Tamara, Alexandra, Marussia, Lisa, Lola, Vera, Manya, Vala, Lily, Mussia and little Tamara.

This chapter of the dance deserves an important place in the history of Isadora Duncan's most important achievements.

And the *Herald Tribune:*

> As their leader and teacher, Irma has found her own valuable niche . . . that she has so successfully instilled into the brains and bodies of the later generation that devotion which is deeper than outward gesture, is sufficient evidence of artistic worthiness in her capacity as heiress and guardian of the Duncan formulae.

We appeared in Philadelphia, Baltimore, Washington, Boston, Montreal, Buffalo, Cleveland, Detroit, Chicago, St. Louis, and Pittsburgh. Later, on our return engagement in New York, when the public had a chance to appraise our work, we danced in Carnegie Hall—scene of my former triumphs as one of the six original Isadora Duncan Dancers—to standing room only. Everything was joy and harmony. How long would it last?

My manager informed me in June that in view of the success we had attained he wished to engage us for another season. I agreed to this, although the Russian girls had obtained permission from their government for only one season. In this respect, I envisioned no difficulties and decided to spend the summer in France for economical reasons. A performance was arranged in Paris in memory of Isadora at the Salle Pleyel. I wrote to Paris Singer and notified him of this, as I very much wanted him to be there. He answered from Bad Nauheim in Germany:

My dearest Irma:

I have been thinking of you for days and wondering if you were back from the U.S.A. and now I have your note. I am so sorry I shall not be there to see you dance, but since I saw you in Paris things have been very bad with my health and I was brought up here on my back by a heart doctor and have been here a month. I have to be here all July also but it has done me a little good and I have great hopes.

Is there any chance of your looking me up on your way to Russia? It is close by Cologne or nearer still to Frankfurt on Main. How was poor old Gus? I feel always so anxious about

him. Au revoir, my dear little Irma, do drop me a little reply
to this—

Your old friend,
Paris

I regretted he could not be present at my performance. I had
so hoped he would take an interest in the furtherance of her
ideas and, by way of a memorial, help endow her school. To
keep her ephemeral art alive from one generation to another,
by means of public performances, was becoming too great a
burden for me to bear alone.

I can't describe with what deep emotion I looked forward to
dancing again in Paris. My artistic association with Isadora always seemed to take on a closer tie here in this beautiful city of
so many wonderful memories. Here, I first appeared with her
as a child in the old Gaité-Lyrique. Then in the Châtelet, and
subsequently—when I was grown up and learned to appreciate
her art fully—we danced together at the beautiful Théâtre des
Champs-Elysées. And then that final wonderful season at the
imposing Trocadéro in January, the year she and I left for Russia. She had choreographed an entire Wagner program. We
girls danced the "Flower-maidens" scene in *Parsifal*, and I recall the garland of flowers I wore that night—fresh anemones,
the large kind, in vivid shades of red, purple, pink, and white, a
lovely combination of colors. I had not danced in Paris since.
Would our French audiences remember me, I wondered? I
thrilled at the idea of being able to show them what she and I
had accomplished in Russia. Our huge posters bearing the announcement: "Isadora Duncan Dancers de Moscou," and in
smaller print underneath: "Sous la direction d' IRMA DUNCAN,"
blazed on every street corner where the advertising columns
stood.

The performance was given at the Salle Pleyel. I can tell of
the French public's reaction and the impression we made only
through newspaper clippings. But I have a letter from Madame
Cécile Sartoris, the same journalist who saw me dance at Isa-

dora's studio before that eventful trip to the land of the Bolsheviks. She wrote:

My dearest Irma:

I did not come round last evening because I saw crowds of people going and my emotions could not be expressed to you. I suffered and was happy at the same time during the performance. The great spirit of Isadora hovered over you all, and she must be proud and pleased with you for what you have accomplished. At moments her breath seemed to pass through you, and the children were beautiful.

I think those last Russian dances remarkable with the singing and it seems to me that you should go towards that expression more and more as it moves with the spirit of today. I was happy that you had such a large and appreciative audience . . . I quite understand you haven't had a minute but I would like to see you. This evening I will call up on chance of making an appointment.

Be proud of yourself, you have done a great work and *you have* Isadora's school. Don't let worries undermine you—yesterday you accomplished a great feat.

Very affectionately yours,
Cécile

That performance on July 2 was the only one we gave in Paris. Later in that month we danced at the Casino Theatre in Le Touquet, where the Prince of Wales spent the summer, and we danced before a very mondaine, chic audience, entirely dressed in black and white. The gentlemen attended in full dress and the ladies all in black evening gowns with ermine wraps. What a contrast to the high boots and shawls of the worker audience in Russia!

It rained every day, and the Hotel Atlantic at the end of the boardwalk had no heat. I had no desire to stay there any longer than I needed to. I returned to the comfortable little hotel on the Rue de Bassano, not far from the Etoile, while the girls with Elisaveta Gregorievna spent the rest of the summer at Pontchartrain in the country. I wrote once more to Singer, who had returned to his lovely house on the Place des Vosges with his wife, his former nurse, whose acquaintance I had made in 1917 at the time of his break with Isadora. Isadora had left a packet of letters he wrote her in my care, and these I now sent back to him. He answered me:

> Many thanks dear, for your letter and for the letters of Isadora's which a nice young man brought to me.
> We are off to Paignton for a month, then Saint-Jean until I have to go to Palm Beach in December. I think I am better but still sleeping very badly.
> Irma darling, I wish you every success in America this time like the last and with better financial results without all those worries. I can always prove Isadora wanted you to take on her school for she told me so in Nice just before her death. With love, dearest Irma,
>
> Your old friend,
Paris Singer

This was the last word I had from my old friend, whom I had known since my childhood days and who gave me that marvelous voyage on the Nile, which remains one of my most treasured memories. He died two years later of a heart attack.

Paris Singer had wished me success in America for my second season and without worries; but, instead of diminishing, my worries mounted and mounted until I was engulfed by nothing but trouble.

There was trouble with my impresario over financial matters. Instead of my suing him for nonpayment of salary due me as per contract, he sued me for $60,000 and also attached my bank account! Some evil forces were conspiring against me. Ill-meaning persons tipped off the unofficial representative of Soviet Russia in Washington. America had not yet recognized the regime in that country. This man, by the name of Borowsky, held a secret meeting with my Russian girls, threatening them with dire reprisals on their relatives in Russia if they refused to return home at once. The girls wanted to remain with me; so they told me during a tearful session in the privacy of my room. But after that talk with Borowsky, they were afraid even to say "How do you do" to me. He had ordered their return to their homeland and, as every Soviet citizen knows, failure to comply means banishment to Siberian concentration camps for those innocent pawns left behind.

Once their government had stepped in, I wielded no more power over them. My strenuous protests were of no further avail. Intimidated and afraid of what might be done to their families, they all meekly obeyed and left on the appointed date for home. Not one of my pupils had the courage to throw in her lot with me, as I had done formerly with Isadora. For I had no intention, especially after having breathed the air of freedom in America, of returning to a country where people are treated as abject slaves. It was a hard decision to make. It meant the loss of all my work that had occupied the best years of my life. But no sacrifice seemed too great for the sake of artistic integrity and the adherence to one's principles that may only flourish in a liberal climate. The same day I saw the girls sail away, I recalled Isadora's words when she once said to me, "Courage, it's a long way but light is ahead . . . these red-tunicked kids are the future, so it is fine to work for them. Plough the ground, sow the seed, and prepare for the next generation that will express the new world."

Well, I had done exactly that. Now it was up to that new generation to sow the seeds. I wished them luck and hoped they would succeed as well as I did with them in trying to propagate Isadora's ideal.

Russia being the iron-walled society it is, I have had no further contact with my former Soviet pupils. Overnight, all the work I had built up at such expense of my young energies and sacrifice fell like a house of cards into the sand. No one knew what untold misery and regret it caused me. Nor did the news item telling of their homecoming in that "Worker's Paradise" help me. Cabled from Moscow by the International Press, it said:

> The twelve young girl dancers who toured the United States last season under the direction of Irma Duncan, and who were forced to return to Russia last winter have been thrown into prison by Soviet authorities, it was learned yesterday. The children were imprisoned, according to reports, because of their failure to send the Soviet authorities all or portions of their American earnings while on tour in this country.
>
> Immediately upon arrival in Moscow from New York, the youngsters' baggage including phonographs, trunks, musical instruments, etc., were confiscated. The girls said shopping tours in America had converted them from Communism to admirers of capitalism. At the conclusion of Miss Duncan's American contract at Christmas time, 1929, local Soviet representatives informed her that the girls must be sent home forthwith. Over the strong objections of Irma Duncan the girls were taken from her and sent back to Russia.

This indictment of that barbaric country speaks for itself. I was relieved to be able to wash my hands of the whole matter. For I was one of the few people in America at that epoch who knew through personal experience—by trying to earn a living in Soviet Russia—that conditions in that country, political and economic as well as ideological, would not improve in time. On the contrary. And therefore I saw no future there for me or my work.

Never one to cry for long over spilt milk (although this was actually a tragic event in my career), I girded myself for further struggles on a new front. I gathered together a group of young American girls, who had had—more or less—some training in the Duncan dance, and worked with them. By magic and sheer hard work, I soon shaped them into a group that could appear with me professionally. Teaching is a gift, and my powers in that field had been early recognized by both Elizabeth and Isadora. We appeared at Lewisohn Stadium in New York and at Robin Hood Dell in Philadelphia in the summertime, dancing out of doors to the music of a large symphony orchestra and to an enthusiastic audience that filled every seat and open space, crowding even into the aisles. My American pupils were as well received as my Russian ones had been by the public and the press. I am not in a position to laud my own efforts. The review in the Minneapolis *Tribune,* where I presented my American group for the first time to the public, had this to say:

> Having seen the magnificent art of Irma Duncan, herself the greatest exponent of the school founded by Isadora Duncan and by many pronounced as even superior to her adopted mother in her power of interpretation, it is a foregone conclusion that whatever group she leads, whether from Moscow, Paris or New York, the result can be but the same, and that is—perfection of the art of interpretive dance as has not been surpassed in this generation.

Of our Lewisohn Stadium performance the *Herald Tribune* of July 14, 1932, remarked in part:

> Miss Duncan, who has done wonders in two years with her first non-Russian pupil group, demonstrated again last night her supremacy as a torch bearer. . . . The girls, at first a little nervous of the platform-edge, soon found themselves at ease and gave an exhibition of intense training and temperamental development which was admirable in every sense.

My press-clipping book is filled with such comments about my art and work. They and a collection of photographs form the only record. The dancer's is an ephemeral art, no sooner performed than it vanishes into thin air. There is nothing left in concrete form for posterity to judge. With this in mind, I thought of doing a documentary film back in 1929, while I was still in my prime and had the Russian pupils of Isadora's school with me. I proposed this scheme to several moving picture producers; but only one, Walter Wanger, showed enough interest at least to discuss the idea with me. He thought we should wait until a story went with it. Well, the story has now been written, but—as always—too late.

In April 1930, while I went through this personal upheaval in my career, I had no one to advise me or protect me. I was still officially a foreigner in this country; my first papers had lapsed, so that I needed to start all over again to apply for citizenship. From out of the blue, I received an invitation from Mr. and Mrs. Silas Newton, whom I had met only once, to be their house guest for a while. I accepted with pleasure, and we became close friends. They had a house on East Sixty-eighth Street between Lexington and Park avenues. He had natural gas and oil wells in Texas. His wife Nancy was a sports writer— golf mainly—for the New York *Journal*.

Those were the days of the speakeasy and, because Silas was a teetotaler, his wife would take an occasional drink with her girl friends at one of the better-known subterranean establishments. One sunny afternoon she invited me to Belle Livingstone's place on Park Avenue. As one of the notorious speakeasy queens, Belle presided over the house in grand style; that is, rowdy in manner and lewd of language. It was the fashionable spot to imbibe forbidden spirits, and much frequented by writers and artists of note. The day I called with Nan the doors had not yet opened for business, since it was too early in the afternoon. We found Belle alone in her negligee taking a rest. She invited us upstairs to her room and offered us a cup of tea! But Nan ordered champagne and the reputation of the speakeasy was saved. Nan, a typical Irish girl with red hair and gray eyes, and the fun and laughter that go with them, liked Belle and invited her to a party at her house.

That party had been secretly planned to take place during her husband's absence in Texas, where he periodically inspected his oil wells. That night, the sixth of April, Belle telephoned beforehand to inquire whether she could bring a couple of men friends along. They had apparently dropped in just as Belle, all dressed in black lace and gardenias for the occasion, was about to leave. Nan told her yes, the more the merrier! And so Belle showed up with her two escorts. They were the writer Cameron Rogers and his older brother Sherman Rogers, who was a lawyer.

I had on a long evening dress in a lovely shade of red, the color of the American Beauty rose. I happened to be pouring the martini cocktails when I was introduced. Cameron remained with Belle, but his brother asked me if he could sit beside me. The sitting room held a crowd of dinner guests, and all we had to sit on was the piano bench. We talked animatedly and he, being so fair with blond hair and blue eyes, gave me the impression he might be a Scandinavian, except for his Harvard accent. He did not leave my side and followed me around everywhere. We sat together at dinner; and afterward, when the guests went upstairs to play roulette or bridge, we repaired to the room where they had music and we danced.

Ten years before, almost to the day, a clairvoyant with a genuine gift for prophecy, a Mademoiselle Berly who lived in Paris, foretold that I would marry. She described my future husband to me, saying he was very blond, had piercing eyes, and was a lawyer. The moment Sherman put his arms about me and we danced, her prophecy came back to me in a flash. "Why," I said to myself, "shades of Mademoiselle Berly! Here he is in the flesh!" The young man, only two years out of law school, apparently had taken a real fancy to me, for he said, "What do you say we go somewhere where we can talk? There are too many people here."

I suggested we go to Belle Livingstone's place, because nobody would be over there. I was right. The place was deserted except for a woman covered with diamonds who had had too much to drink; she was telling the captive audience in the person of the bartender all her troubles. Up in the room with the silver mattresses on the floor, Dwight Fiske played softly the tune of the hour, "What is this thing called love?" We talked till dawn. He told me he had been separated from his wife of two years, but that the divorce had not yet been instituted.

A son of California, he was born in a house in Mission Canyon, Santa Barbara. Of pioneer stock, he came of a distinguished family that traced its ancestry to the *Mayflower*. His father also belonged to the legal profession, but was at heart a poet. He was the author of "The Rosary." These lovely words, written to his wife, became world famous when Ethelbert Nevin set them to music. By a strange coincidence, when that song was given its first public performance at a concert by Nevin at the Carnegie Lyceum in 1898, Isadora Duncan appeared on the same program. I was delighted to discover that Sherman too possessed the soul of a dreamer.

At dinner one wonderful night in May at the restaurant "21," he wrote on the back of the menu the following lines to me:

A REVERY

Music and laughter—a single flower glows
Bright crimson in the darkness of your hair;
Behind the jade-green of your eyes, who knows
What pagan Goddess beckons to me there.

Pagan Goddess or Hamadryad?
Two thousand years ago you danced for Pan,
Danced while he piped, white limbs with ivy clad;
What brings you here to dance for mortal man?

Let us enjoy your dancing; it is not long
I feel, before the shaggy one returns
To claim you. Even now his song
Shrills wild and in your hair a crimson flower burns.

Our attachment grew stronger with each day that passed. He left for Paris that winter to obtain his divorce. But quite a few more years had to pass before he was professionally established and we could think of marriage. This supreme happiness came to me at last, somewhat late in life, but better late where the right man is concerned than never.

In the early part of 1933, I lived in a women's hotel on Mitchell Place, near the East River. I held my dancing classes there, as I now taught—for the first time in my career—paying pupils. I had a livelihood to earn. One rainy morning, sitting by the window in my room, I made a watercolor sketch of the view in the distance—the Queensborough Bridge over the river and Ward's Island in the center. I had not sketched since school days and had no idea I had any talent for this art. Just then the telephone rang. It was the secretary of Walter Damrosch. Damrosch, who was then nearly eighty, had conducted for Isadora. The secretary made an appointment for me to see the old gentleman, since he had something important to discuss with me. The next day he told me of his plan to present the Ninth Symphony of Beethoven as a huge pageant to Peace. He wanted me to stage the choreography for the last movement, which contains Schiller's "Ode to Joy." I remembered Isadora's lifelong ambition of dancing the Ninth. I enthusiastically agreed to his plan. Isadora had written of her vision:

> I was possessed by the idea of a school—vast ensemble—dancing in the Ninth Symphony of Beethoven. At night I had only to shut my eyes and these figures danced through my brain in mighty array, calling on me to bring them to life. "We are here! You are the one at whose touch we might live! . . ." I was possessed by the dream of Promethean creation that, at my call, might spring from the Earth, descend from the Heavens, such dancing figures as the world had never seen.*

Damrosch told me, "Isadora Duncan's delineation of Beethoven's Seventh Symphony, twenty-five years ago, helped to open my eyes and mind to the significant connection between the art of music and dance. When I started to work on the scenario of the dramatization of the Ninth, it was as if Beethoven's music controlled me and prevented me from introducing any element which smacked of the theatrical or artificial."

* *Life*, p. 213.

The scenario, which Walter Damrosch worked out for me to follow in staging the last movement with its stupendous choral "Ode to Joy," gives an indication of what we tried to express. I will append it here the way he wrote it:

First, war and the desolation of war. The unhappy restlessness of the world. Then remonstrance by the Priest of the Temple of Peace with some hopeful pleading in pantomime, after which comes the soft beginning by the orchestra only playing the Hymn of the brotherhood of man, gradually increasing in strength as if coming nearer and nearer from a great distance—indicating a world awakening. During this music the dancer might begin to decorate the altar and the temple with garlands. The stage becomes brighter and at the fortissimo reiteration of the hymn, the dance becomes more and more joyous and triumphant in character. A short interruption by the renewed loud dissonance of battle as the High Priest comes forward and slowly sings:

"O Friends, no longer these sounds of war, let us intone more peaceful and joyful ones!"

The great chorus now begins to chant the Hymn of Joy. Representatives of all the nations of the world in their native costumes begin to pour in through the two side entrances of the auditorium and march up the middle of the aisle with their banners, garlands, etc., towards the steps leading to the altar of Peace. As the chorus chants the words: "And the cherub stands before God," there is a great devotional climax from the entire multitude.

To the music that follows this devotional climax a march of youths, half-naked like athletes with garlands and banners symbolizing the joyousness of youth in a world freed from war come dancing forward. They ascend the stage and together with the maidens execute a wild dance of joy. To the words: "Be embraced O Ye Millions, this kiss to the whole world!" they all embrace and in pantomime express the symbolical words chanted by the chorus:

"Brothers! over yonder starry tent a loving Father must be dwelling! O ye millions, ye fall down, feel ye not the Creator?

Search Him above the starry tent, far above the stars he must dwell."

Then the chorus chants the Hymn of Joy in quicker time and new accentuations accompanied by dancing by the multitude. The banner bearers and the soldiers carrying arms deposit them around the altar on which a flame of eternal Peace had been lighted followed by a general expression of joy.

The night dedicated to the grand music and dance festival at Madison Square Garden in New York, at a time when warlike rumbles were heard once more in Europe, was that of January 25, 1933. Damrosch conducted the orchestra of a hundred men and a mixed chorus of a hundred voices in a magnificent rendering of Beethoven's mighty symphony. I danced at the head of a group of fifty men, women, and children—all humanity—as my great teacher had always envisioned it. As the theme of the "Ode to Joy" began, that hymn of the brotherhood of man, played very softly by the strings alone, I stepped out onto the big stage—a single figure dancing. As the grandiose melody built higher with the whole orchestra coming in, two others joined me, then more and more, until the entire stage was filled with dancing figures in mighty array, exactly as Isadora Duncan had dreamed it. Before the dance had ended, I surreptitiously stole away from the whirling mass of dancing figures and stood quietly in the shadow of the wings to watch them dance the closing measures. No one had noticed my departure.

Among that crowd of eighteen thousand spectators filling every seat in that vast auditorium, there was only one person, the man I was going to marry, who knew that this was my swan song—my last dance in public. As I stood and watched, I suddenly sensed a presence near, hovering over me, and seemed to hear these whispered words: "I see the Future, it is there—and we will dance the Ninth Symphony yet!"

I had come a long way. In my mind's eye I saw the little girl in Hamburg, skipping along the darkened street with a red paper torch light in her hand. This light had turned into a brighter flame as I had to uphold the torch of an ideal. All things must come to an end. I had had my own share of public acclaim during nearly thirty years of dancing on the stage. I did not regret leaving the glaring spotlights for the obscurity of a private existence. Life, at that moment, seemed to prove that wonders never cease; that out of the hardship and miseries of existence should bloom the marvel of a great, true love.

And so, with a fervent heart, I thanked Providence for all the blessings I had received and—at the end—for giving me this unique opportunity to close that part of my life in harmony and beauty and artistic fulfillment. For being able, through Beethoven's immortal music and Schiller's inspired poem to the brotherhood of mankind—for which all men of good will must strive—to say a glorious and joyful farewell to my dance career.

Index of Names

Adamson, Fire Commissioner, 154
Alexander, King of Greece, 198
Alexandra, Queen, 81–82, 212
André Vladimirovitch, Grand Duke, 66–68
Arts of the Theatre, The, 79
Aubert, Johnny, 181–182
Auguste Victoria, Empress, 42, 78
Axen, Mrs. Anna, 247, 306–308

Bach, Johann Sebastian, 168, 182, 205
Bacchae, The, 158
Baker, Josephine, 199
Baker, Miss, 148, 150
Balashova, Alexandra, 226, 232
Baltanic, S.S., 218–219, 221
Bara, Theda, 161, 179
Bauer, Harold, 200
Baumgarten, Otto, 179–180, 184
Beethoven, Ludwig von, 20, 119, 168, 173, 193, 197, 205, 241, 251, 339, 341, 342
Begas, Mrs. Reinhold, 39
Bentley, Alys, 170
Benson, Stuart, 160, 180–181
Bérault, Count and Countess de, 122–123
Berly, Mademoiselle, 337
Black Crook, The, 326
Blake, William, 115
Bloch, Mr. and Mrs. Ernest, 156
Boissevain, Eugen, 160, 182–184, 186
Bonaparte, Jerôme, 89, 99
Borodin, Mrs. Fanny, 289–293, 300–301, 314

DANCE

A Books for Libraries Collection

Ashihara, Eiryo. **The Japanese Dance.** 1964

Bowers, Faubion. **Theatre in the East.** 1956

Brinson, Peter. **Background to European Ballet.** 1966

Causley, Marguerite. **An Introduction to Benesh Movement Notation.** 1967

Devi, Ragini. **Dances of India.** 1962

Duggan, Ann Schley, Jeanette Schlottmann and Abbie Rutledge. **The Teaching of Folk Dance.** Volume 1. 1948

_____. **Folk Dances of Scandinavia.** Volume 2. 1948

_____. **Folk Dances of European Countries.** Volume 3. 1948

_____. **Folk Dances of the British Isles.** Volume 4. 1948

_____. **Folk Dances of the United States and Mexico.** Volume 5. 1948

Duncan, Irma. **Duncan Dancer.** 1966

Dunham, Katherine. **A Touch of Innocence.** 1959

Emery, Lynne Fauley. **Black Dance in the United States from 1619 to 1970.** 1972

Fletcher, Ifan Kyrle, Selma Jeanne Cohen and Roger Lonsdale. **Famed for Dance.** 1960

Gautier, Théophile. **The Romantic Ballet as Seen by Théophile Gautier.** 1932

Genthe, Arnold. **Isadora Duncan.** 1929

Hall, J. Tillman. **Dance! A Complete Guide to Social, Folk, & Square Dancing.** 1963

Jackman, James L., ed. **Fifteenth Century Basse Dances.** 1964

Joukowsky, Anatol M. **The Teaching of Ethnic Dance.** 1965

Kahn, Albert Eugene. **Days with Ulanova.** 1962

Karsavina, Tamara. **Theatre Street.** 1950

Lawson, Joan. **European Folk Dance.** 1953

Martin, John. **The Dance.** 1946

Sheets-Johnstone, Maxine. **The Phenomenology of Dance.** 1966